Springer-Verlag Berlin Heidelberg GmbH

G. Germann · R. Sherman · L. S. Levin

Decision-Making
in Reconstructive Surgery

Upper Extremity

Forewords by W. P. Cooney and G. Foucher

With 109 Algorithms
and 194 Figures, Mostly in Color

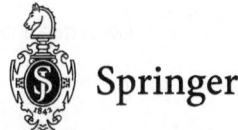 Springer

G. Germann, M. D., Ph. D.
Professor of Surgery
Chief – Department of Plastic and Hand Surgery –
Burn Center – BG – Trauma Center
Plastic and Hand Surgery – University of Heidelberg
Ludwig-Guttmann-Str. 13
D-67071 Ludwigshafen
Germany

R. Sherman, M. D.
Professor of Surgery
Chief – Division of Plastic and Reconstructive Surgery
University of Southern California (USC)
1450 San Pablo Street, Suite 2000
Los Angeles, CA 90033
USA

L. S. Levin
Associate Professor of Plastic and Orthopedic Surgery
Chief – Division of Plastic, reconstructive,
maxillofacial and oral Surgery
DUKE University
DUKE University Medical Center
P. O. Box 3945
Durham, NC 27710
USA

ISBN 978-3-642-64037-7   ISBN 978-3-642-59585-1 (eBook)
DOI 10.1007/978-3-642-59585-1
Library of Congress Cataloging-in-Publication Data

Germann, G. (Günter), 1952. Decision-making in reconstructive surgery : upper extremity / G. Germann, R. Sherman, L.S. Levin ; forewords by Walter P. Cooney and Guy Foucher.   p.   cm. Includes bibliographical references and index.
  ISBN-13: 978-3-642-64037-7
  1. Shoulder–Wounds and injuries–Surgery. 2. Elbow–Wounds and injuries–Surgery. 3. Wrist–Wounds and injuries–Surgery. 4. Surgery, Plastic–Decision making. I. Sherman, R. (Randolph) II. Levin, L. Scott. III. Title.
[DNLM: 1. Arm Injuries–surgery. 2. Algorithms. 3. Decision Making. 4. Hand Injuries–surgery. 5. Reconstructive Surgical Procedures.   WE 805 G373d 1998]   RD557.G43 2000   627.5'7059–dc21   DNLM/DLC   for Library of Congress   99-36189 CIP

© Springer-Verlag Berlin Heidelberg 2000
Softcover reprint of the hardcover 1st edition 2000

Drawings: Katharina Arns-Germann, Ludwigshafen
Algorithms: Günther Hippmann, Nürnberg
Cover design: Erich Kirchner, Heidelberg
Reproduction of the drawings: AM-productions, Wiesloch
Typesetting and page composition: Fotosatz-Service Köhler GmbH, Würzburg

SPIN 10530918   24/3135 – 5 4 3 2 1 0

Foreword I

In dealing with reconstructive surgery of the upper extremity, conditions such as rheumatoid arthritis and even congenital anomalies may some day have a cure or be substantially altered by genetic engineering. Traumatic injury to the upper extremity, however, will always be with us in the fast-paced world that we live in. It is in this regard that the algorithmic-based text by Drs. Gunter Germann, Randy Sherman, and Scott Levin becomes so important in providing a straightforward guide to injuries of the upper extremity for the trauma surgeon. These authors have produced a modern-day guide to reconstructive surgery for a variety of conditions affecting the hand itself and associated important functions of the upper extremity. It serves as a twenty-first century guide to the traumatically injured upper extremity, much like Rank, Wakefield, and Huston's classic text served after World War II. The book serves to help guide the decision-making process by the evaluating surgeon and importantly highlights the surgical exploration as an essential part of the extended physical examination. By surgical exploration, the surgeon has great knowledge and flexibility in determining various options for initial treatment and subsequent reconstruction.

In this well-organized text, the reader can move succinctly and with clarity through the principles of injured limb management: (1) skeletal fixation (2) vascular reconstruction of the injured extremity, and (3) delicate tissue handling involved in soft tissue reconstruction and wound coverage. Beginning first with a statement of principles and a general strategy for treatment, the authors take us through all of the different types of potential upper limb injuries and proceed with specific treatment algorithms related to the bone, ligaments, flexor and extensor tendons, vascular reconstruction, and finally, soft tissue integument coverage. In particular, their use of case histories provides practical day-to-day information to the operative surgeon. Finally, and most importantly, well-established operative procedures related to soft tissue coverage with an atlas of skin and muscle flaps provides the upper limb reconstructive surgeon with all of the essentials in a single bound volume of how to address the simple to the complex salvage of the injured upper extremity. The authors are to be congratulated by combining the talents of two continents in producing a universal guide to decision-making in traumatic upper limb reconstructive surgery. It is simple to use, very effective in design, and practical on a day-to-day basis to all surgeons in the advanced field of upper limb reconstructive surgery.

September 1999

W. P. Cooney, M. D.

Chair, Division of Hand Surgery,
Mayo Clinic and Mayo Foundation
Professor of Orthopedics, Mayo Medical School
Rochester, Minnesota, USA

Foreword II

In a small country such as France, a recent survey showed that each year around 500 000 individuals sustain an injury just of the hand. Even if not all of them are major injuries, in such conditions, the existing network of the European Federation of Emergency Hand Units (FESUM), which I am proud to have founded 20 years ago with the late professors Vilain and Michon, is not able to cope with such numbers of patients. Even if it remains ideal to convey patients to a specialized unit, we have to accept that a lot of them are treated in orthopedic and plastic surgery departments where, sometimes, trainees are on duty. These young surgeons have to face a wide variety of apparently simple or even more complex injuries of the upper extremity. They already have a plethora of surgical textbooks to consult and so it could seem senseless to published another one.

However, this book will be their Bible as it is not a traditional textbook in any sense. It was written for them by three busy and dedicated surgeons young enough to spend their days and nights on duty but experienced enough to have been able to summarize their experience in a simple way, which is easy and fast to review at 2 o'clock in the morning when confronted with an unfamiliar case. Evidently this collection of algorithms and illustrative cases has some oversimplifications and will give rise to healthy controversies. However, it has the major advantage of avoiding the pitfall of the kind of book in which a group of surgeons provide conflicting opinions. It is a practical book with a uniform presentation of reliable and versatile guidelines and techniques which take into account the myriad of factors influencing the decision. These guidelines are oriented to the philosophy we have adhered to for nearly a quarter of a century, the so-called OSREM ("One Stage Repair with Early Mobilisation"). In an era when decreasing cost is a major concern in combination with increased expectations from the patients, it is relevant to select the most appropriate technique to solve a specific reconstructive problem even through it may sometimes be a sophisticated compound flap performed in one stage on an outpatient basis due to its reliability and low complication rate.

I am honored by the request of the authors to write the foreword to such a book, which will be an exceptional investment with early and rewarding returns for each unit interested in the acute care of upper extremity injuries. If it is geared chiefly to residents, it would be a mistake for the senior surgeon to overlook its power as a teaching tool to better the functional and cosmetic result, cut expenses, and save time. I hope that the authors will continue to work in this field and could envisage an interactive CD-ROM version.

September 1999

G. Foucher, M.D.

Hand Surgeon – Plastic and Reconstructive Surgeon
Director – SOS Main – Emergency Hand Unit
Strasbourg, France

Preface

The assembly of dedicated upper extremity surgeons with different backgrounds from both Europe and North America has brought together concepts, philosophies, and approaches that have been integrated to fabricate a text that will share modern thinking as it relates to reconstructive surgery of the upper extremity for trauma, sepsis and tumor. What began as a vision has evolved into reality that is a unique work given the abundance of literature and textbooks that relate to upper extremity surgery. The purpose of this book is to guide the uninitiated through thought processes related to upper extremity problems and to point the direction towards solutions using an algorithm format. This textbook is illustrated in order to augment and elucidate thinking processes with technical details and to demonstrate principles and practices of reconstructive upper extremity surgery. The authors hope that this textbook will be a contribution to upper extremity surgery and assist complex bone and soft tissue management in an integrated approach for care of the upper limb.

The artistry of hand surgery is beautifully illustrated by Katharina Arns-Germann, whose creative interpretations significantly enhanced the text.

September 1999

G. Germann
R. Sherman
L. S. Levin

The authors would like to express their gratitude to the Borchard Foundation.

Contents

Glossary

AO/ASIF:	Association for Stable Internal Fixation	FTSG:	full thickness skin graft
APL:	abductor pollicis longus	IP:	interphalangeal joint
APB:	abductor pollicis brevis	IPJ:	interphalangeal joint
AP:	adductor pollicis	LT:	lunotriquetral
AR:	axial radial	MCI:	midcarpal instability
ARI:	axial radial instability	MCPJ:	metacarpo-phalangeal joint
AROM:	active range of motion	MM:	malignant melanoma
AU:	axial ulna	MP:	metacarpophalangeal
AUI:	axial ulnar instability	MVA:	motor vehicle accident
AxRI:	axial radial instability	ORIF:	open reduction/internal fixation
AxUI:	axial ulnar instability	OT:	occupational therapy
BCC:	basal cell carcinoma	PIN:	posterior interosseous nerve
CIC:	carpal instability complex	PIP:	proximal interphalangeal
CID:	carpal instability dissociative	PIPJ:	proximal interphalangeal joint
CIND:	carpal instability non-dissociative	PL:	palmaris longus
CL:	capito-lunate	PLD:	perilunate dislocation
CLIP:	capito-lunate instability pattern	PT:	palmar translation (carpal instability)
CMC:	carpo-metacarpal	PT:	physical therapy
DD:	differential diagnosis	PT:	pronator teres
DIP:	distal interphalangeal	RC:	radiocarpal
DIPJ:	distal interphalangeal joint	RMCI:	radio-midcarpal instability
DISI:	dorsal intercalated segment instability	ROM:	range of motion
DMCA:	dorsal metacarpal artery	RT:	radial translation
DT:	dorsal translation	SCC:	squamous cell carcinoma
ECRB:	extensor carpi radialis brevis	SIEA:	superficial inferior epigastic artery
ECRL:	extensor carpi radialis longus	SL:	scapholunate
ECU:	extensor carpi ulnaris	SLAC:	scapholunate advanced collapse
EDC:	extensor digitorum communis	SLD:	scapholunate dissociation
EDM:	extensor digiti minimi	SNAC:	scaphoid non-union advanced collapse
EDQ:	extensor digiti quinti	SRD:	sympathetic reflex dystrophy
EI:	extensor indicis	STA:	superficial temporal artery
EIP:	extensor indicis proprius	STSG:	split thickness skin graft
EMG:	electro myogram	STT:	scapho-trapezio-trapezoidal
EPL:	extensor pollicis longus	STV:	superficial temporal vein
EPB:	extensor pollicis brevis	TBSA:	total body surface area
FCR:	flexor carpi radialis	TFCC:	triangular fibro-cartilage complex
FCU:	flexor carpi ulnaris	TPF:	temporo-parietal fascia
FDP:	flexor digitorum profundus	UT:	ulnar translation
FDS:	flexor digitorum superficialis	VISI:	volar intercalated segment instability
FPL:	flexor pollicis longus		

Introduction

The hand is one of the most extraordinary tools in nature. A combination of strength, dynamic stability, and precision movements provide the hand within the composity of the upper extremity with the capacity to attain a broad range of technical skills that are hardly reached by the most sophisticated electronic equipment.

Hand surgery is functional restorative surgery. The hand is one of our most important points of contact with our environment and possesses a myriad of important functions such as cognitive discrimination, tactile gnosis, and the ability to transmit and receive emotional signals. The hand serves as the eye for the blind, the ears for the deaf, and the mouthpiece for the mute. Character virtues are often attributed to size, shape, and appearance of a person's hands. Galen considered the hand an instrument of human ratio and as a mirror image of the human soul. The monks of the middle ages used their fingers as a help in mathematic calculations (*"Si tria digita scribunt, totum corpus laborat"*). This tradition has now evolved to the "digital era" in which the hand is used to press buttons on a keyboard, operate a mouse, or use a cellular phone.

"Hand surgery is also aesthetic surgery". The significance of this statement by Dr. Guy Foucher, a well-recognized hand surgeon and author, becomes clear if we consider that the face and hands are usually the only points of contact in the western civilization with the exception of warmer days when, through more casual dressing, other body parts become visible. If one observes individuals with mutilated hands carefully, it becomes obvious that the majority of these patients attempt to conceal their injured and disfigured hands.

In such cases this may lead to psychological disturbances in some patients whose professions require frequent contact with the public. Reconstruction of this complicated biomechanical tool with restoration of appearance, functional structures, and tactile gnosis are goals in order to reconstitute general well-being achieving simultaneous professional and social re-integration.

Specific tactics and overall strategy depend on many variables that evolve as the surgeon's experience increases. They have to be integrated into a complex decision making process which has to compare and evaluate all influencing factors that affect outcome.

Reconstructive procedures should be tailored to the individual needs of the patient. For example, application of only one coverage technique to different lesions and circumstances may result in solutions that may not match the patient's specific requirements. The principle of "one technique fits all" has little place in hand and upper extremity reconstruction. The main goal of the reconstructive surgeon should be to achieve functional reconstruction with the greatest similarity of tissues possible, to preserve or restore hand aesthetics, and to return the individual back to a normal life of work, play, and family as reasonably soon as possible.

This book will help to elucidate decision making processes developed by the authors throughout many years of clinical practice. The method of using algorithms has been selected to achieve the greatest possible clarity. This book does not claim completeness; there will always be exceptions and particular clinical situations that do not fit into one of the categories described.

The Key to the Map – How to Use the Book

As the cover implies, this text is designed to be a guide to decision-making through the labyrinth of problems we face in treating patients with hand and upper extremity problems. Using **Algorithms** (step-by-step procedures used to solve particular problems) specific injuries and clinical situations can be addressed in a logical, deductive fashion. These algorithms constitute the centerpiece of the book. They serve as a map to move you from point of origin to your intended destination. The various sections on Classifications, Techniques of Structure Repair, and Atlas of Flaps are designed to support your use of the Algorithms. As you focus on a particular alogrithm, their utility will be maximized if you understand the symbology used to construct each diagram. The following display should be frequently referenced until you are comfortable with the flow of each page.

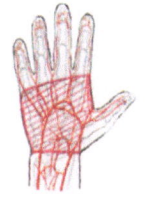

Anatomic Designator

In the inner or outer corner of each algorithm will appear a pictoral representation of the anatomic location and particular structure being covered. A barber poll (angled and striped) overlay will highlight the pertinent anatomy.

Contractures I

This large bolded heading will describe the specific problem addressed in the algorithm.

**Nail/Joints/
Tissue Loss**

These small bolded headings will describe decision **waypoints**, or those identifiable places where a choice must be made to discriminate different paths for diagnosis and/or therapy.

Light red boxes will hold different parameters used for decision-making, either anatomic discriminators or supplemental information used as a navigational aid.

Medium red boxes will give additional explanations, treatment options, or guidelines.

Dark red boxes are for warnings, precautions or pitfalls.

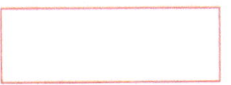

This red outlined box will be used to emphasize particular waypoints.

CHAPTER I
General Principles

General Principles of Upper Extremity Reconstruction

Reconstructive surgery of the upper extremity as it relates to trauma, tumor, or sepsis has experienced significant progress during the last two decades. The introduction of microsurgical techniques, a wide variety of new flaps, functional free muscle transfer, and sophisticated treatment concepts have greatly enhanced the armamentarium of reconstructive procedures. The philosophy of treatment has evolved from the mere coverage of defects with secondary functional reconstruction, to the concept of "one-stage" reconstructions using compound flaps of skin, tendon, nerve, vessel, and bone for the total reconstructive surgery goal.

This total reconstructive surgery plan can be executed immediately during the first operative exploration or after a second look procedure during definitive wound closure. Primary or "postponed primary" reconstruction not only saves time, but allows for an early and total patient rehabilitation. Thereby, this strategy not only saves treatment costs but of utmost importance, prevents social and professional isolation of the patient. In addition studies have shown that primary reconstruction is highly cost effective reducing insurance expenditures and positively affects society by restorating the worker.

Secondary reconstructions while occasionally necessary are frequently performed in scarred tissue. Despite serious efforts it is not always possible to keep joints and soft tissues mobile by passive motion exercise while awaiting secondary reconstruction.

The ultimate treatment goal is now to maximize the reconstruction of gliding, functional structures to restore form and function, and to achieve rapid professional and social reintegration. However, the application of flaps or any other reconstructive procedure has to be embedded in sound concepts that are individually tailored to the needs of the patients.

Treatment goals

- Extremity salvage
- Preservation and restoration of function
- Correction of acquired defects (trauma or tumor)
- Optimal aesthetic appearance
- Social and professional reintegration
- Cost-effective therapy

Following injury the decision for a specific treatment concept and the choice of preferred reconstructive procedures is based on a thorough analysis that includes the areas:

- Clinical evaluation of the patient
- Pertinent medical and demographic profile
- Wound assessment including tissue loss and functional impairment
- Injury classification to guide management

Compliance with these guidelines will lead to

- Standard Treatment Protocols with sufficient flexibility to select the best operative procedure for each patient and each injury.

The rationale for this concept is the idea that the upper extremity should be thought of as a functional organ. Soft tissues, functional structures such as tendons or nerves, and the skeleton should not be thought of as isolated structures, but should be recognized as interacting parts of a highly complex machine. Subsequently, reconstructive procedures for complex defects should not be directed towards repair of isolated structures, but to restore the integrity of a functional entity of the hand and the upper extremity.

Patient Evaluation

Patients with severe injuries to the upper extremity should be routinely checked for accompanying injuries, which may be life threatening in some cases. Approximately 10%–15% of all polytraumatized patients suffer injuries to the hand or the upper extremity. The injury severity score (ISS) or a similar score can be performed during the initial patient evaluation. These scoring systems try to predict the survival of severely injured patients but do not describe the type and extent of a complex injury to the upper extremity.

Patient Profile – Vocation and Rehabilitation Issues

It is important to acquire a patient's medical and social history since the decision regarding the appropriate therapy is based on factors such as:

- Age
- Medical conditions
- Occupation
- Social environment
- Compliance of the patient

Equally important are the following vocational requirements:

- Technical skills
- Endurance
- AROM
- Grip strength
- Sensitivity and coordination
- Socioeconomic issues (length of rehabilitation etc.)
- Psychological effects on patient (i.e., can the injured machinist return to same machine)

Assessment and Management Strategy

The injury wound should be first assessed by clinical examination on admission and a primary operative exploration is performed as soon as the condition of the patient permits. A standard algorithm for patient admission and primary surgical strategy is recommended. The examination and the judgement of the wound is one of the most critical problems in the evaluation of an injury. Surgery serves not only as a method of treatment of the injured limb but in our thinking, an important and essential element of extended physical examination and assessment of the patient. Since many detrimental decisions are based on lack of experience and compromised judgement in this phase, special algorithms will be devoted to this particular problem (see below).

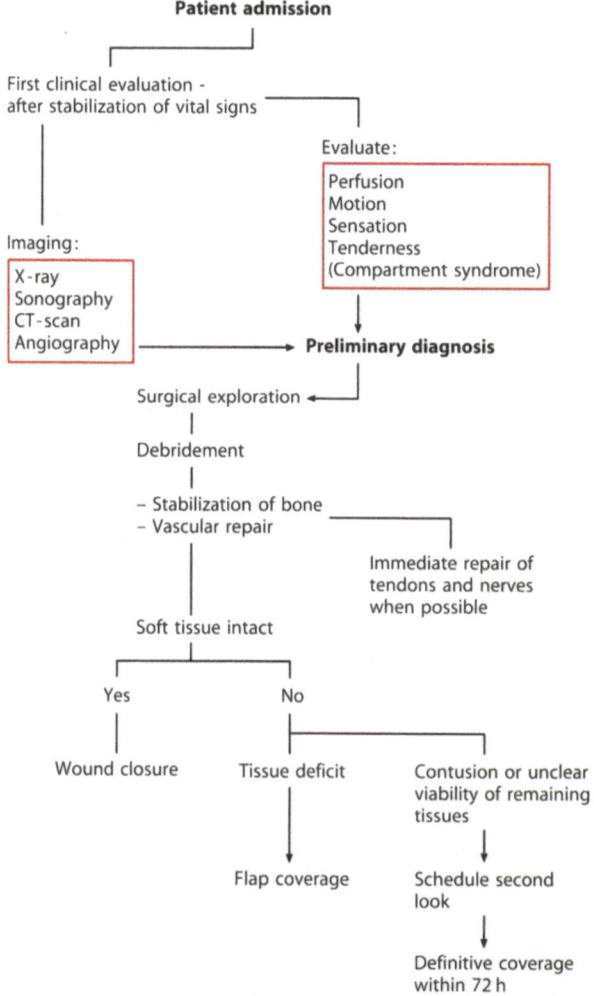

During the first surgical exploration, all nonvital tissue is debrided. The skeleton must first be stabilized and blood flow returned to all devitalized tissue. Vital structures such as vessels, nerves, tendons, and bones are repaired primarily, whenever possible. Depending on the mechanisms of injury, the condition of the patient, and the options available, primary wound closure is preferred. If there is any doubt about the viability of tissues remaining in the wound, the wound is managed temporarily using synthetic skin substitutes which can maintain a moist wound environment for 48–72 hours, and a second look is scheduled for the next day or 48 hours at the latest.

Definitive coverage is then performed. Only in rare cases such as crush or avulsion injuries as well as burns or electrical inuries, if a "second look" may not allow determination about the viability of tissues, a delayed closure is preferred within the first 5–7 days.

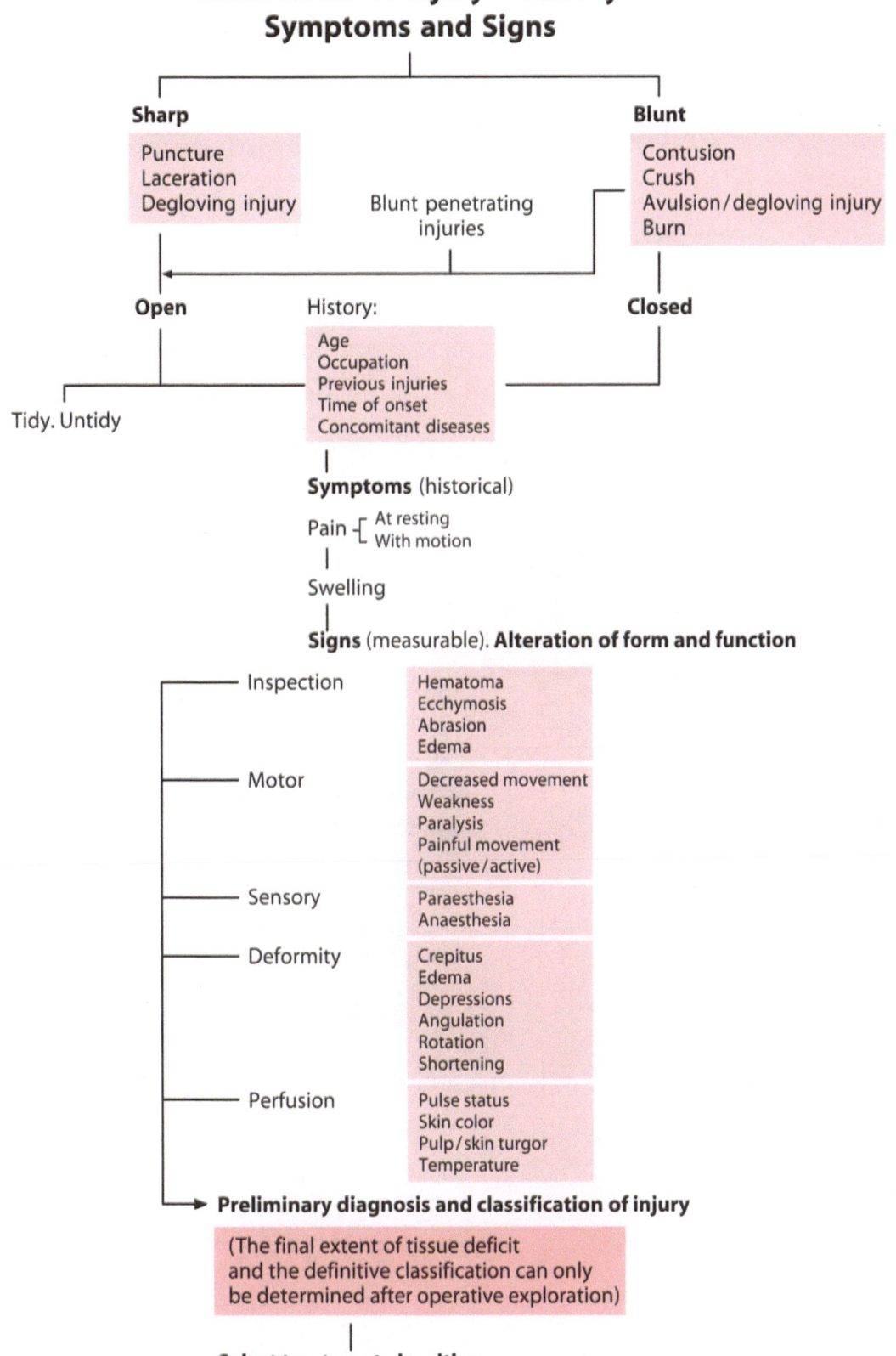

Mechanism of Injury – History
Symptoms and Signs

Sharp
Puncture
Laceration
Degloving injury

Blunt penetrating
injuries

Blunt
Contusion
Crush
Avulsion/degloving injury
Burn

Open   History: **Closed**
Age
Occupation
Previous injuries
Time of onset
Concomitant diseases

Tidy. Untidy

Symptoms (historical)

Pain ⌠ At resting
      ⌡ With motion

Swelling

Signs (measurable). **Alteration of form and function**

Inspection
Hematoma
Ecchymosis
Abrasion
Edema

Motor
Decreased movement
Weakness
Paralysis
Painful movement
(passive/active)

Sensory
Paraesthesia
Anaesthesia

Deformity
Crepitus
Edema
Depressions
Angulation
Rotation
Shortening

Perfusion
Pulse status
Skin color
Pulp/skin turgor
Temperature

Preliminary diagnosis and classification of injury

(The final extent of tissue deficit
and the definitive classification can only
be determined after operative exploration)

Select treatment algorithm

Swelling

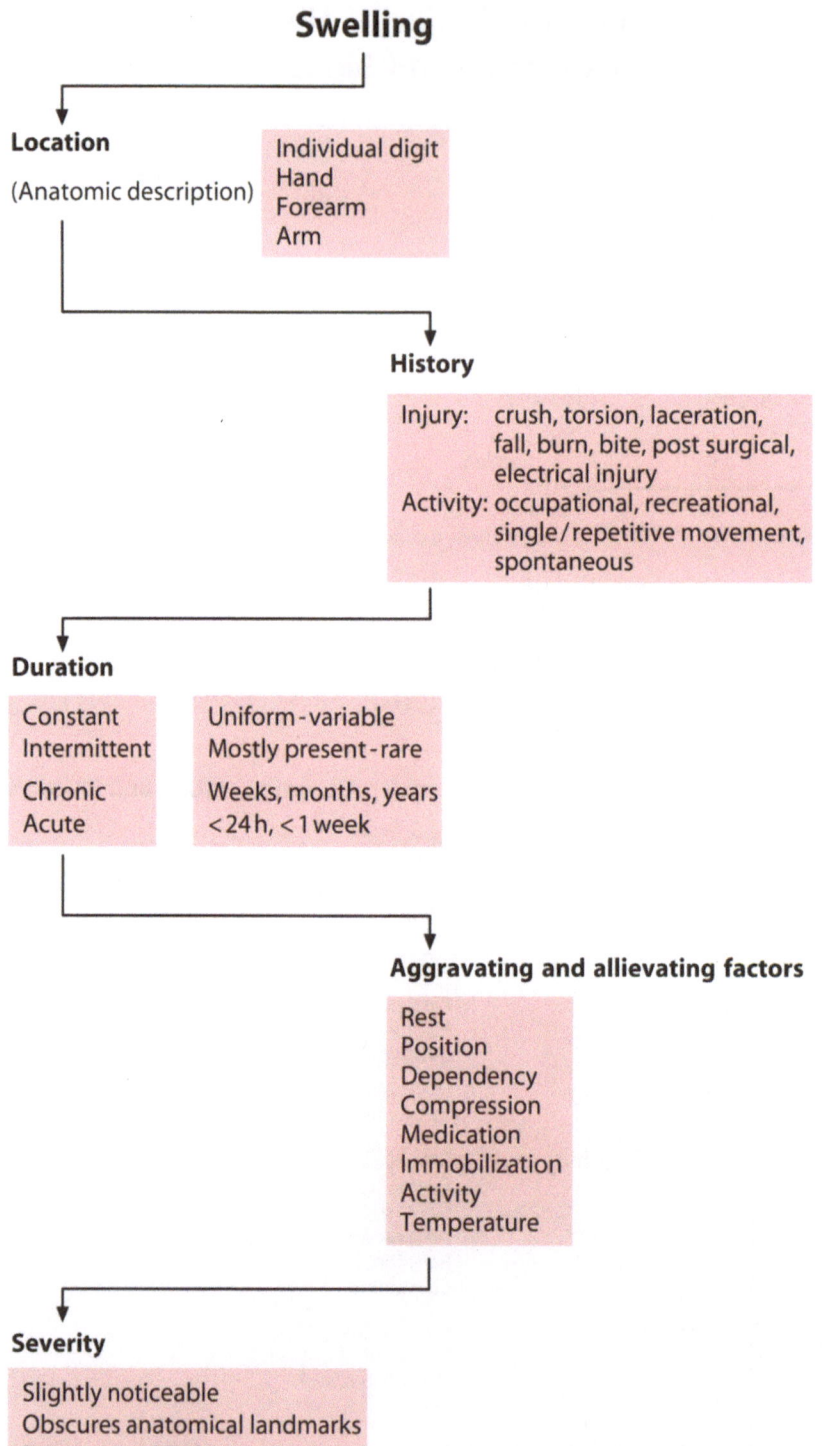

Location

(Anatomic description)

Individual digit
Hand
Forearm
Arm

History

Injury: crush, torsion, laceration,
          fall, burn, bite, post surgical,
          electrical injury
Activity: occupational, recreational,
          single / repetitive movement,
          spontaneous

Duration

Constant   Uniform - variable
Intermittent   Mostly present - rare

Chronic   Weeks, months, years
Acute   < 24 h, < 1 week

Aggravating and allievating factors

Rest
Position
Dependency
Compression
Medication
Immobilization
Activity
Temperature

Severity

Slightly noticeable
Obscures anatomical landmarks
Decreases AROM

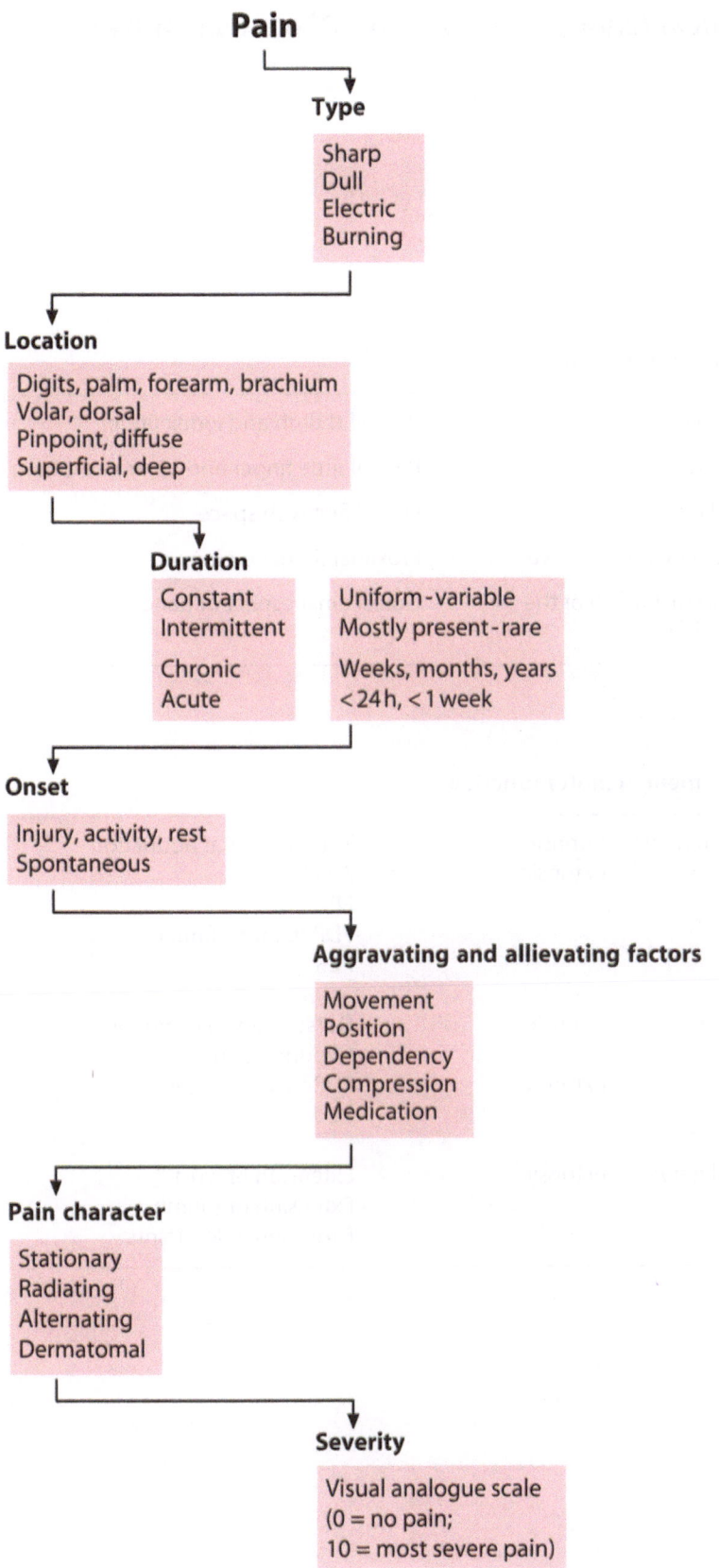

Physical Examination for the Diagnosis of Nerve Injuries

Sensory assessment

Median nerve	Pulp of thumb and index finger
Ulnar nerve	Pulp of little finger and ulnar half of ring finger
Radial nerve	Dorsal first web space
Palmar cutaneous nerve	Proximal thenar eminence
Dorsal cut. branch of the ulnar nerve	Dorsal ulnar aspect of hand

Assessment of motor function

Median nerve:	intrinsic	Thumb palmar abduction
	extrinsic	All FDS
		FPL
		FDP to index finger
		FCR
Ulnar nerve:	intrinsic	Dorsal interossei muscles
		Hypothenar muscles
	extrinsic	FDP to little finger
		FCU
Radial nerve:	extrinsic	Extension of wrist
		Extension of thumb
		Extension of MP joints

Classification and Zones of Injury

The definitive extent of an injury can only be determined after a thorough history, physical examination, and the initial operative exploration. A descriptive scoring system has been developed by AO/ASIF for both bone and soft tissues. Other scoring systems that are predominantly used for the lower extremities are the MESI or the MESS (Mangled Extremity Severity Score). A Hand Injury Severity Score (HISS) has been recently published. We found all systems suitable for scientific purposes, but too complicated for practical use on a routine basis. However, classification systems are useful for comparison of treatment results and guidance for selected therapy.

- AO/ASIF fracture classification
- Salter Harris classification of pediatric physeal fractures
- AO/ASIF soft tissue injury classification
- Mangled Extremity Severity Score (MESS)
- Hand Injury Severity Score (HISS)
- Verdan's zone of flexor tendon injuries
- Zone of extensor tendon injuries
- Mackinnon's classification of nerve injuries
- Mayfield's classification for injuries of the carpal ligaments
- SLAC/SNAC wrist – CIND/CID (Mayo, Viegas, Green)
- Classification of burn injuries

AO/ASIF Fracture Classification
Phalanges and Metacarpals

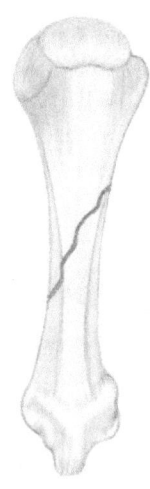 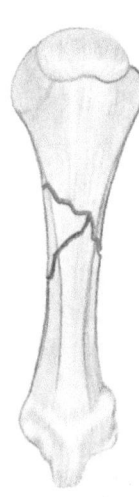 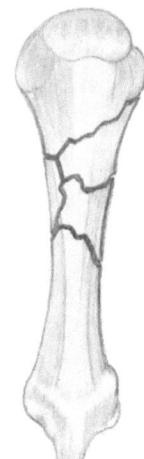

A1
Simple oblique diaphyseal fracture

A2
Diaphyseal butterfly fracture

A3
Comminuted diaphyseal fracture

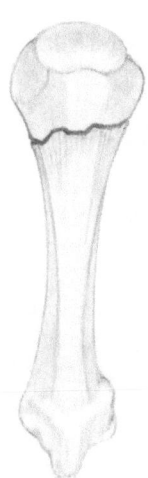 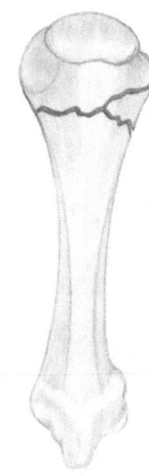 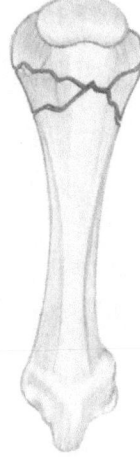

B1
Simple oblique metaphyseal fracture

B2
Metaphyseal butterfly fragment fracture

B3
Metaphyseal comminuted fracture

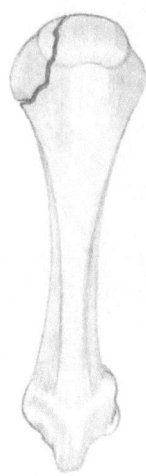 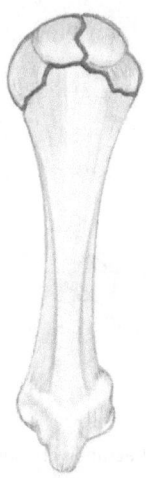 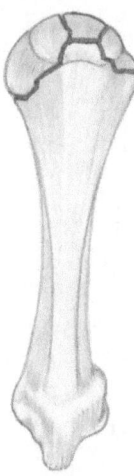

C1
Unicondylar intra-articular fracture

C2
Bicondylar intra-articular fracture

C3
Comminuted intra-articular fracture

Radius – Distal Forearm

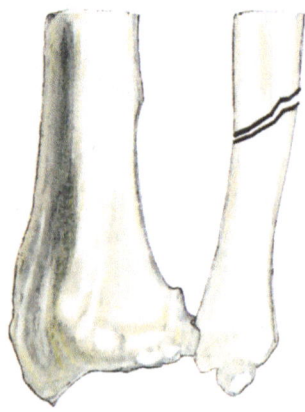

A 1
Simple extraarticular ulna fracture

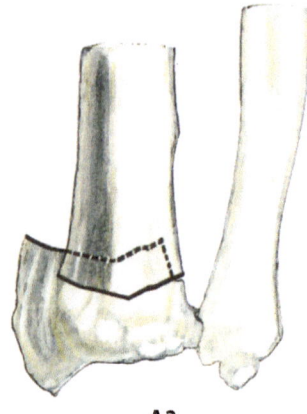

A 2
Extraarticular radius fracture

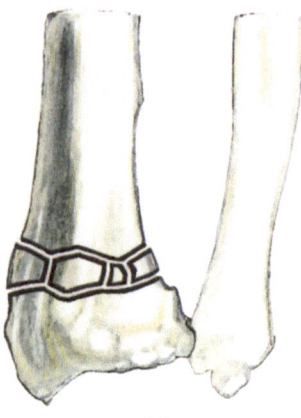

A 3
Comminuted extraarticular fracture

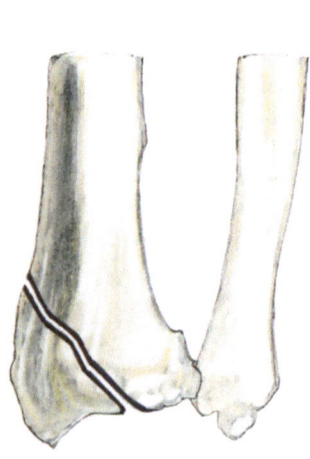

B 1

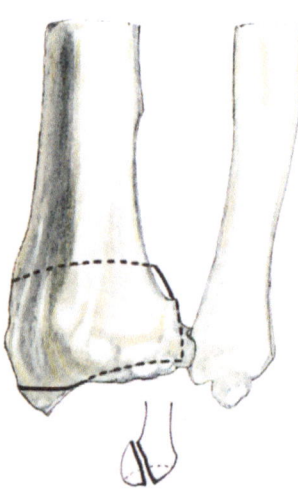

B 2
Simple intraarticular fracture

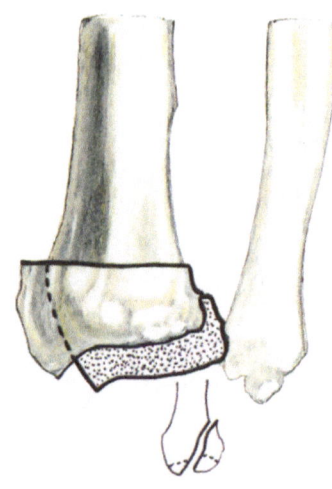

B 3

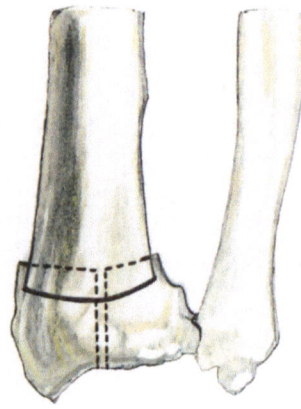

C 1

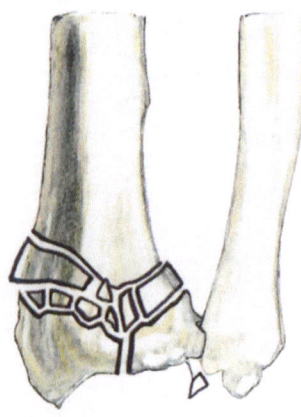

C 2
Complex intraarticular fracture with metaphyseal extension

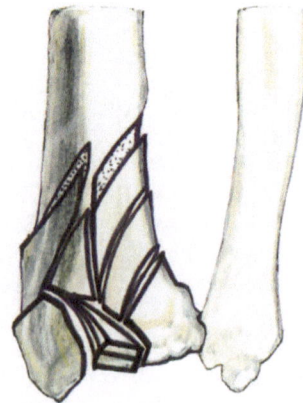

C 3

Forearm Shaft

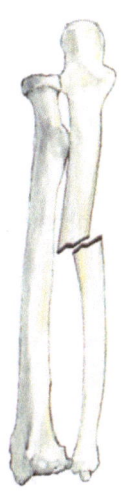

A 1
Transverse diaphyseal ulna fracture

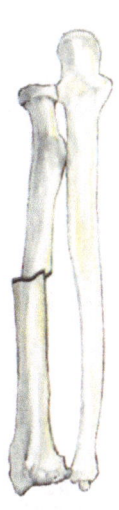

A 2
Transverse diaphyseal radius fracture

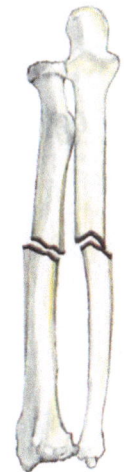

A 3
Both bones forearm fracture

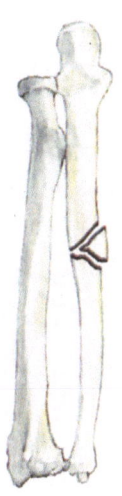

B 1
Diaphyseal butterfly ulna fracture

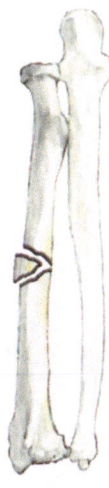

B 2
Diaphyseal butterfly radius fracture

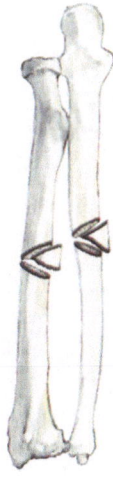

B 3
Both bones diaphyseal butterfly fractures

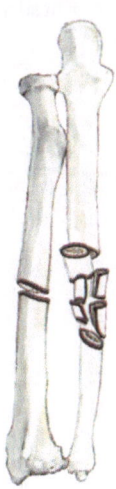

C 1

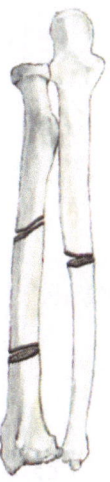

C 2
Comminuted forearm fractures

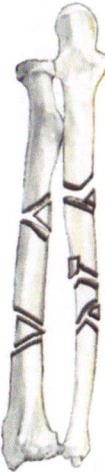

C 3

Proximal Forearm – Elbow

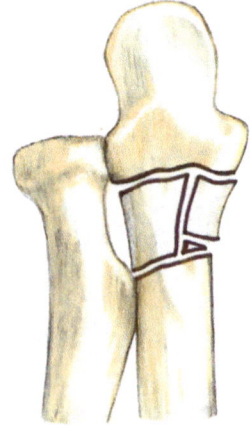

A1
Extraarticular ulnar fracture

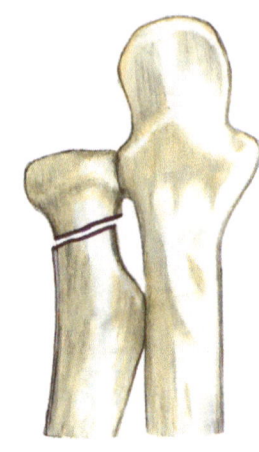

A2
Extraarticular radial head fracture

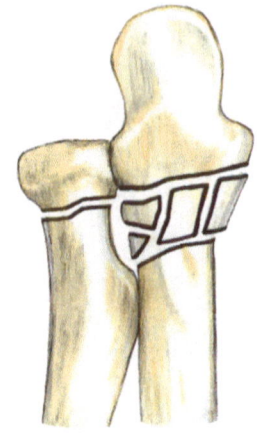

A3
Both bones extraarticular fracture

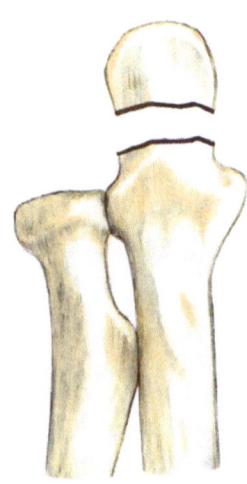

B1
Simple olecranon fracture

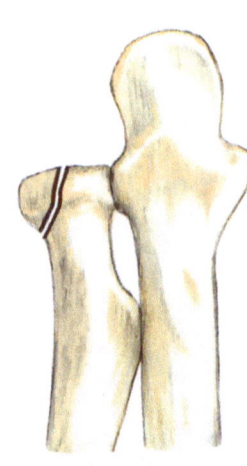

B2
Radial head fracture

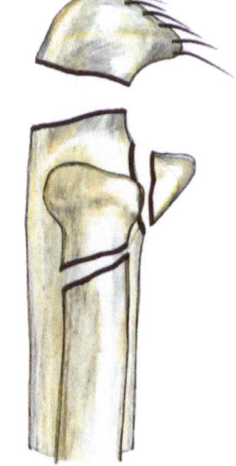

B3
Dislocated olecranon fracture
with radial head fracture

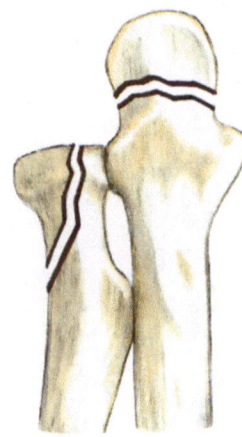

C1

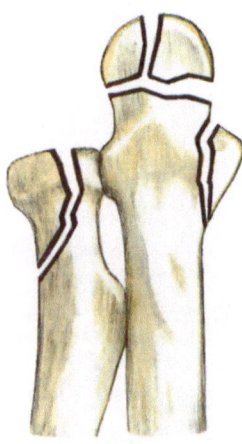

C2
Comminuted both bones intraarticular fracture

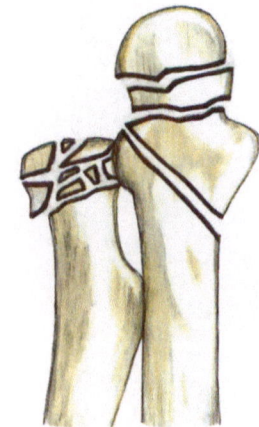

C3

Distal Humerus – Elbow

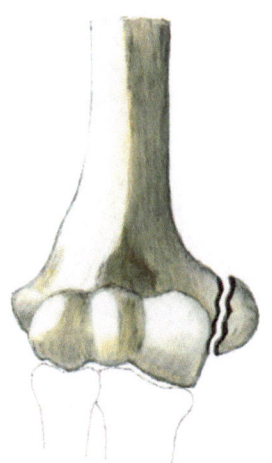

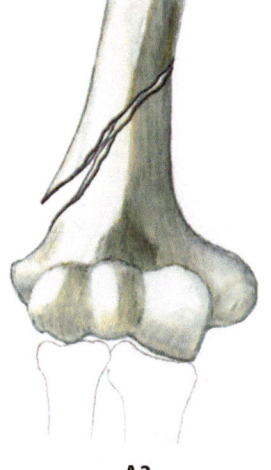

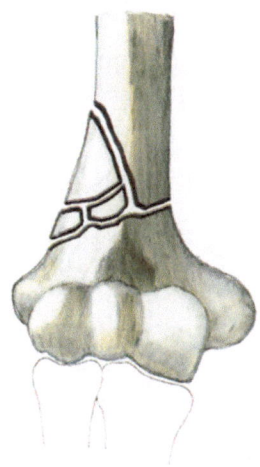

A1

A2
Supracondylar extraarticular fracture

A3
Comminuted supracondylar
extraarticular fracture

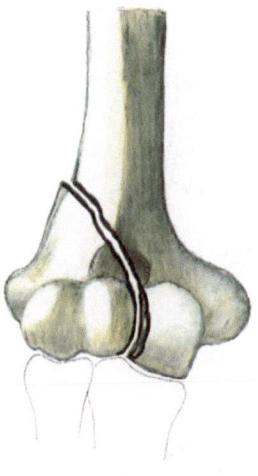

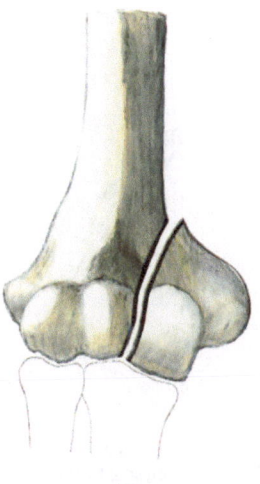

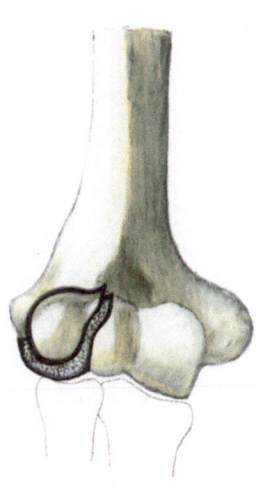

B1

B2
Simple intraarticular fracture

B3

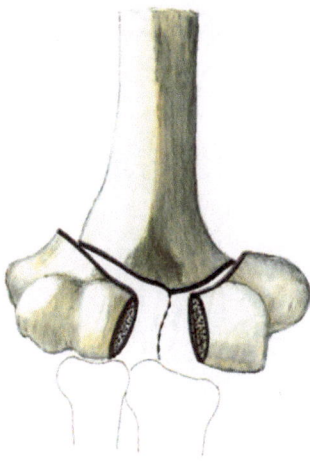

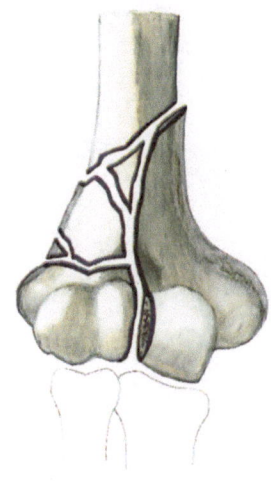

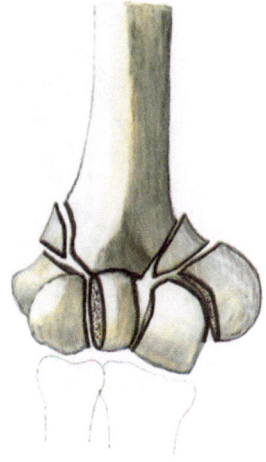

C1

C2
Comminuted intraarticular fracture

C3

Humerus – Shaft

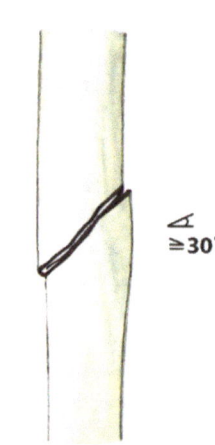

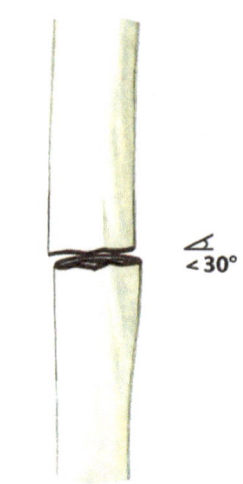

A1
Spiral diaphyseal fracture

A2
Oblique diaphyseal fracture

A3
Transverse diaphyseal fracture

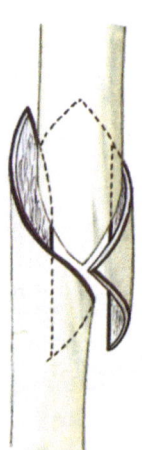

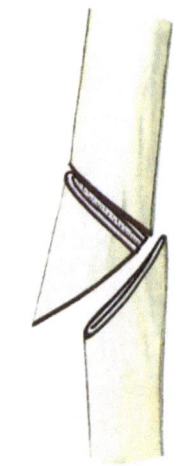

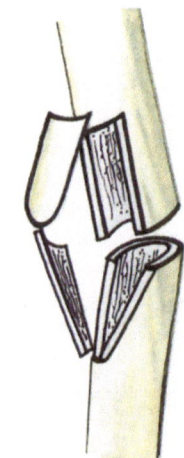

B1
Spiral diaphyseal butterfly fracture

B2
Oblique diaphyseal butterfly fracture

B3
Transverse diaphyseal butterfly fracture

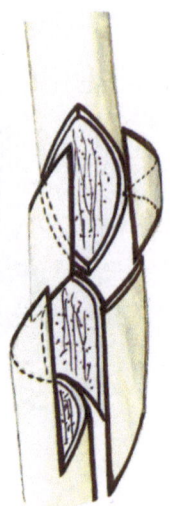

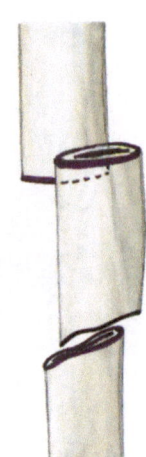

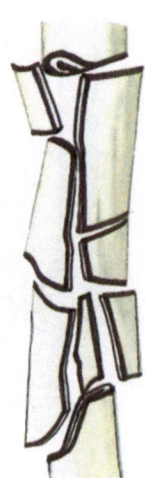

C1

C2
Segmental or comminuted diaphyseal fracture

C3

Proximal Humerus

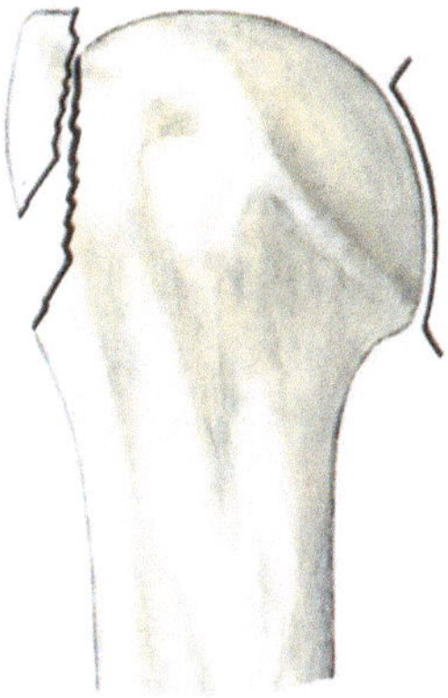

A1
Avulsion of the tuberosity

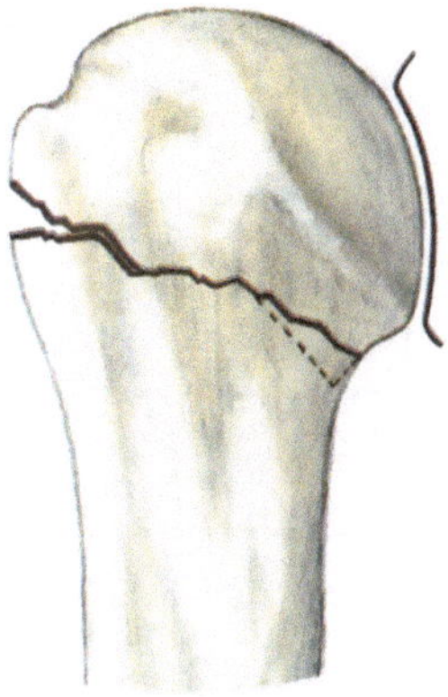

A2

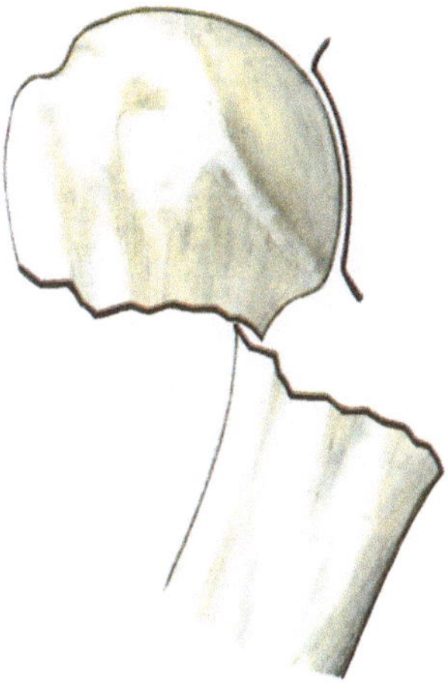

A3

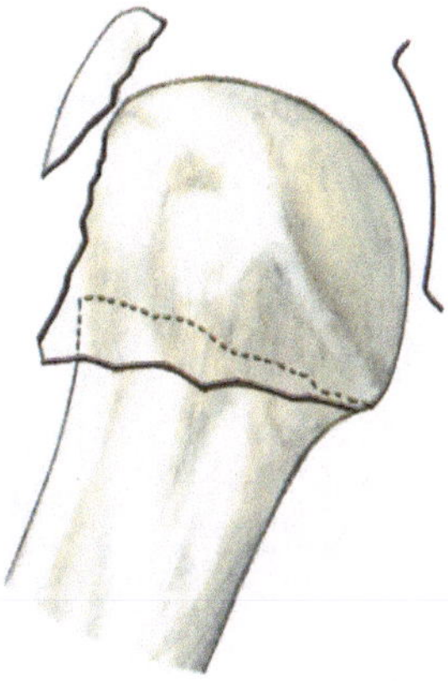

B1

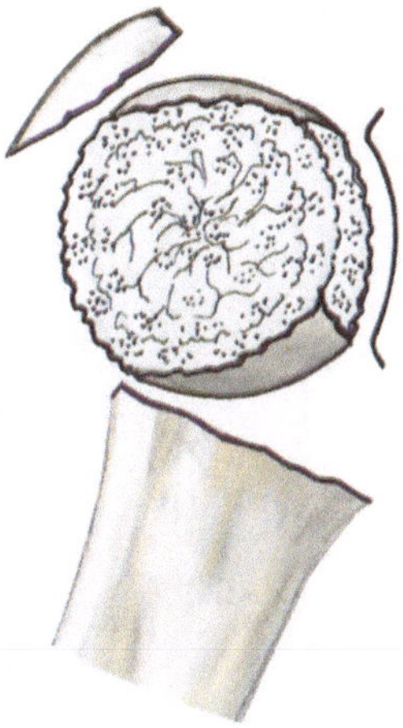

B2
Three part simple fracture

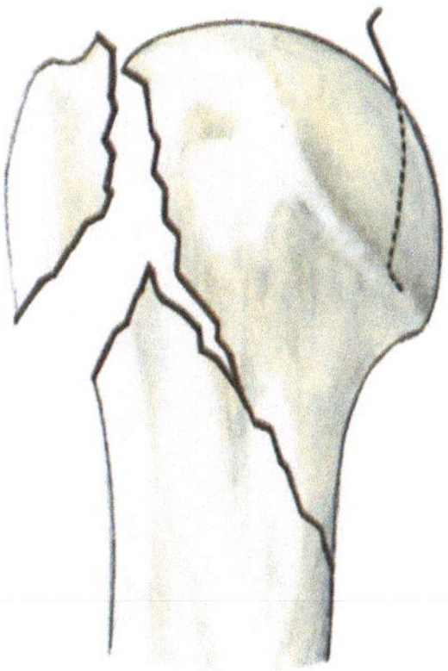

B3

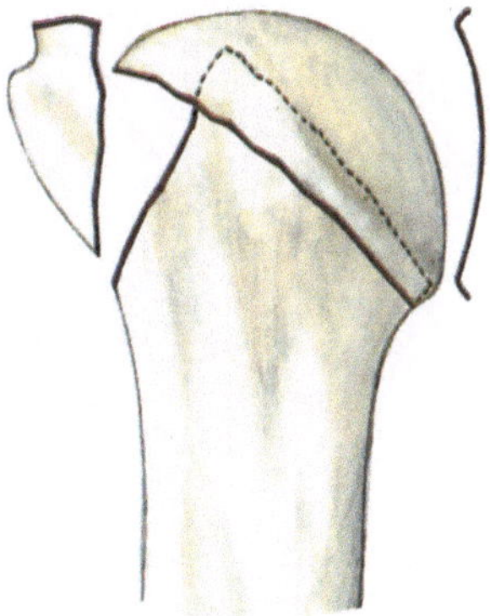

C1

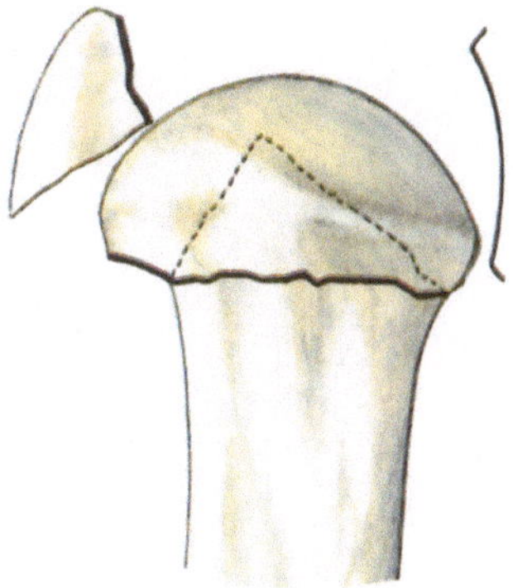

C2
Three part complex fracture

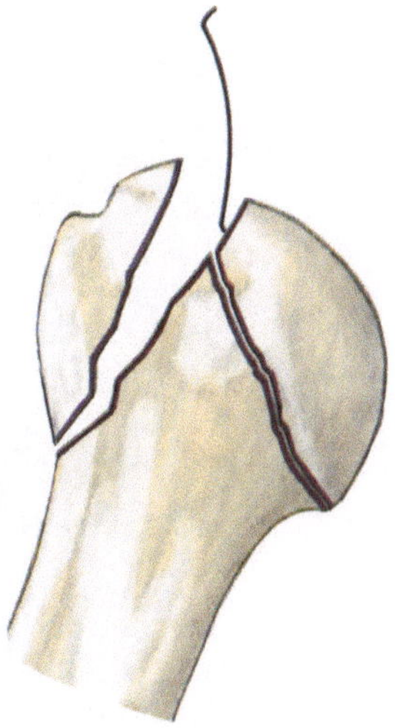

C3

AO/ASIF Classification of Scaphoid and Carpal Fractures

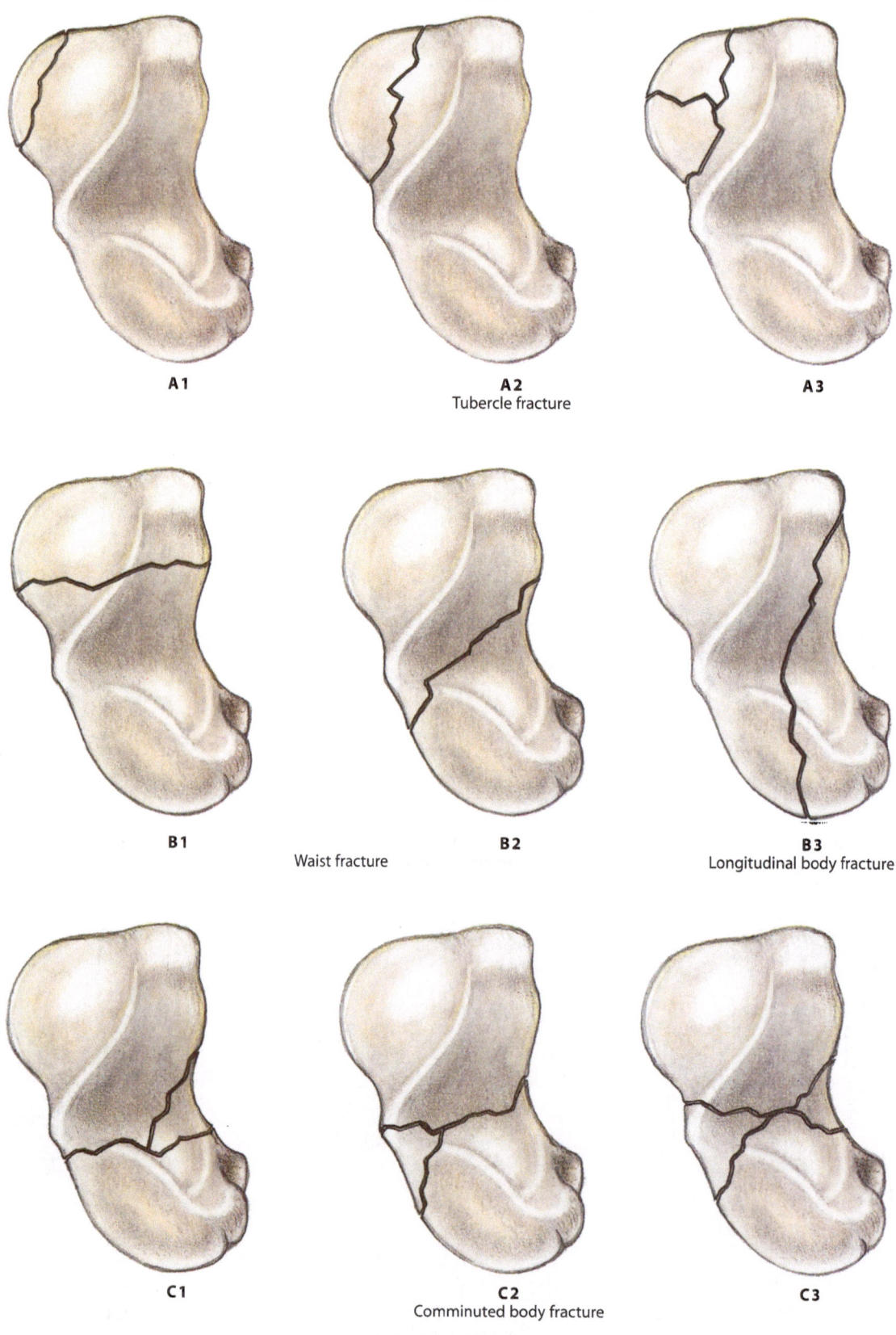

A1

A2
Tubercle fracture

A3

B1

B2
Waist fracture

B3
Longitudinal body fracture

C1

C2
Comminuted body fracture

C3

Herbert's Classification – Scaphoid Fractures

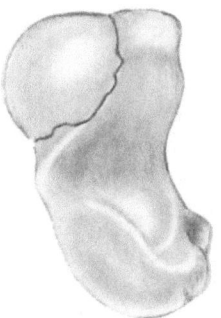

A 1
Fracture of tubercle

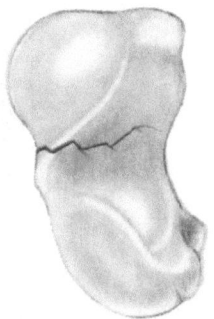

A 2
Incomplete fracture through waist

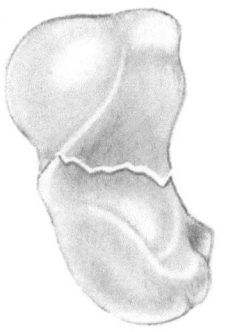

B 1
Distal oblique fracture

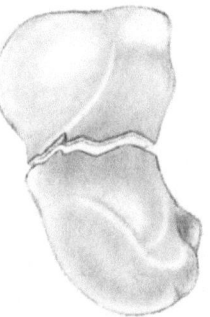

B 2
Complete fracture of waist

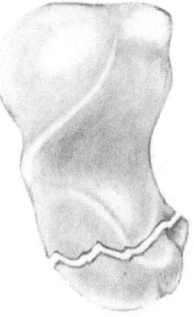

B 3
Proximal pole fracture

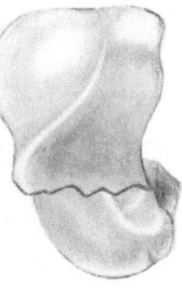

B 4
Trans-scaphoid
perilunate fracture –
dislocation of carpus

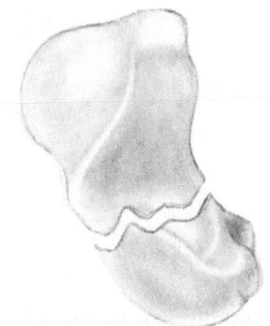

C
Delayed union

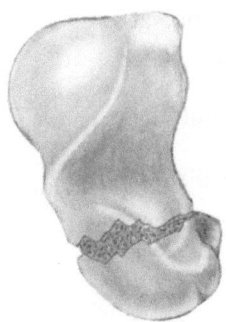

D 1
Fibrous union

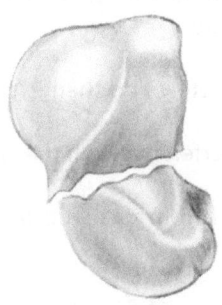

D 2
Pseudarthrosis
Early deformity

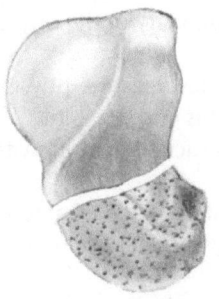

D 3
Sclerotic pseudarthrosis
Advanced deformity

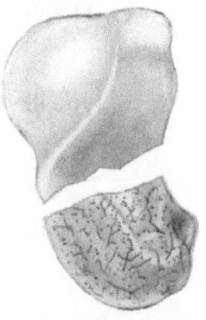

D 4
Avascular necrosis
Fragmented proximal pole

Salter-Harris Classification of Pediatric Growth Plate Fractures

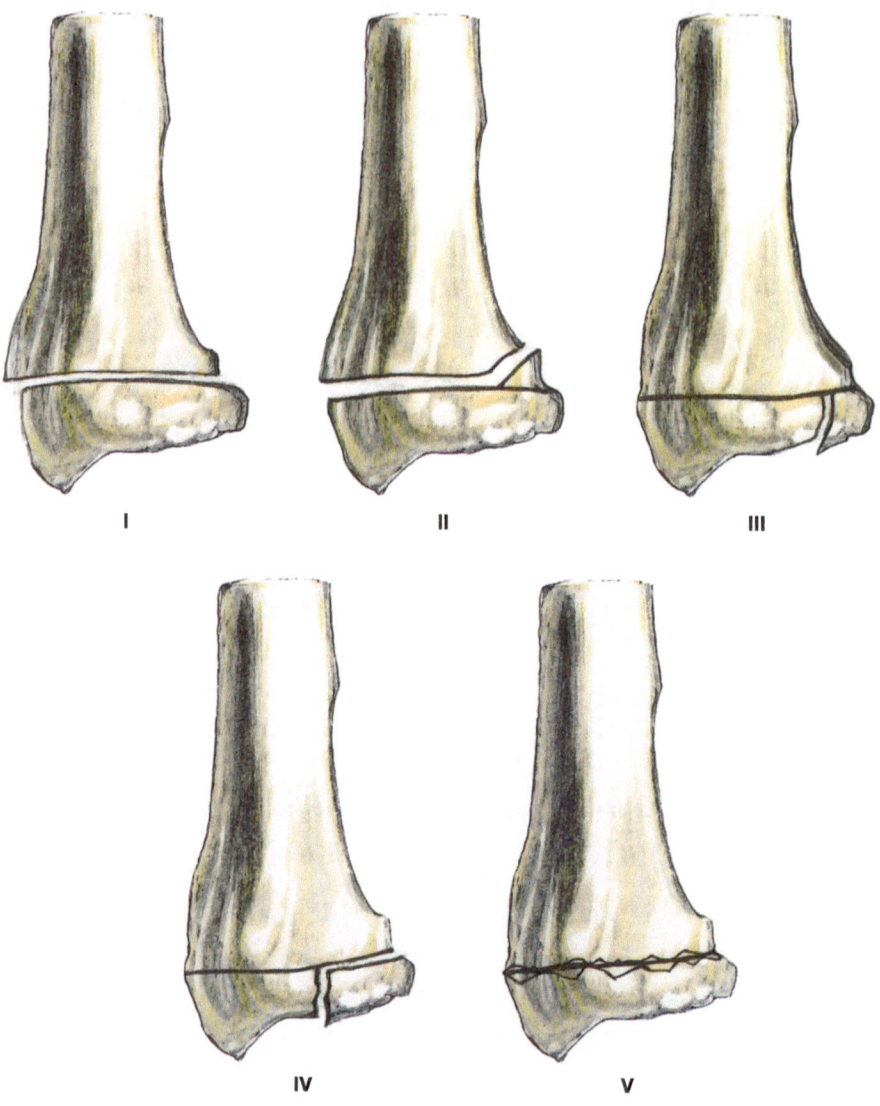

Type I: Injury traverses horizontally across the physis (separation of the epi-physis)

Type II: Injury includes separation of a triangular piece of metaphyseal bone at one boundary of the physeal fracture

Type III: Injury traverses the physis incompletely and then extends through the epiphysis into the joint
(Intra-articular fracture without interference with the epiphyseal plate)

Type IV: Vertical, displaced fracture passing from the articular surface through epiphysis, plate, and metaphysis.

Type V: Injury involves crushing of the physis without a bony fracture

AO/ASIF Soft Tissue Injury Classification

Scale

1   = normal (except open fractures)
2–4 = increasing severity of lesion
5   = a special situation

Skin lesions (closed fractures)

IC 1   = No skin lesion
IC 2   = No skin laceration, but contusion
IC 3   = Circumferential degloving
IC 4   = Extensive, closed degloving
IC 5   = Necrosis from contusion

Skin lesions (open fractures)

IO 1   = Skin breakage from inside out
IO 2   = Skin breakage < 5 cm, edges contused
IO 3   = Skin breakage > 5 cm, devitalized edges
IO 4   = Full thickness contusion, avulsion, soft tissue defect Muscle/tendon injury

Muscle-Tendon injury

MT 1 = No muscle injury
MT 2 = Circumferential injury, one compartment only
MT 3 = Considerable injury, two compartments
MT 4 = Muscle defect, tendon laceration, extensive contusion
MT 5 = Compartment syndrome/crush injury

Neurovascular injury

NV 1 = No neurovascular injury
NV 2 = Isolated nerve injury
NV 3 = Localized vascular injury
NV 4 = Extensive segmental vascular injury
NV 5 = Combined neurovascular injury, including subtotal or complete amputation

Mangled Extremity Severity Score (MESS)

Injury	Score
A. Skeletal/soft tissue injury	
Low energy (stab, simple fracture, civilian GSW)	1
Medium energy (open or multiple Fxs, dislocation)	2
High energy (close range shotgun, military GSW, crush injury)	3
Very high energy (above plus gross contamination, soft tissue avulsion)	4
B. Limb ischemia	
Pulse reduced or absent but perfusion normal	1
Pulseless, paraesthesia, diminished capillary refill	2
Cool, paralyzed, insensate, numb	3
Score is doubled for ischemia lasting > 6 h	
C. Shock	
Systolic pressure always > 90 mm Hg	0
Transient hypotension	1
Persistent hypotension	2
D. Age (years)	
< 30	0
30–50	1
> 50	2
Cut-off point = 7	
Critical score > 7; suggest amputation	

Hand Injury Severity Score (HISS)

Injury				Score
Integument				
Skin loss	Absolute values (hand)	Dorsum	< 1 cm	5
			> 1 cm	10
			> 5 cm	20
		Palm	Dorsum × 2	
	Weighed values (digit)	Dorsum	< 1 cm	2
			> 1 cm	3
		Pulp	< 25 %	3
			> 25 %	5
Skin laceration		< 1 cm		1
If extends across more than one ray, include in both ray scores		> 1 cm		2
Nail damage				
Skeletal				
Fractures	Simple shaft			1
	Comminuted shaft			2
	Intraarticular DIPJ			3
	Intraarticular PIP/IPJ of thumb			5
	Intraarticular MCPJ			4
Dislocation	Open			4
	Closed			2
Ligament injury	Sprain			2
	Rupture			3
Motor				
Extensor tendon	Proximal to PIPJ			1
	Distal to PIPJ			3
Flexor profundus	Zone 1			6
	Zone 2			6
	Zone 3			5
Flexor superficialis				5
Intrinsics				2
Neural				
Absolute values	Recurrent branch of the median nerve			30
	Deep branch of the ulnar nerve			30
Weighed values	Digital nerve × 1 (simple)			3
	Digital nerve × 2 (multiple)			4

The absolute point values are translated into grades developed by expert opinions.

Grade	HISS points
I – Minor	< 20
II – Moderate	21–50
III – Severe	51–100
IV – Major	> 100

Classification of Nerve Injuries

Seddon and Sunderland Classification of Nerve Injuries

Seddon	Sunderland
Neuropraxia	I
Axonotmesis	II
	III
	IV
Neuronotmesis	V
	IV (combination of any of Sunderland)

Mackinnon Classification of Nerve Injuries

Degree of injury	Histopathologic changes					Tinel sign	
	Myelin	Axon	Endo-neurium	Peri-neurium	Epi-neurium	Present	Progresses distally
I Neuropraxia	+/--	--	--	--	--	--	--
II Axonotomesis	+	+	--	--	--	+	+
II	+	+	+	--	--	+	+
IV	+	+	+	+	--	+	--
V Neuronotmesis	+	+	+	+	+	+	--
VI Various fibers and fascicles demonstrate various pathologic changes						+	+/--

Zones of Flexor Tendon Injuries

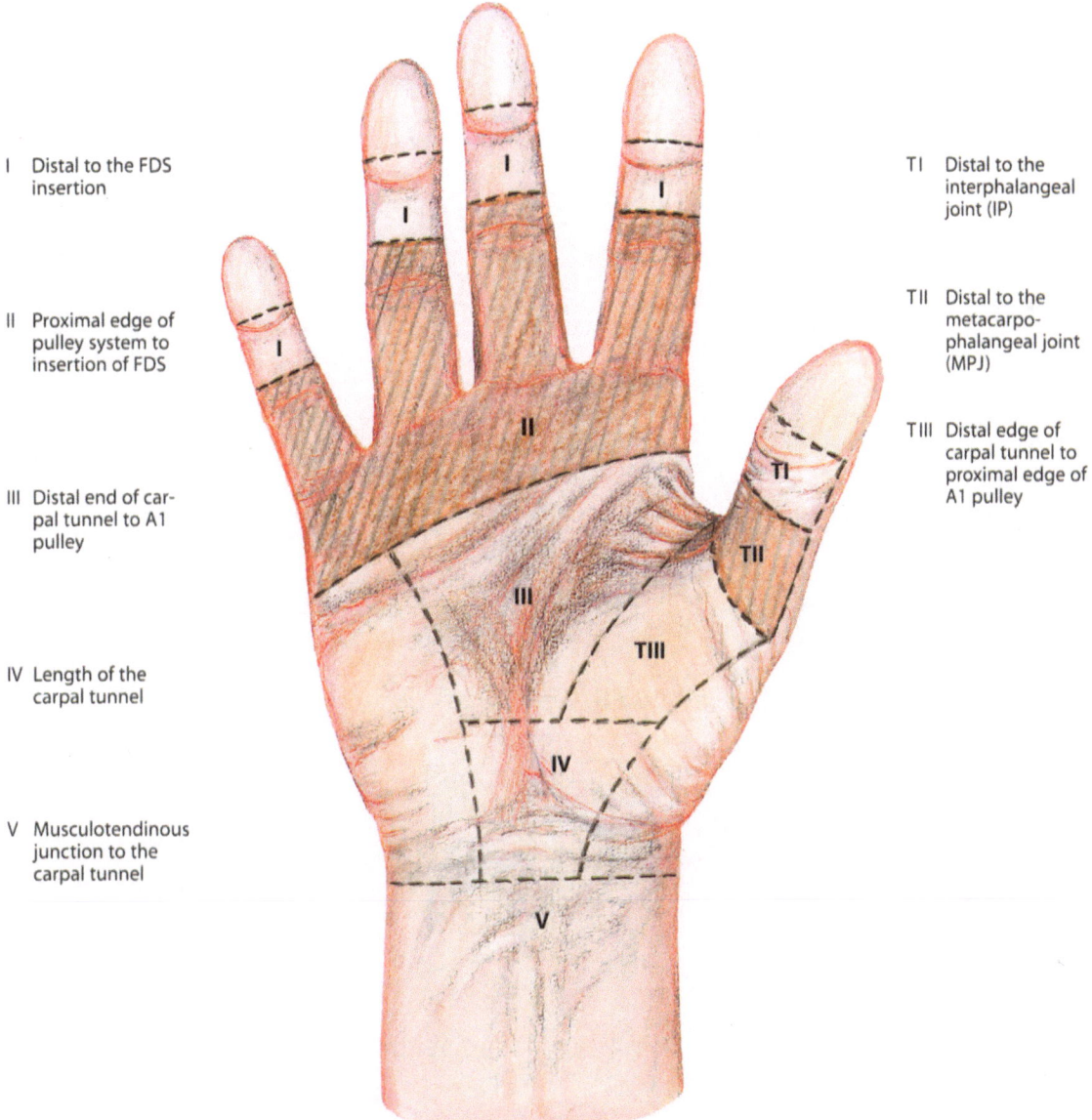

I   Distal to the FDS insertion

II Proximal edge of pulley system to insertion of FDS

III Distal end of carpal tunnel to A1 pulley

IV Length of the carpal tunnel

V   Musculotendinous junction to the carpal tunnel

T I   Distal to the interphalangeal joint (IP)

T II Distal to the metacarpo-phalangeal joint (MPJ)

T III Distal edge of carpal tunnel to proximal edge of A1 pulley

After the Committee on Tendon Injuries,
International Federation of Societies for Surgery of the Hand

Zones of Extensor Tendon Injuries

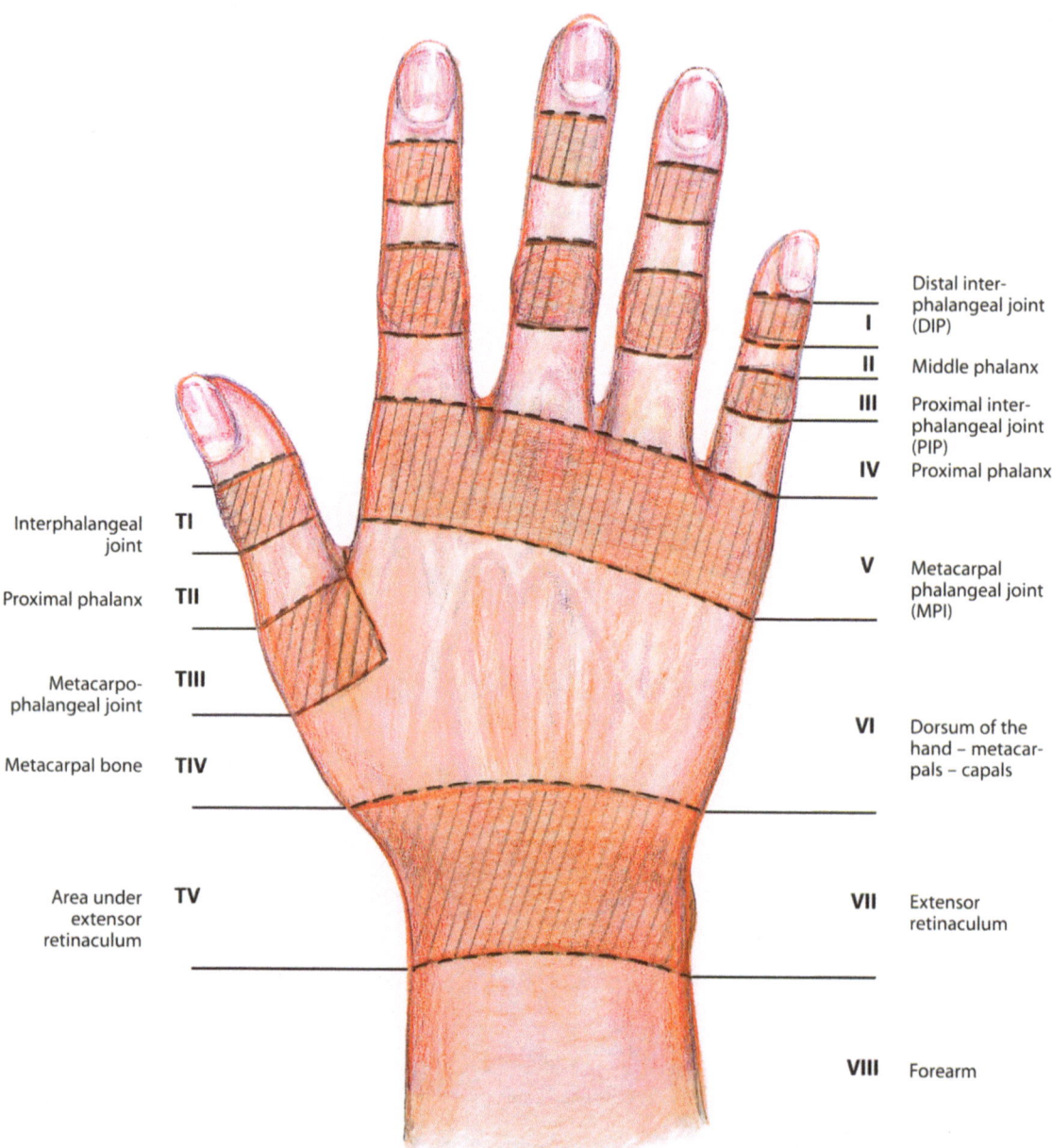

	I	Distal inter-phalangeal joint (DIP)
	II	Middle phalanx
	III	Proximal inter-phalangeal joint (PIP)
	IV	Proximal phalanx
Interphalangeal joint	TI	
Proximal phalanx	TII	
		V	Metacarpal phalangeal joint (MPI)
Metacarpo-phalangeal joint	TIII	
Metacarpal bone	TIV	
		VI	Dorsum of the hand – metacar-pals – capals
Area under extensor retinaculum	TV	VII	Extensor retinaculum
		VIII	Forearm

After the Committee on Tendon Injuries,
International Federation of Societies for Surgery of the Hand

Carpal Instability
Viegas' Classification of Carpal Instabilities

I.   **Ulnar-sided perilunate instability**

   A. **Stage I:**   partial to complete triquetrolunate tear (no VISI)

   B. **Stage II:**   complete tear of lunotriquetral ligaments, interosseus and palmar (dynamic VISI)

   C. **Stage III:**   as in stage II plus disruption of the dorsal radiotriquetral ligament (static VISI)

II. **Radial-sided perilunate instability**

   A. **Stage I:**   partial to complete scapholunate tear (no DISI)

   B. **Stage II:**   complete scapholunate interosseus ligament tear plus tear of attenuation of volar ligaments (dynamic DISI)

   C. **Stage III:**   complete disruption of the ligaments of stage II plus dorsal ligament disruption, radiotriquetral (static DISI)

   D. **Stage IV:**   complete disruption of all ligaments noted in stage III (static DISI)

III. **Dissociative:** ligament lesion, usually between bones of the proximal carpal row but occasionally between bones of the distal carpal row, the metacarpals, or even the radius and ulna

Taleisnik's Classification of Carpal Instabilities

Static		Dynamic	
Lateral	**Medial**	**Proximal**	
Scapotrapezium	Triquetrohamate (dynamic "central")	Radiocarpal Ulnar translocation	
Scapocapitate	DISI without SLD VISI	Dorsal translocation Volar translocation	
Scapholunate (DISI with SLD)	Triquetrolunate (static VISI)	Midcarpal (secondary DISI without SLD)	
Location	**Cause**	**Type**	**Other information**
By joint SL, LT, CL, RC, UT	Primary (intrinsic) Isolated Residual Associated	Static (constant) Dynamic (intermittent)	Direction: DISI, VISI, Carpal translocation
By area Lateral Medial Proximal	Secondary	Potential	Dissociation CID CIND

Mayo Classification of Carpal Instabilities

Type, site and name	Radiographic pattern
I. CID	
1.1 Proximal row CID	
a. Unstable scaphoid fracture	**DISI**
b. Scapholunate dissociation	**DISI**
c. Lunotriquetral dissociation	**VISI**
1.2 Distal carpal row CID	
a. AR disruption	**RT, PT**
b. AU disruption	**UT, PT**
c. Combined AR and AU disruption	
1.3 Combined proximal and distal CID	
II. CIND	
2.1 Radiocarpal CIND	
a. Palmar ligament rupture	**DISI, UT** of entire proximal row **UT** with increased SL space
b. Dorsal ligament rupture	**VISI, DT**
c. After radius malunion, Madelung's deformity, scaphoid malunion, lunate malunion	
2.2 Midcarpal CIND	
a. Ulnar MCI from palmar ligament damage	**VISI**
b. Radial MCI from palmar ligament damage	**VISI**
c. Combined UMCI and RMCI, palmar ligament damage	**VISI**
d. MCI from dorsal ligament damage	**DISI**
2.3 Radiocarpal – midcarpal CIND	
a. Clip	**VISI, DISI** alternating
b. Disruption of radial and central ligaments	**UT** with or without **VISI** or **DISI**
III. CIC	
a. Perilunate with radiocarpal instability	**DISI** and **UT**
b. Perilunate with axial instability	**AxUI** and **UT**
c. Radiocarpal with axial instability	**AxRI** and **UT**
d. Scapholunate dissociation with UT	**DISI** and **UT**
IV. "Adaptive carpus"	
a. Malposition of carpus with distal radius malunion	**DISI** or **DT**
b. Malposition of carpus with scaphoid nonunion	**DISI**
c. Malposition of carpus with lunate malunion	**DISI** or **VISI**
d. Malposition of carpus with Madelung's deformity	**UT, DISI, PT**

Green's Modification of the Mayo Classification of Carpal Instabilities

I.   Carpal instability dissociative (CID)
   A. Dorsiflexion (DISI) – scapholunate
   B. Palmar flexion (VISI) – triquetrolunate

II. Carpal instability non-dissociative (CIND)
   A. Radiocarpal
   B. Midcarpal
   C. Ulnar translocation

III. Carpal instability complex (CIC)
   A. Perilunate dislocation
      1. Dorsal perilunate/volar lunate
      2. Trans-scaphoid perilunate

IV. Carpal instability longitudinal
   A. Axial ulnar (AU)
      1. Capitate – hamate diastasis
   B. Axial radial
   C. Axial ulnar-radial (AUR) combined

Severity grade:
I.   Dynamic instability (Normal plain x-rays, diagnosis made on the basis of stress or motion studies and/or cineradiographs)
II. Static (fixed) instability (seen on plain x-rays)
III. Dislocation or fracture dislocation

Mayfield's Classification of Perilunate Dislocations

Stage	Radiographic findings
I: Perilunate dissociation at scapholunate joint	Scapholunate diastasis, foreshortened scaphoid, dorsal subluxation of proximal scaphoid pole
II: Dissociation at lunocapitate joint	Same as stage I plus dorsal dislocation of the capitate
III: Dissociation of lunotriquetral joint	Volar triquetral fracture (avulsion of volar radiotriquetral ligament and/or ulnotriquetral ligaments)
IV: Complete lunate dislocation	Triangular lunate, volarly rotated lunate

Posttraumatic Arthritis

SLAC: scapholunate advanced collapse
SNAC: scaphoid non-union advanced collapse
STT: scaphotrapezial trapezoidal arthritis

Stage I:	Arthritis localized to the lateral (radial) side of the scaphoid and the radial-styloid region of the distal radius
Stage II:	Arthritis extending to the entire radiscaphoid joint with progressive radioscaphoid changes (**II A**) or arthritis from the radioscaphoid joint secondarily involving the STT joint (**II B**)
Stage III:	Arthritis extending in a periscaphoid distribution and involving the radioscaphoid and lunocapitate joints

Principles of Treatment and Management

General Strategy

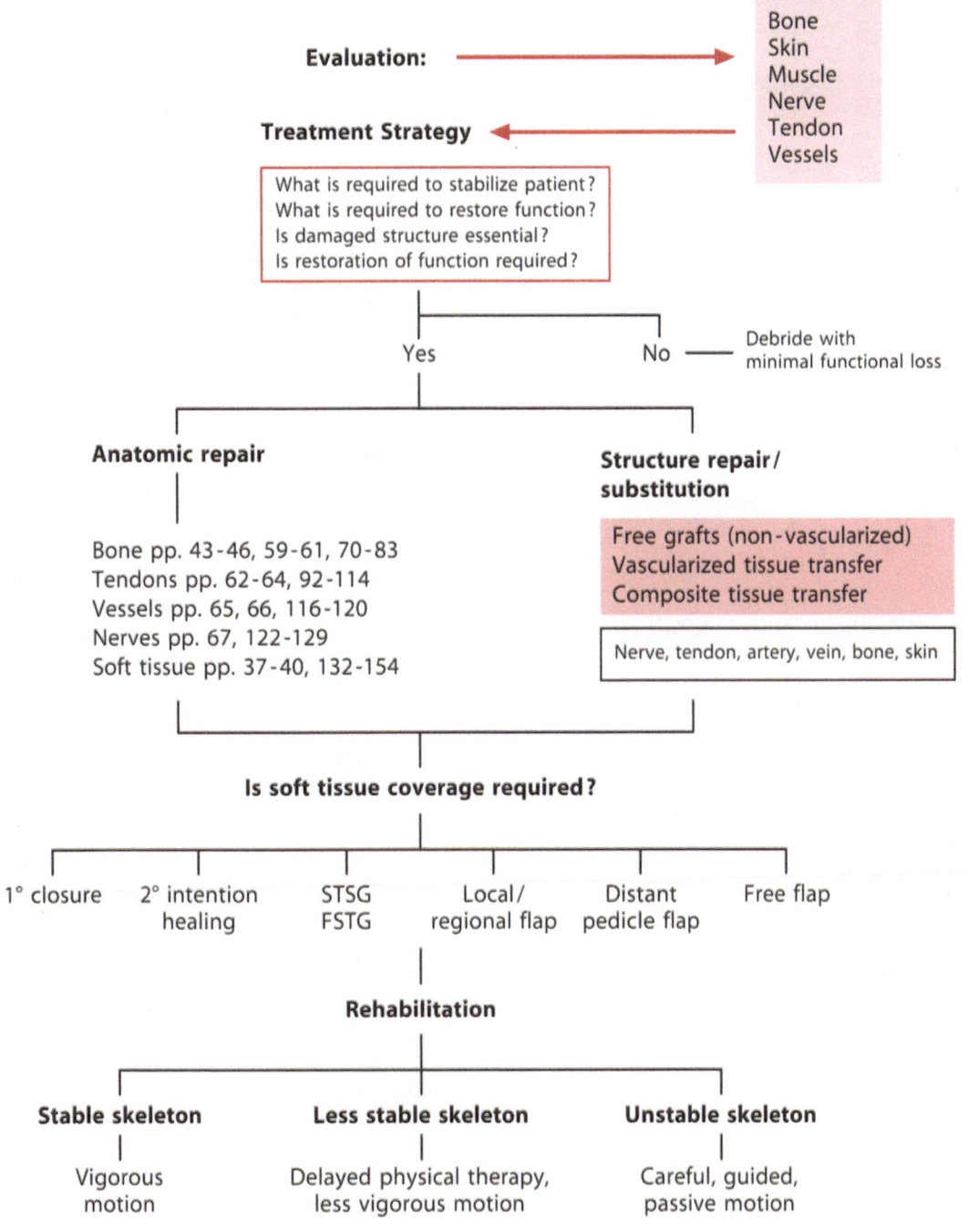

Evaluation: ⟶ Bone
Skin
Muscle
Nerve
Treatment Strategy ⟵ Tendon
Vessels

What is required to stabilize patient?
What is required to restore function?
Is damaged structure essential?
Is restoration of function required?

Yes   No —— Debride with
minimal functional loss

Anatomic repair   **Structure repair/
substitution**

Bone pp. 43-46, 59-61, 70-83   Free grafts (non-vascularized)
Tendons pp. 62-64, 92-114   Vascularized tissue transfer
Vessels pp. 65, 66, 116-120   Composite tissue transfer
Nerves pp. 67, 122-129
Soft tissue pp. 37-40, 132-154   Nerve, tendon, artery, vein, bone, skin

Is soft tissue coverage required?

1° closure   2° intention   STSG   Local/   Distant   Free flap
healing   FSTG   regional flap   pedicle flap

Rehabilitation

Stable skeleton   **Less stable skeleton**   **Unstable skeleton**

Vigorous   Delayed physical therapy,   Careful, guided,
motion   less vigorous motion   passive motion

Skin and Soft Tissue Loss

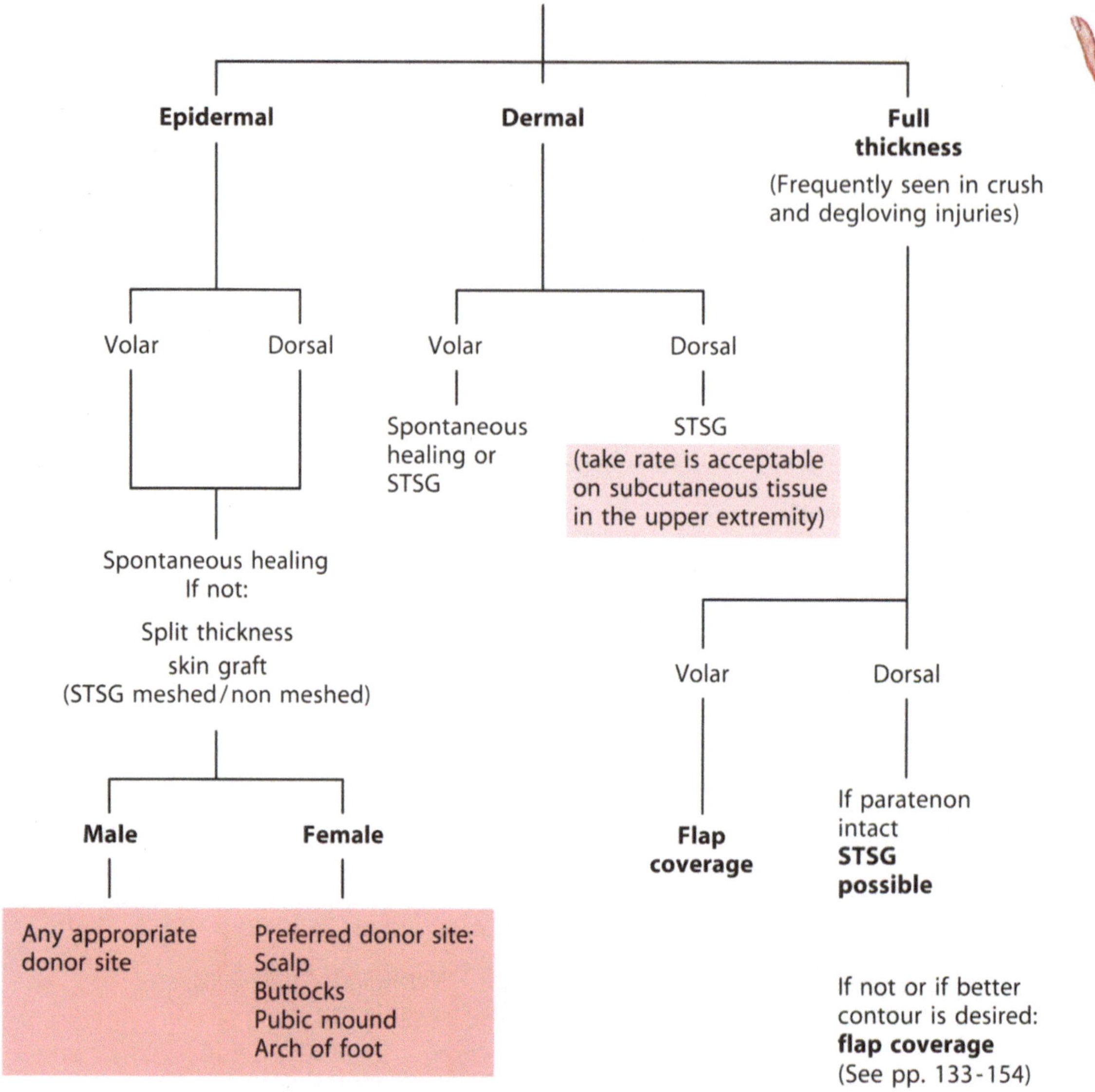

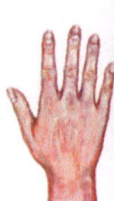

Epidermal

Dermal

Full thickness

(Frequently seen in crush and degloving injuries)

Volar   Dorsal

Volar

Dorsal

Spontaneous healing or STSG

STSG

(take rate is acceptable on subcutaneous tissue in the upper extremity)

Spontaneous healing
If not:

Split thickness skin graft
(STSG meshed/non meshed)

Volar

Dorsal

Male

Female

Flap coverage

If paratenon intact **STSG possible**

Any appropriate donor site

Preferred donor site:
Scalp
Buttocks
Pubic mound
Arch of foot

If not or if better contour is desired: **flap coverage** (See pp. 133-154)

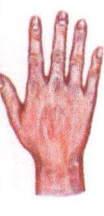

Skin and Soft Tissue – Closed Injury

Cutaneous manifestation of injury

No

Yes
Bruises
Signs of contusion/crush,
marginal skin perfusion

Signs of
compartment —— | Pain
syndrome | Paraesthesia
                 | Pulselessness
                 | Swelling
                 | Skin tense to palpation
                 | Pain on hyperextension

Signs of
compartment
syndrome

No   **Yes**

Proceed with
care of specific
injuries
as described in
pertinent protocols

Verify suspicion

| Compartment pressure
| measurement > 30 mmHg

Exploration by fasciotomy ——

Nerve release (i.e., carpal
tunnel)

Determination of extent
of injury

Debridement of skin and
muscle necrosis

Perfusion intact

Yes   No

Consider second look   Vascular
                                  reconstruction
          if not

Defect reconstruction   Secondary closure

| STSG, dermal advancement,
| delayed primary closure

Skin and Soft Tissue Injuries
Open injuries

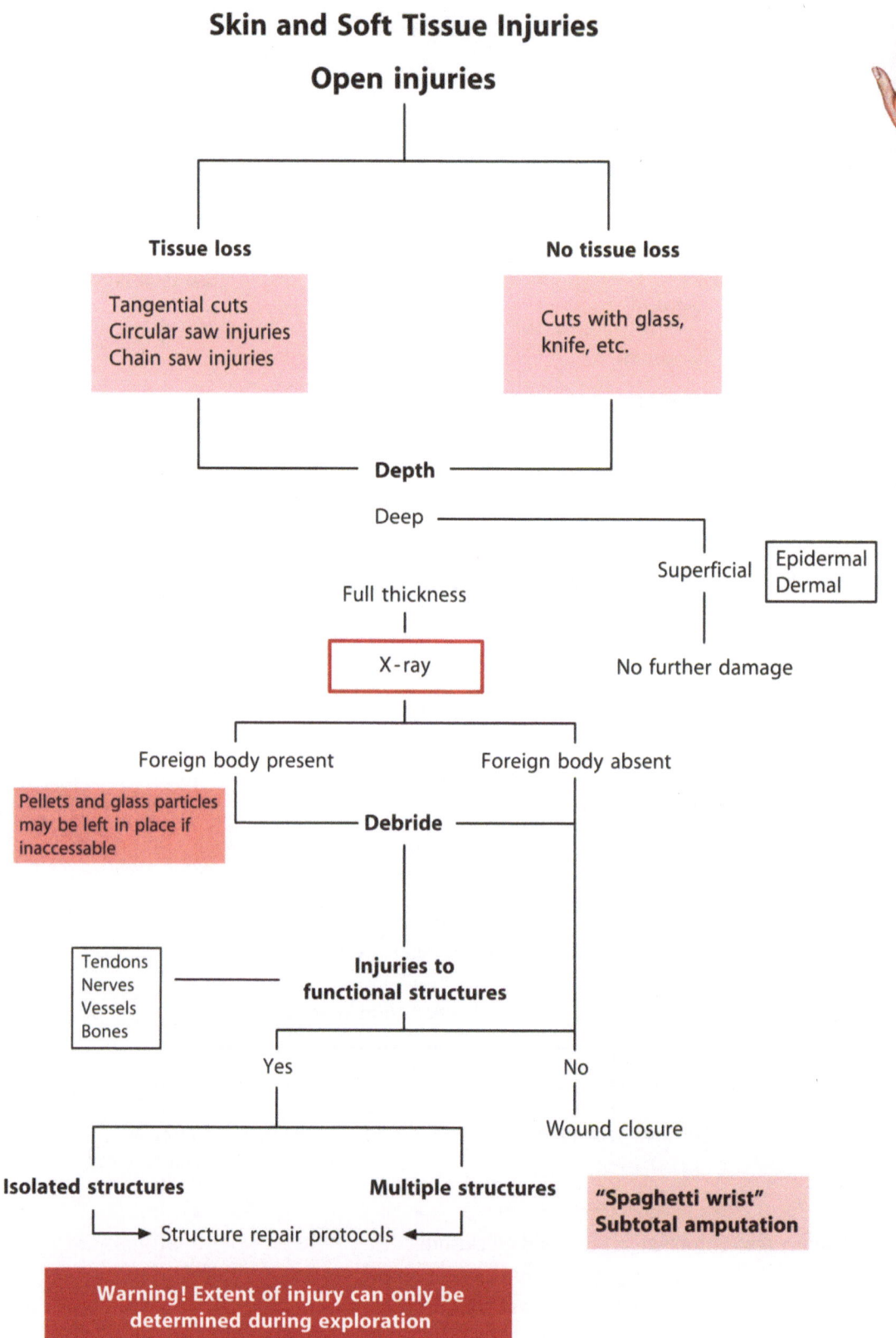

Tissue loss

Tangential cuts
Circular saw injuries
Chain saw injuries

No tissue loss

Cuts with glass,
knife, etc.

Depth

Deep

Superficial

Epidermal
Dermal

Full thickness

No further damage

X-ray

Foreign body present

Foreign body absent

Pellets and glass particles
may be left in place if
inaccessable

Debride

Tendons
Nerves
Vessels
Bones

**Injuries to
functional structures**

Yes

No

Wound closure

Isolated structures

Multiple structures

**"Spaghetti wrist"
Subtotal amputation**

Structure repair protocols

**Warning! Extent of injury can only be
determined during exploration**

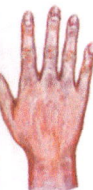

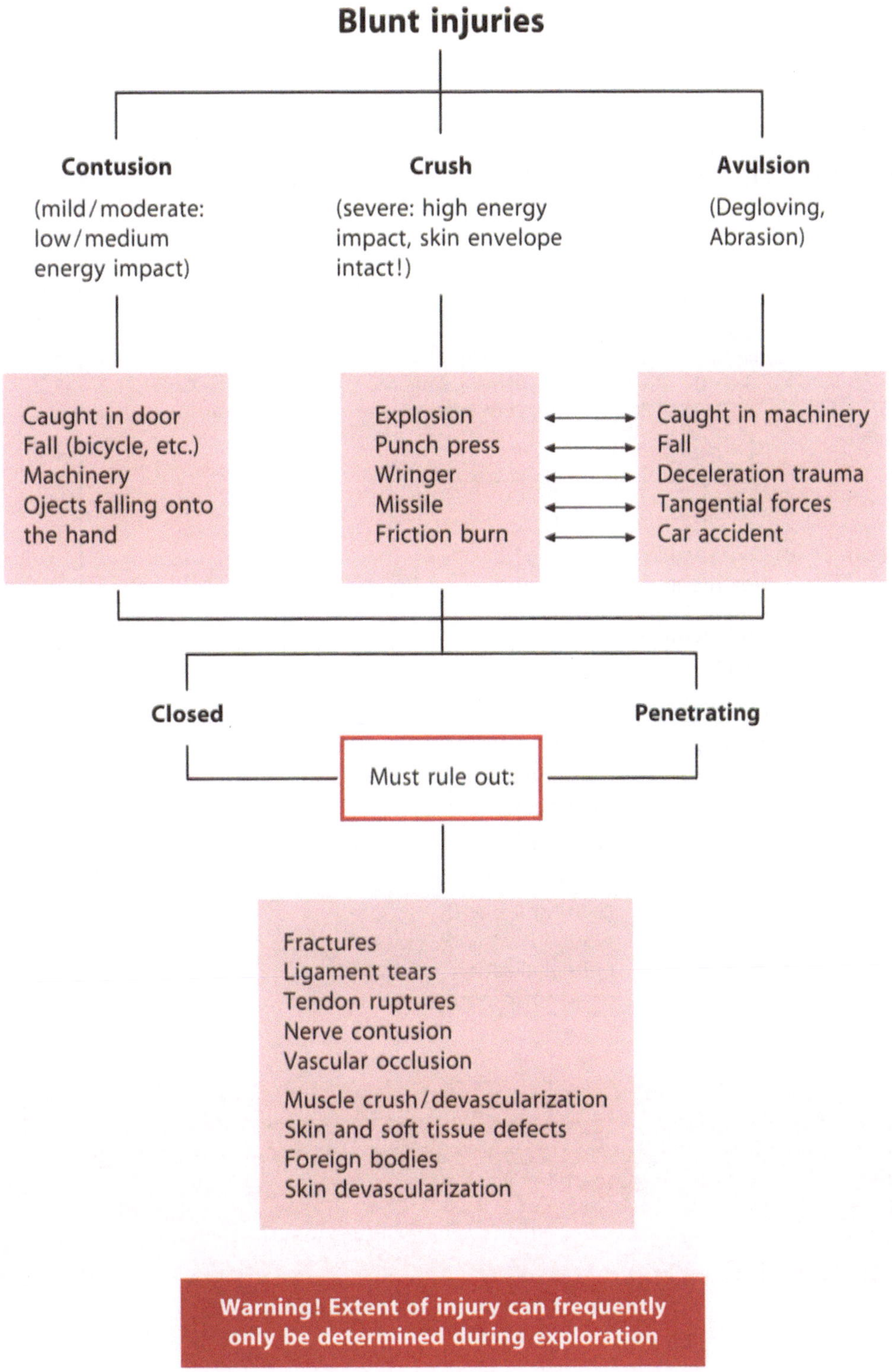

Blunt injuries

Contusion	**Crush**	**Avulsion**
(mild/moderate: low/medium energy impact)	(severe: high energy impact, skin envelope intact!)	(Degloving, Abrasion)

Caught in door Fall (bicycle, etc.) Machinery Ojects falling onto the hand	Explosion Punch press Wringer Missile Friction burn	Caught in machinery Fall Deceleration trauma Tangential forces Car accident

Closed   **Penetrating**

Must rule out:

Fractures
Ligament tears
Tendon ruptures
Nerve contusion
Vascular occlusion

Muscle crush/devascularization
Skin and soft tissue defects
Foreign bodies
Skin devascularization

**Warning! Extent of injury can frequently
only be determined during exploration**

Thermal Burns

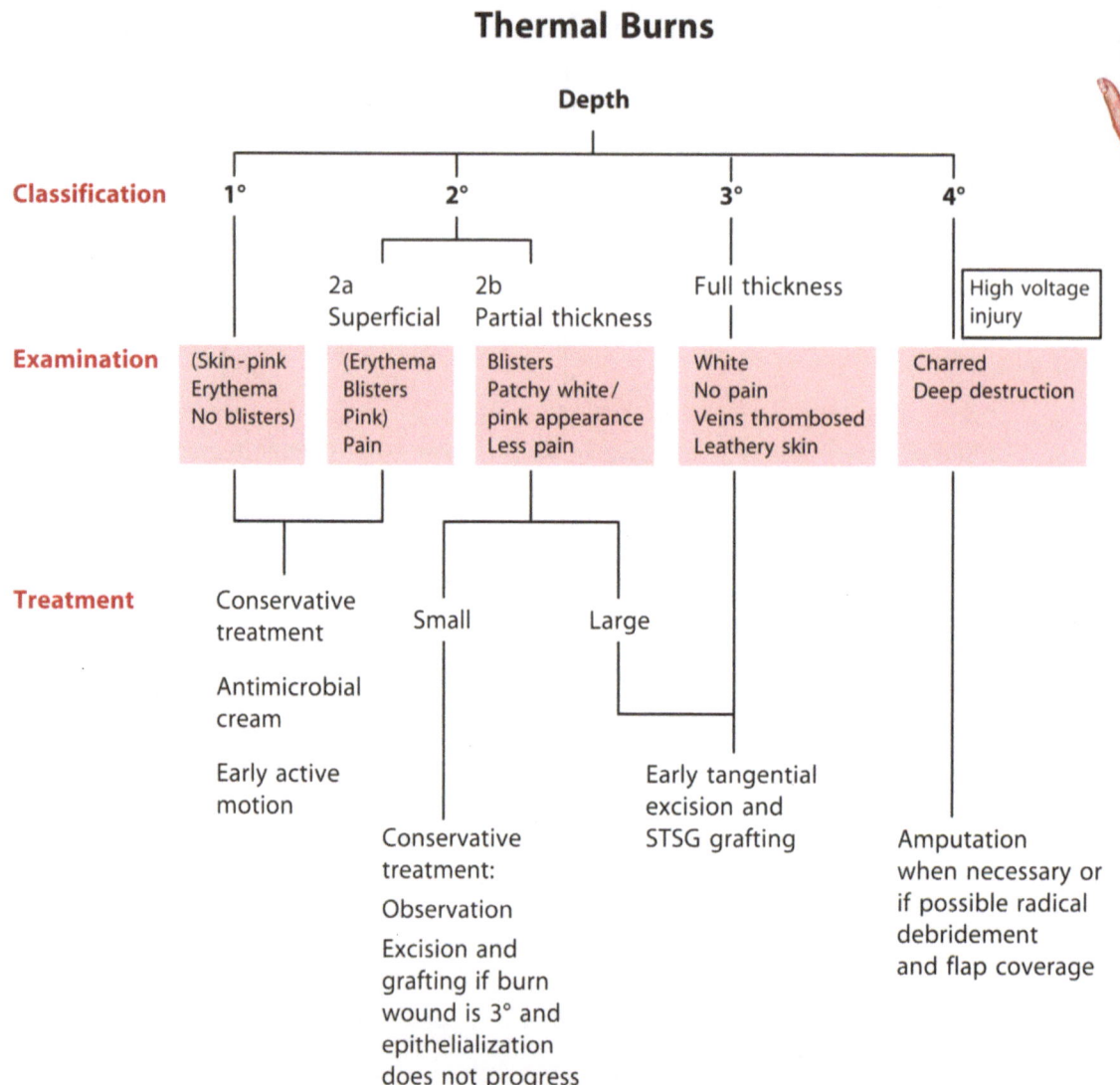

Depth

Classification

1°	2°		3°	4°
	2a Superficial	2b Partial thickness	Full thickness	High voltage injury

Examination

(Skin-pink Erythema No blisters)	(Erythema Blisters Pink) Pain	Blisters Patchy white/ pink appearance Less pain	White No pain Veins thrombosed Leathery skin	Charred Deep destruction

Treatment

Conservative treatment

Antimicrobial cream

Early active motion

Small   Large

Early tangential excision and STSG grafting

Conservative treatment:

Observation

Excision and grafting if burn wound is 3° and epithelialization does not progress

Amputation when necessary or if possible radical debridement and flap coverage

Note: In volar hand burns, conservative treatment is encouraged due to the tremendous capacity for re-epitheliailization and the difficulty of adequate reconstruction. Indications for excision only are: non-healing 2°, 3° and definitive 4° burns. Criteria of referral to Burn Center:
More than 15 % TBSA – Face – Genital area – Hands involved – Inhalation trauma – Full thickness burns

Chemical Lesions

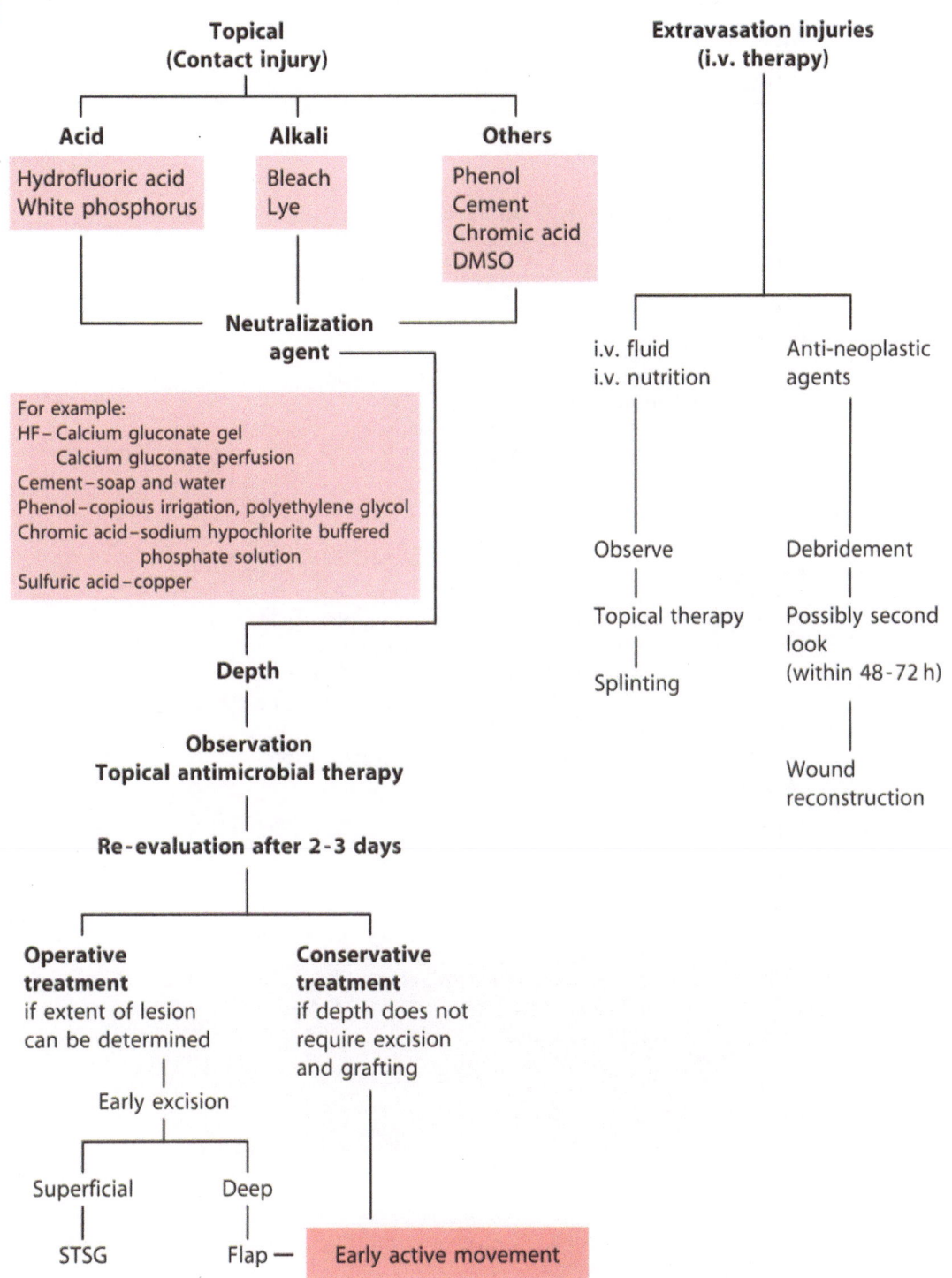

**Topical
(Contact injury)**

**Extravasation injuries
(i.v. therapy)**

Acid

Hydrofluoric acid
White phosphorus

Alkali

Bleach
Lye

Others

Phenol
Cement
Chromic acid
DMSO

**Neutralization
agent**

For example:
HF – Calcium gluconate gel
       Calcium gluconate perfusion
Cement – soap and water
Phenol – copious irrigation, polyethylene glycol
Chromic acid – sodium hypochlorite buffered
                        phosphate solution
Sulfuric acid – copper

Depth

**Observation
Topical antimicrobial therapy**

Re-evaluation after 2-3 days

**Operative
treatment**
if extent of lesion
can be determined

**Conservative
treatment**
if depth does not
require excision
and grafting

Early excision

Superficial   Deep

STSG   Flap —   **Early active movement**

i.v. fluid
i.v. nutrition

Anti-neoplastic
agents

Observe

Debridement

Topical therapy

Possibly second
look
(within 48-72 h)

Splinting

Wound
reconstruction

Management of Open Fractures

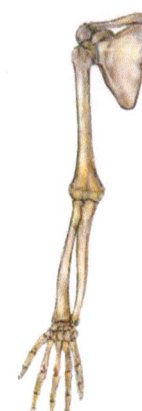

Assessment

Patient profile
Medical risk factors
Classification
(AO / ASIF, HISS, MESS, etc.)
Mechanism of injury
Delay between injury and hospital admission

Bone

X-ray: Simple, complex, degree of comminution
Joints above and below
Bone loss: Yes, no (see algorithm pp. 44, 45)
Associated injuries (abdomen, spine, pelvis)

Soft tissue

Skin:	Laceration simple, complex
	Defect: skin, skin and muscle
	Incomplete, complete amputation
Contamination:	Dirt, grease, organic material (grass, twigs), metal (filing, wadding)
Neurovascular injury:	Artery, vein, nerve, combination
Motor system:	Tendon – Laceration, defect

Treatment

1. Debridement (see pp. 47, 48)
2. Fracture fixation (see p. 46)
3. Wound care after 1 + 2

| Definitive | Non-definitive |
| see algorithm pp. 44, 45 | Bead pouch, porcine allograft, topical, wound vacuum |

Fractures

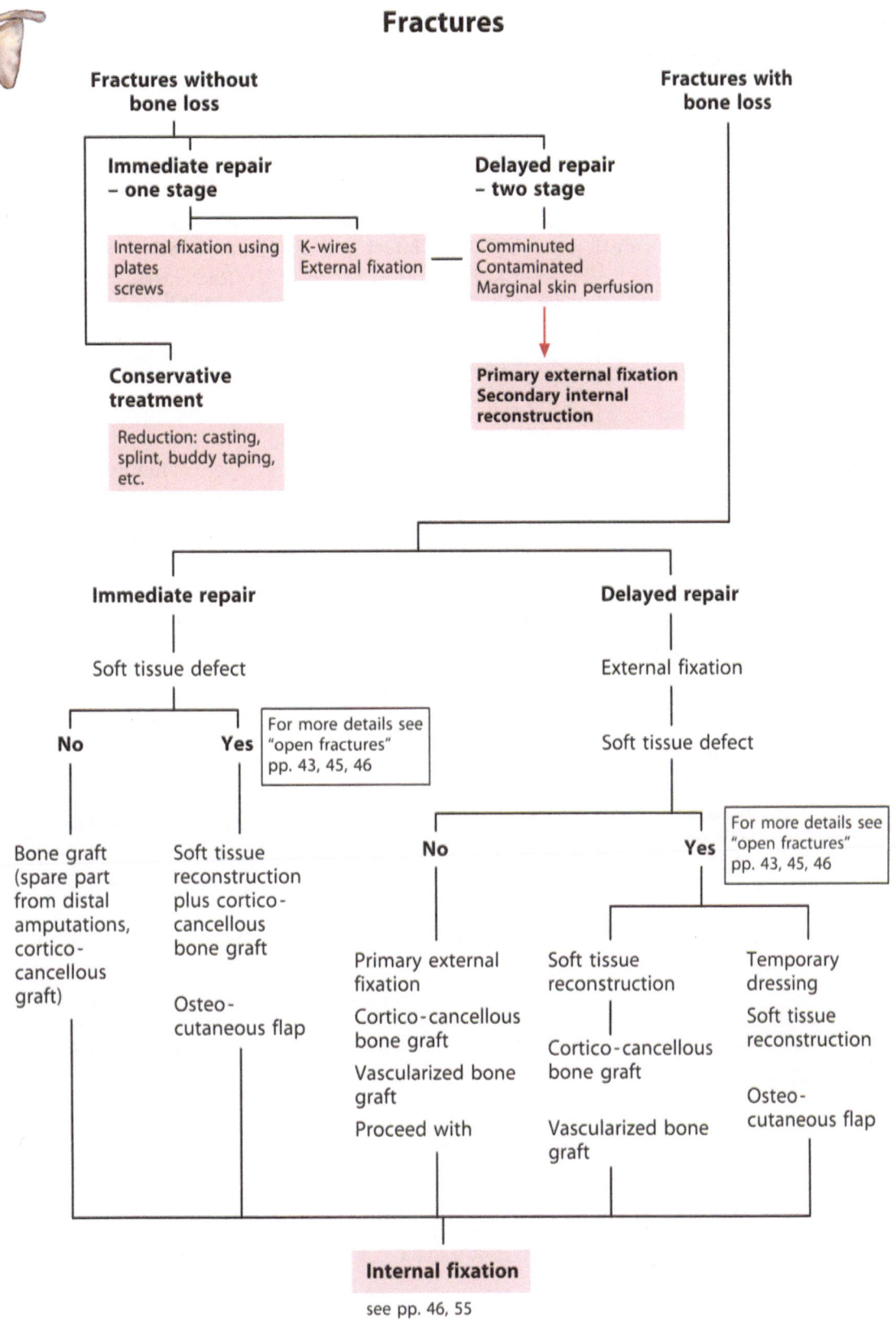

Fractures without bone loss

Fractures with bone loss

Immediate repair – one stage

Internal fixation using plates screws

K-wires
External fixation

Delayed repair – two stage

Comminuted
Contaminated
Marginal skin perfusion

Primary external fixation
Secondary internal reconstruction

Conservative treatment

Reduction: casting, splint, buddy taping, etc.

Immediate repair

Soft tissue defect

No

Bone graft (spare part from distal amputations, cortico-cancellous graft)

Yes

Soft tissue reconstruction plus cortico-cancellous bone graft

Osteo-cutaneous flap

For more details see "open fractures" pp. 43, 45, 46

Delayed repair

External fixation

Soft tissue defect

No

Primary external fixation

Cortico-cancellous bone graft

Vascularized bone graft

Proceed with

Yes

Soft tissue reconstruction

Cortico-cancellous bone graft

Vascularized bone graft

Temporary dressing

Soft tissue reconstruction

Osteo-cutaneous flap

For more details see "open fractures" pp. 43, 45, 46

Internal fixation

see pp. 46, 55

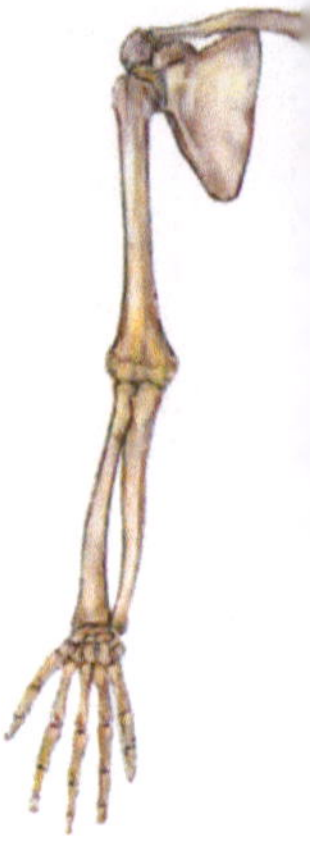

Management of Fractures
with Associated Soft Tissue Involvement

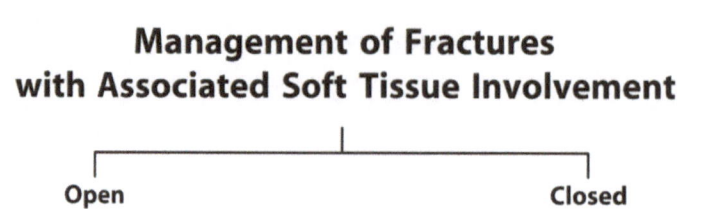

Open

Closed

Adequate soft tissue 1° / 2°

Inadequate soft tissue 3°

Soft tissue intact

Soft tissue not intact

(Contusion, swelling)

Appropriate bone treatment including bone graft if necessary (see open fractures)

Closed reduction

Percutaneous pins
or
External fixation
Reduction and secondary reconstruction in case of significant bone loss

Bone loss

Yes

No

Immediate bone graft + ORIF

Proceed with appropriate bone treatment

Internal or external fixation

Soft tissue healing

Secondary bone reconstruction

Bone loss

Yes

No

ORIF + immediate soft tissue reconstruction

External fixation
Temporary wound closure

Scheduled second look

ORIF or external fixation

Soft tissue reconstruction during second look within 48-72 h post trauma

External fixation temporary wound coverage

Scheduled second look

ORIF or external fixation including bone reconstruction

Soft tissue reconstruction during second look within 48-72 h post trauma

Consider vascularized bone grafts in large intercalated defects
Consider one-stage primary or delayed bone / soft tissue reconstruction with osteo-cutaneous flaps

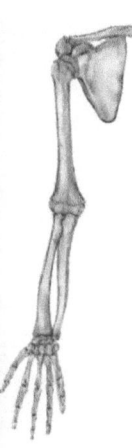

Choice of Fracture Fixation

External fixation

Bone comminuted

Severe contamination

Long delay from
injury to OR

If unable to achieve wound
closure in a timely fashion

If second look and debridement
is required

If bone or soft tissue
is devascularized

Major soft tissue defects

Internal fixation

Intact soft tissue

Fracture accessible with minimum
stripping (in open injuries)

Clean wounds

Internal fixation possible

Closure possible

Bridge or span plate:
can be used with bone graft after
wound closure (i.e., flap)

Intraarticular inujries – absolute
indications even in open injuries

Debridement

All wounds in the upper extremity at some point in time will require debridement to optimize wound conditions that will allow for wound closure. In cases of open fractures, debridement and stabilization are the most important prophylaxis against sepsis.

Sequence

I. **Timing**

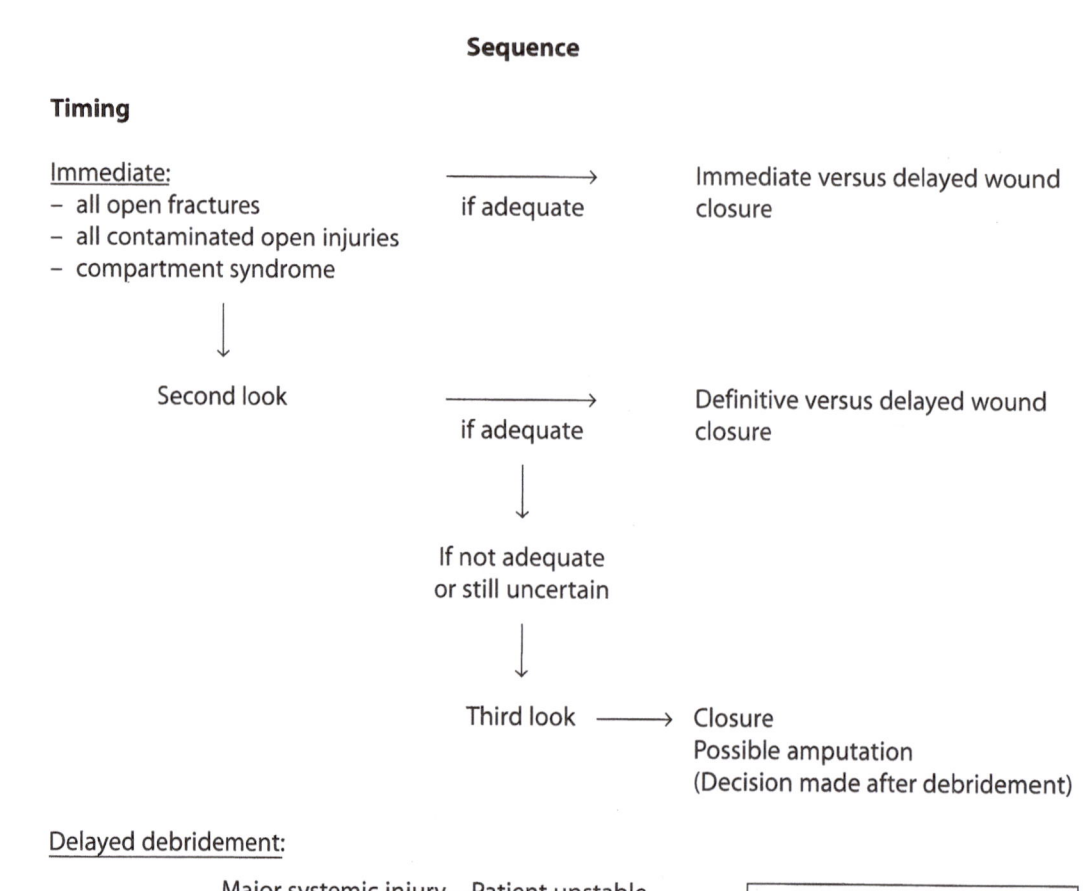

Immediate:
– all open fractures
– all contaminated open injuries
– compartment syndrome

if adequate ⟶ Immediate versus delayed wound closure

Second look

if adequate ⟶ Definitive versus delayed wound closure

If not adequate
or still uncertain

Third look ⟶ Closure
Possible amputation
(Decision made after debridement)

Delayed debridement:

Major systemic injury – Patient unstable

Contusion injury – amount and extent of dermal/subcutaneous infarction cannot be determined

Burn injury – deep 2°, superficial 3°

If delaying debridement set time tolerance to OR

II. **Tourniquet inflation**

III. **Wound inspection**

IV. **Centripetal debridement by structure**

Debridement – Structures

Skin, Subcutis	Sharp knife dissection to bleeding dermis. Trim edges 1–2 mm to create clean wound edge. Cut fat back to healthy fat. Punctuate bleeding, minimal hemosiderin staining.
Fascia	May be debrided sharply and should always be removed if not vascularized. Liberal opening/extensive exploration of compartment.
Muscle	Debride to contractile muscle. Color – pink; bleeding from cut myosomes.
Bone	All fragments devoid of significant soft tissue attachments should be removed.
Nerve	Be aware of cutaneous nerves – they may cause painful neuromas. Epineurium can be removed if contaminated (median, radial, and ulnar nerve) with fascicles remaining. If nerve is not vascularized it can remain, provided it does not desiccate, and wound closure is achieved early.
Vessels	Remove any perforated, thrombosed segments. Identify main vascular trunks. If not intact and if there is no flow, segmental vascular debridement; ligate major vessels, clip minor. Identify, mark, and protect major viable vessels that can be used for vascular access during immediate/delayed free tissue transfer.

V. **Pulsatile irrigation**

Caveat: avoid implosion of foreign material, hydrodissection of tissue planes and insufflation of tissues.

VI. **Deflate tourniquet**
Evaluate structures for bleeding

VII. **Decision making on wound closure**

Infections – Overview

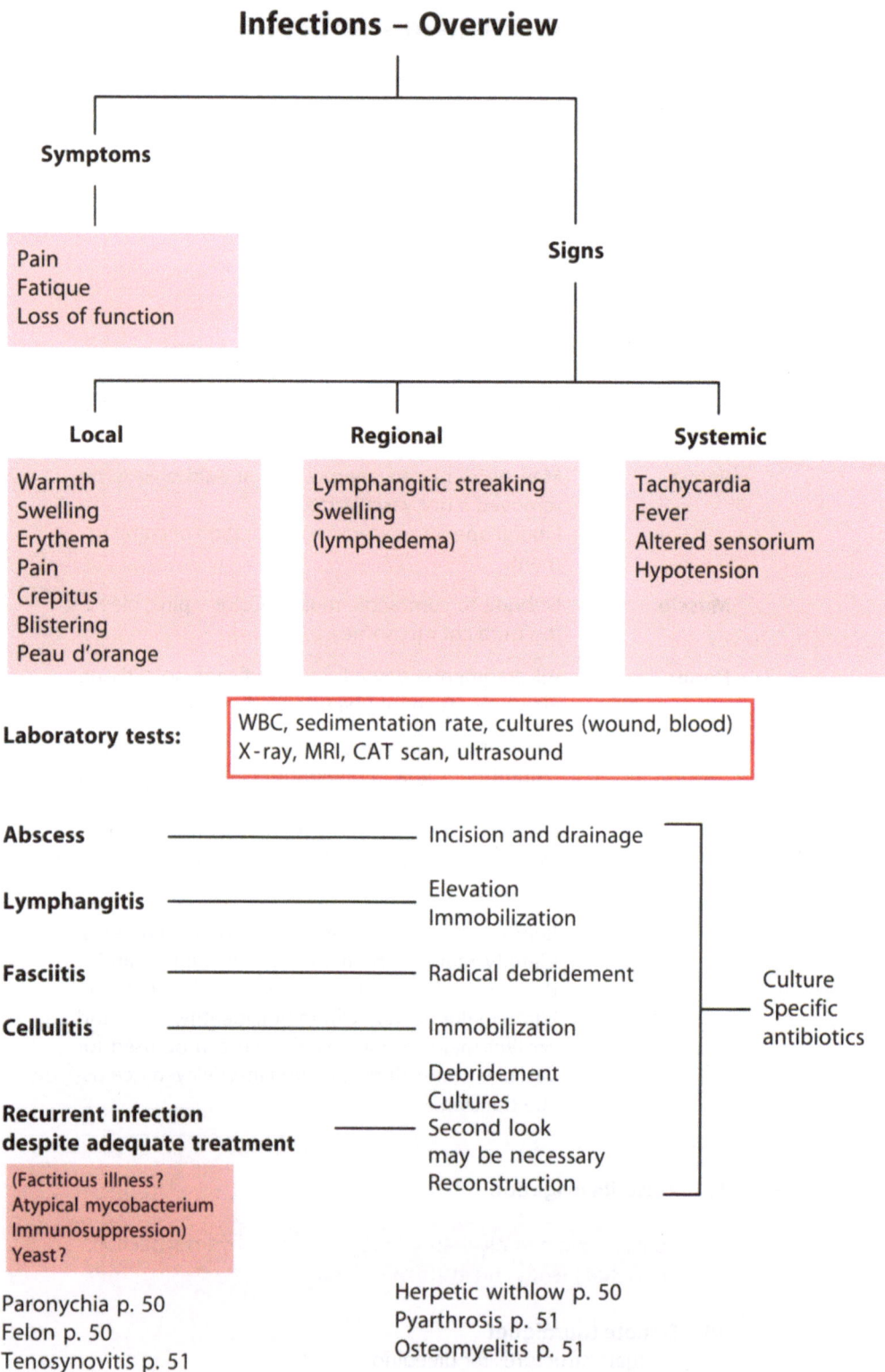

Symptoms

Pain
Fatique
Loss of function

Signs

Local

Warmth
Swelling
Erythema
Pain
Crepitus
Blistering
Peau d'orange

Regional

Lymphangitic streaking
Swelling
(lymphedema)

Systemic

Tachycardia
Fever
Altered sensorium
Hypotension

Laboratory tests: WBC, sedimentation rate, cultures (wound, blood)
X-ray, MRI, CAT scan, ultrasound

Abscess ———————————— Incision and drainage

Lymphangitis ———————————— Elevation
Immobilization

Fasciitis ———————————— Radical debridement

Cellulitis ———————————— Immobilization

**Recurrent infection
despite adequate treatment** ——— Debridement
Cultures
Second look
may be necessary
Reconstruction

Culture
Specific
antibiotics

(Factitious illness?
Atypical mycobacterium
Immunosuppression)
Yeast?

Paronychia p. 50
Felon p. 50
Tenosynovitis p. 51

Herpetic withlow p. 50
Pyarthrosis p. 51
Osteomyelitis p. 51

Infections

Fingertip

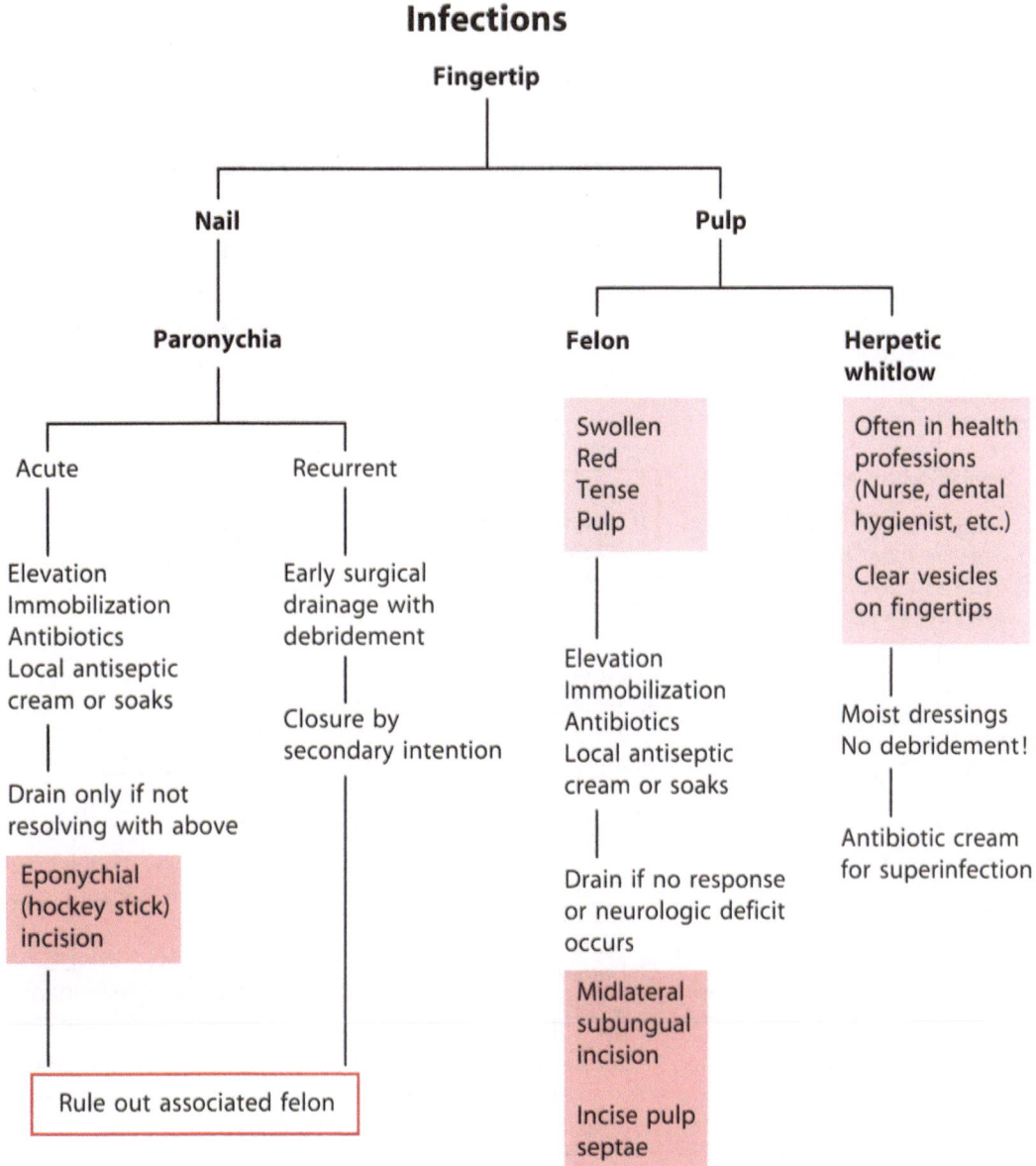

Nail

Paronychia

Acute

Elevation
Immobilization
Antibiotics
Local antiseptic
cream or soaks

Drain only if not
resolving with above

Eponychial
(hockey stick)
incision

Recurrent

Early surgical
drainage with
debridement

Closure by
secondary intention

Rule out associated felon

Pulp

Felon

Swollen
Red
Tense
Pulp

Elevation
Immobilization
Antibiotics
Local antiseptic
cream or soaks

Drain if no response
or neurologic deficit
occurs

Midlateral
subungual
incision

Incise pulp
septae

**Herpetic
whitlow**

Often in health
professions
(Nurse, dental
hygienist, etc.)

Clear vesicles
on fingertips

Moist dressings
No debridement!

Antibiotic cream
for superinfection

Infections

Tendon, bones and joints

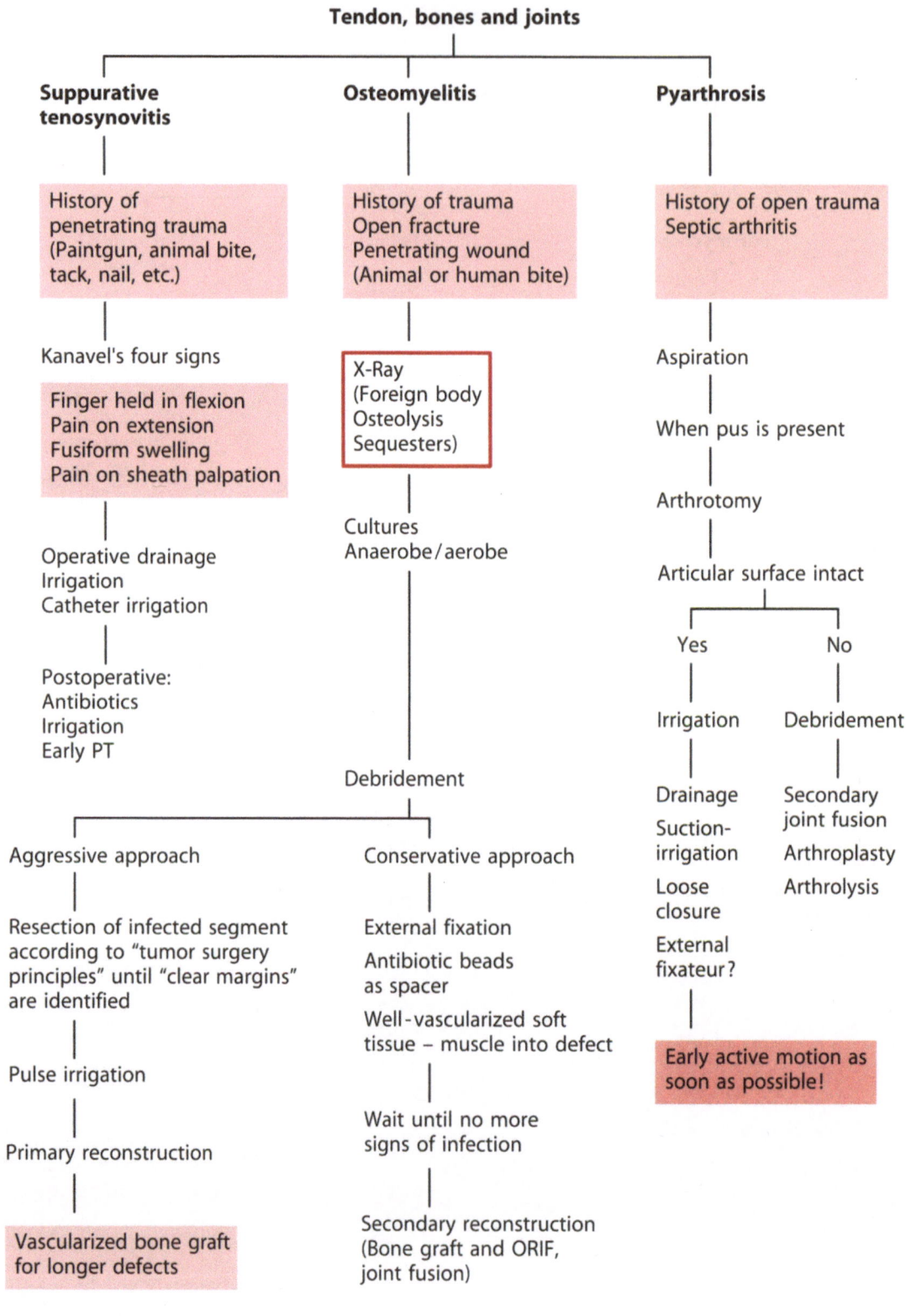

Suppurative tenosynovitis	**Osteomyelitis**	**Pyarthrosis**
History of penetrating trauma (Paintgun, animal bite, tack, nail, etc.)	History of trauma Open fracture Penetrating wound (Animal or human bite)	History of open trauma Septic arthritis

Suppurative tenosynovitis:

Kanavel's four signs

Finger held in flexion
Pain on extension
Fusiform swelling
Pain on sheath palpation

Operative drainage
Irrigation
Catheter irrigation

Postoperative:
Antibiotics
Irrigation
Early PT

Osteomyelitis:

X-Ray
(Foreign body
Osteolysis
Sequesters)

Cultures
Anaerobe / aerobe

Debridement

Aggressive approach

Resection of infected segment according to "tumor surgery principles" until "clear margins" are identified

Pulse irrigation

Primary reconstruction

Vascularized bone graft
for longer defects

Conservative approach

External fixation

Antibiotic beads
as spacer

Well-vascularized soft
tissue – muscle into defect

Wait until no more
signs of infection

Secondary reconstruction
(Bone graft and ORIF,
joint fusion)

Pyarthrosis:

Aspiration

When pus is present

Arthrotomy

Articular surface intact

Yes   No

Irrigation   Debridement

Drainage   Secondary
Suction-   joint fusion
irrigation   Arthroplasty
Loose   Arthrolysis
closure
External
fixateur?

Early active motion as
soon as possible!

Contractures I

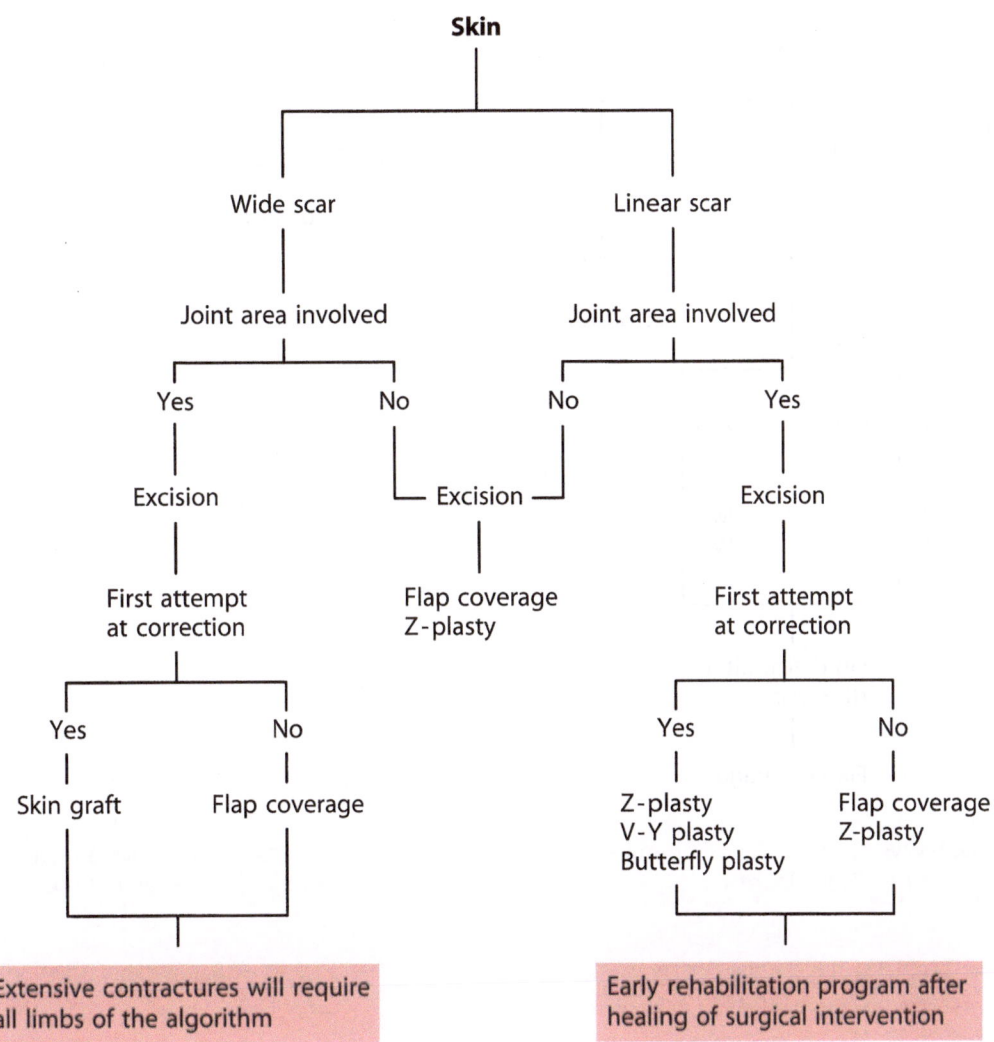

Skin

Wide scar

Joint area involved

Yes — Excision
No — Excision

Flap coverage
Z-plasty

First attempt at correction
Yes — Skin graft
No — Flap coverage

Extensive contractures will require all limbs of the algorithm

Linear scar

Joint area involved

No — Excision
Yes — Excision

Flap coverage
Z-plasty

First attempt at correction
Yes — Z-plasty / V-Y plasty / Butterfly plasty
No — Flap coverage / Z-plasty

Early rehabilitation program after healing of surgical intervention

Contractures II

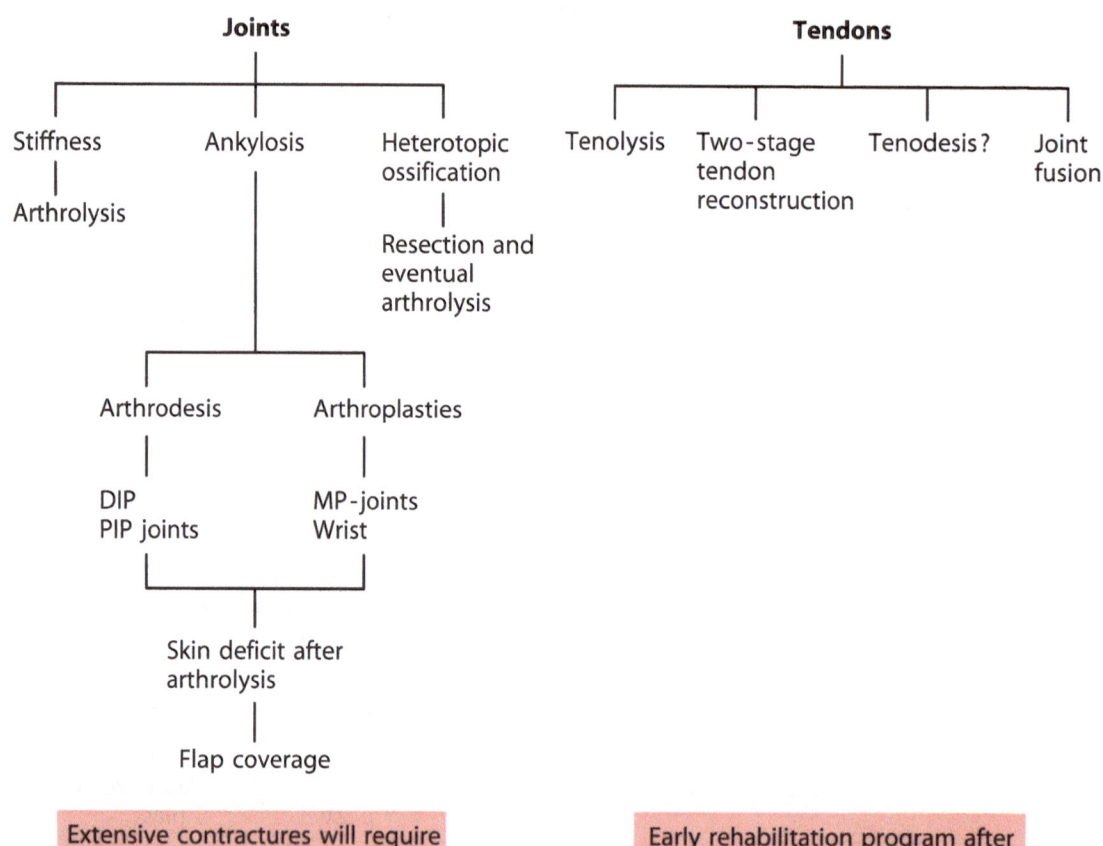

Joints

Stiffness   Ankylosis   Heterotopic
ossification

Arthrolysis

Resection and
eventual
arthrolysis

Arthrodesis   Arthroplasties

DIP   MP-joints
PIP joints   Wrist

Skin deficit after
arthrolysis

Flap coverage

Tendons

Tenolysis   Two-stage   Tenodesis?   Joint
tendon   fusion
reconstruction

Extensive contractures will require
all limbs of the algorithm

Early rehabilitation program after
healing of surgical intervention

Tumors

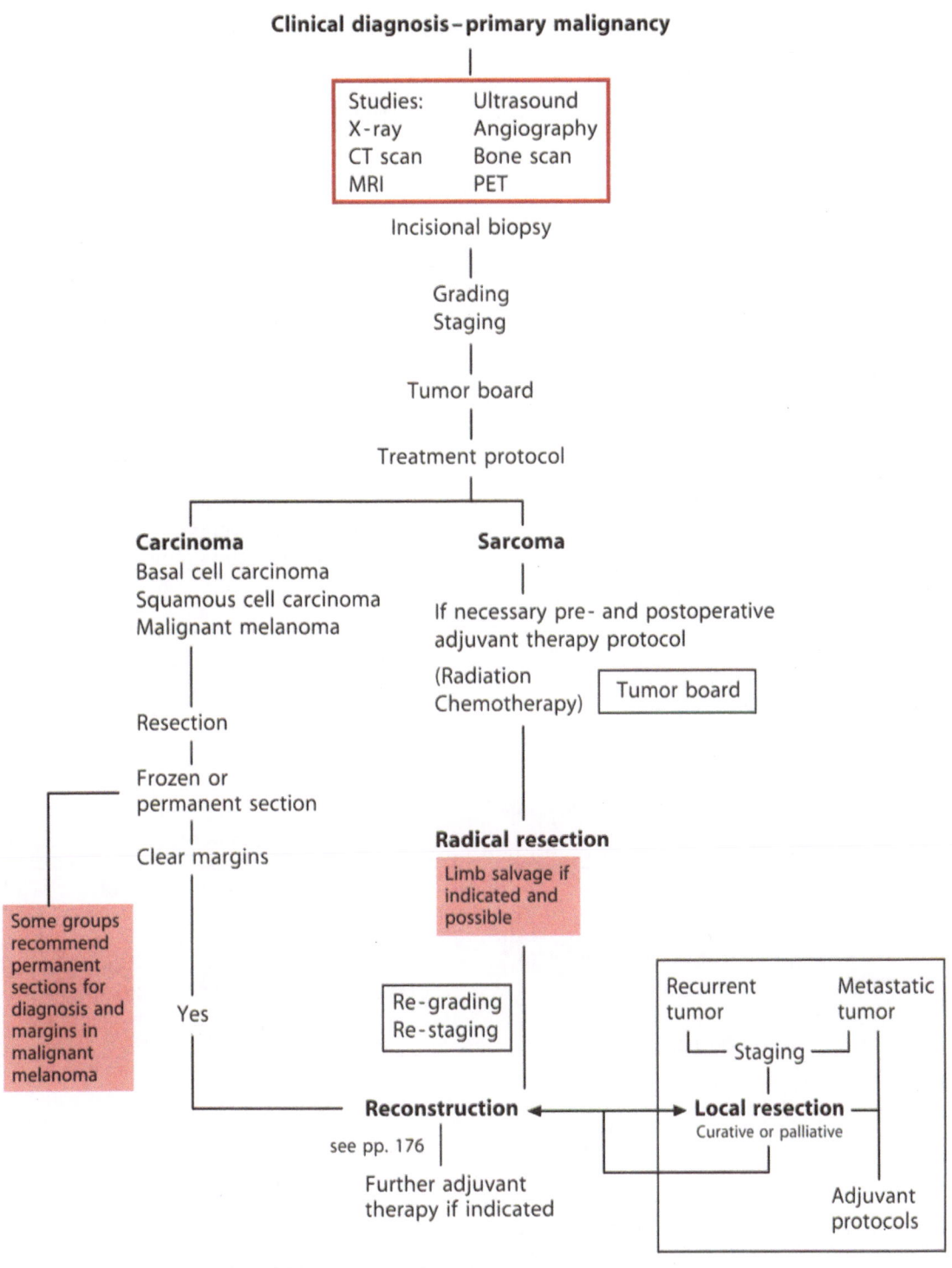

Clinical diagnosis – primary malignancy

Studies: Ultrasound
X-ray   Angiography
CT scan   Bone scan
MRI   PET

Incisional biopsy

Grading
Staging

Tumor board

Treatment protocol

Carcinoma   **Sarcoma**
Basal cell carcinoma
Squamous cell carcinoma   If necessary pre- and postoperative
Malignant melanoma   adjuvant therapy protocol

                                       (Radiation
Resection   Chemotherapy)   Tumor board

Frozen or
permanent section   **Radical resection**

Clear margins   Limb salvage if
                                       indicated and
                                       possible

Some groups
recommend
permanent   Re-grading   Recurrent   Metastatic
sections for   Re-staging   tumor   tumor
diagnosis and
margins in   Yes   Staging
malignant
melanoma   **Reconstruction** ◄───────► **Local resection**
                                                                    Curative or palliative
                       see pp. 176

                                       Further adjuvant   Adjuvant
                                       therapy if indicated   protocols

Monitoring of Flaps and Impending Flap Failure

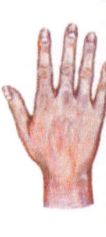

	Signs of regular perfusion	**Signs of abnormal perfusion**	
		Venous compromise	Arterial compromise
Skin:	Pink, warm normal capillary refill	Patchy, blueish fast capillary refill; cool	Pale; slow capillary refill; cool
Muscle:	Normal color, brisk bleeding when scarificized; normal Doppler signal; pink adherent skin graft	Dark; dark red bleeding; skin graft not adherent	Pale; no brisk bleeding; skin graft not adherent; no Doppler signal
Fascia:	Normal Doppler signal; palpable pulse in pedicle; pink adherent skin graft	Dark; grayish Doppler signal may remain normal for a longer period	No palpable pulse; skin graft not adherent; no Doppler signal

Possible Causes for Impaired Perfusion

Pedicle flaps

Inflow	Outflow	Both
Arterial kinking	Venous occlusion	
Inset too tightly	Tunnel too tight	
Damage to pedicle	Inset to tight	
Arterial insufficiency	Venous thrombosis in major vein	
Thrombosis in extremity	Kinking of pedicle	

Hematoma under flap

Free flaps

Inflow (arterial compromise)	Outflow (venous compromise)	Both

See pedicle flaps + check for thrombus
in anastomosis

Emergency measures

**Release bandages and dressing
Optimize blood pressure and
intravascular volume
Elevate room temperature
Change position of extremity and flap**

**All measures described in pedicle
flaps – but most important**

**Early surgical revision if perfusion
does not normalize within a short
period!**

if no change

Release sutures
Open tunnel

Evacuate hematoma
Suture flap back into bed

Delayed venous insufficiency
in small flaps:
Leeches - scarification +
heparin gauze

Venous insufficiency in larger flaps:
Turbocharging by microsurgical
venous anastomoses

CHAPTER II
Techniques of Structure Repair

Skin Graft

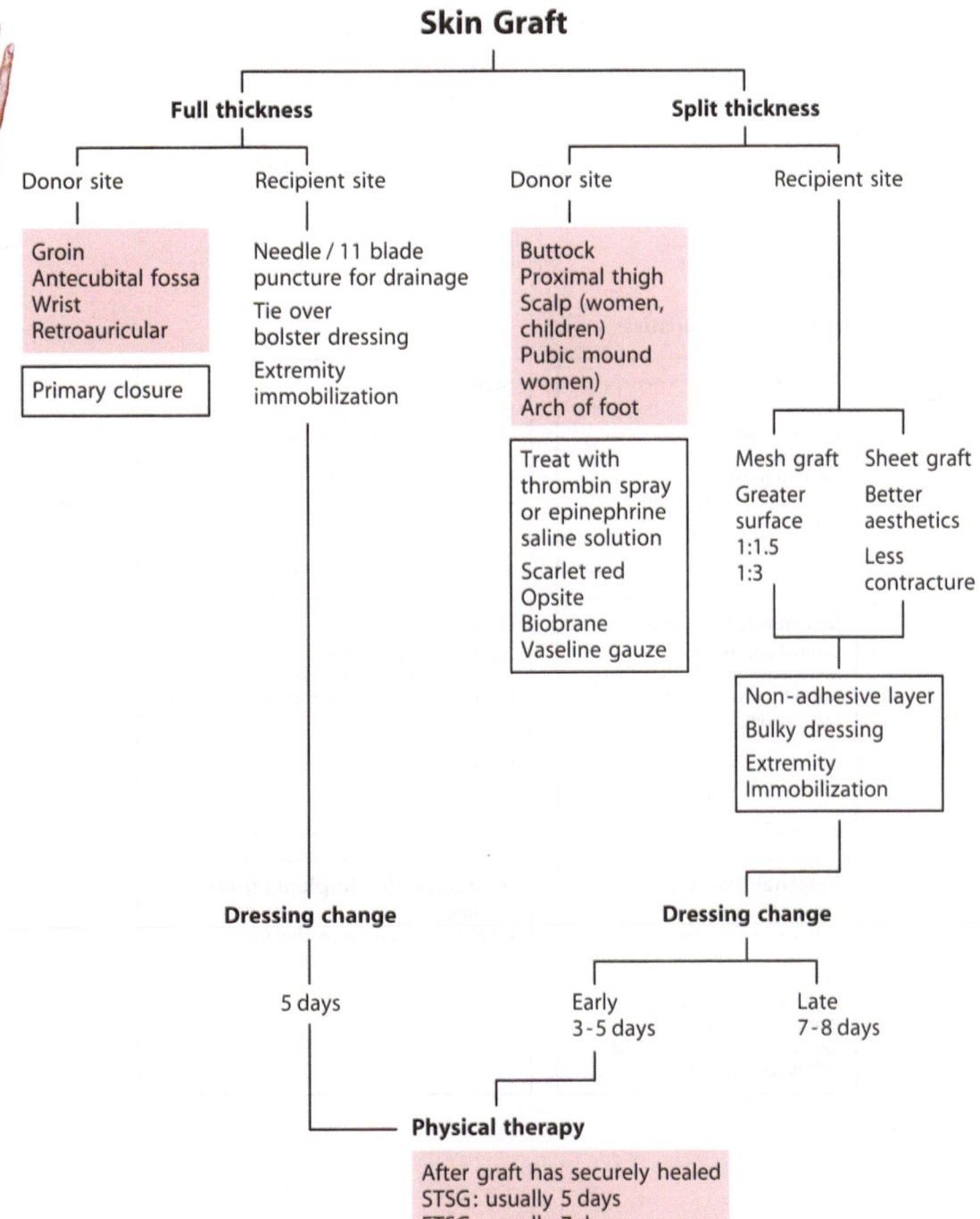

Full thickness

Donor site

> Groin
> Antecubital fossa
> Wrist
> Retroauricular

> Primary closure

Recipient site

Needle / 11 blade
puncture for drainage

Tie over
bolster dressing

Extremity
immobilization

Split thickness

Donor site

> Buttock
> Proximal thigh
> Scalp (women,
> children)
> Pubic mound
> women)
> Arch of foot

Treat with
thrombin spray
or epinephrine
saline solution

Scarlet red
Opsite
Biobrane
Vaseline gauze

Recipient site

Mesh graft

Greater
surface
1:1.5
1:3

Sheet graft

Better
aesthetics

Less
contracture

Non-adhesive layer
Bulky dressing
Extremity
Immobilization

Dressing change

5 days

Dressing change

Early
3-5 days

Late
7-8 days

Physical therapy

> After graft has securely healed
> STSG: usually 5 days
> FTSG: usually 7 days

Options - Osteosynthesis

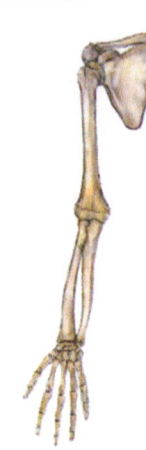

Internal	**External**	**Combination**
K-wire	Traction	ExFix + plate
Plate / screws	Casting	ExFix + screws
Rod	Frame	K-wire + ExFix
Biodegradable pins	- Unilateral	
Suture (ligaments)	- Delta	

Implant characteristics:

K-wire
Simple
Percutaneous
Less rigid
Tension possible
(in tension band wiring)
Rapid
Easy removal

Screws
Neutralization device
Compression device (lag screw)
Alone or with plate
For interfragmental compression,
a 3:1 ratio is desired

Intramedullary rod
Limited approach
Minimum soft tissue stripping
Good for gross alignment
Compression limited

Plate
Rigid if combined with screw
Requires soft tissue stripping
Hazardous if used in inadequate soft tissue
Compression
Neutralization
Spanning
Bridging
Buttress

External fixation
Helpful in open fractures
with contamination
Stabilizes comminuted fractures
Less rigid
Helpful in skin contusion
Pins can cause infections
Can be combined with ORIF if
soft tissue is stable

Biodegradable implants (pins)
Not rigid
Good for small osteocondral fragments
Early mobilization may be delayed

Techniques of Osteosynthesis
Lag Screw Principle-Plate – External Fixation – K-Wire-Fixation

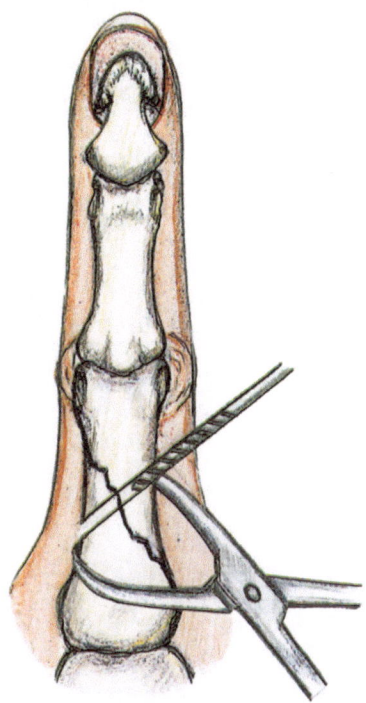

Bicortical drilling after fracture reduction

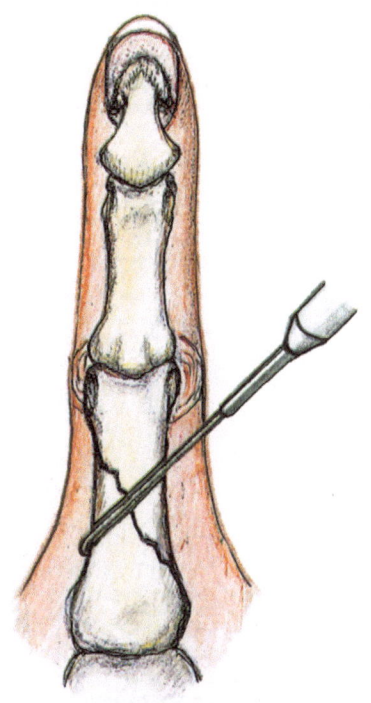

Measurement of screw length with depth gauge

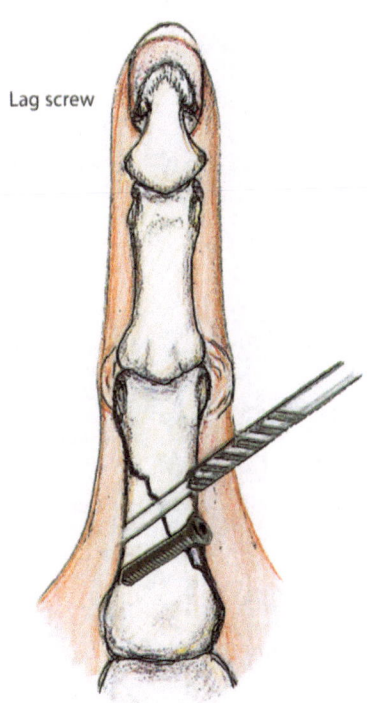

Lag screw

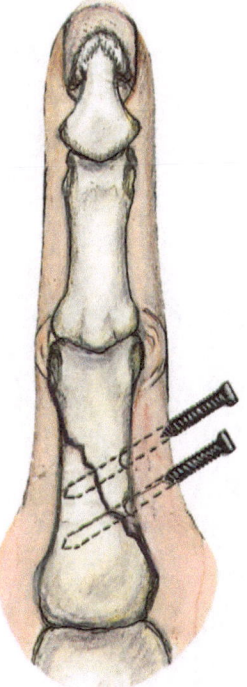

Oblique fractures can also be fixed with interfragmentary compression screws. Application of the lag screw principle yields maximal compression and stability. After bicortical drilling with the screw-size driller, the proximal cortex is over-drilled with the next size driller. Self tapping screws are used in the hand, with the exception of metacarpal fractures in young males with thick cortices

Screw placement should not be too close to the tip of the bone spikes to avoid splitting of the bone.

Plate fixation of horizontal or comminuted fractures.

Plates are frequently placed dorsally after splitting the extensor tendons. This can lead to adhesions and extensor lags. Ideally, the plate should be placed latero-dorsally or latero-medially to reduce undesired adhesions

After reduction of the fracture, the plate is held with reduction forceps. The screws closest to the fractures are set first. In digital fractures, neutralization plates are used. In metacarpal fractures, dynamic compression plates may be appropriate. Here, the holes closest to the fracture are drilled "eccentrically".

After drilling the holes, screw length is determined by a depth gauge. After setting the first screws proximal and distal to the fracture site, the reduction forceps can be removed

Plate

Reduction is maintained by an assistant. The first pin is inserted close to the joint on either side. The fracture is then permanently reduced with all screws still loose. After best possible reduction and desired joint position, screws are fixed. Insertion of two more pins – completion

If a horizontal fracture is stabilized with pins – avoid crossing of the pins in the fracture line

Oblique fracture treated with percutaneous pins. The pin tips can either be cut off and bent just under the skin or bent outside the skin. Occasionally, percutaneous pins can migrate and penetrate other structures such as the extensor mechanism

Best access to metacarpals and phalanges is latero-dorsal to avoid grasping the extensor mechanism with the pins

Insertion of two pins on either side of the fracture. Reduction by assistant and fixation under amplification. Insertion of additional pins – completion

External fixator

K-wire

Techniques of Tendon Repair

Basic technique is a rectangle suture which has undergone numerous modifications after Kirchmayer's first description in 1917

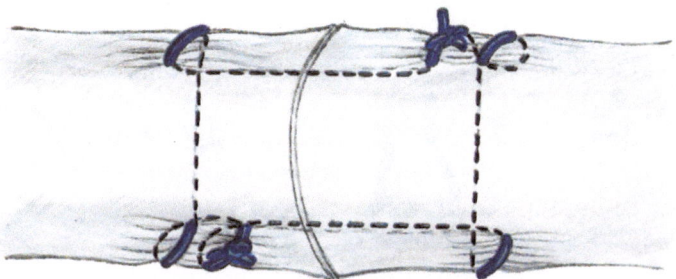

Original Kirchmayer/ Kessler:
Two sutures (two-strand) with knots buried in the tendon outside the suture line

A two-strand core suture with knots in the suture line or buried in the tendon outside the suture line. Intratendinous knots may have better gliding properties, but have more suture material in the tendon gap. Theoretically, sutures should be placed insofar as possible at the volar aspect of the tendon to avoid disturbance of the dorsally situated vessels. Too much compression at the suture line should be avoided to prevent bulging of the tendon repair with subsequent impairment of gliding

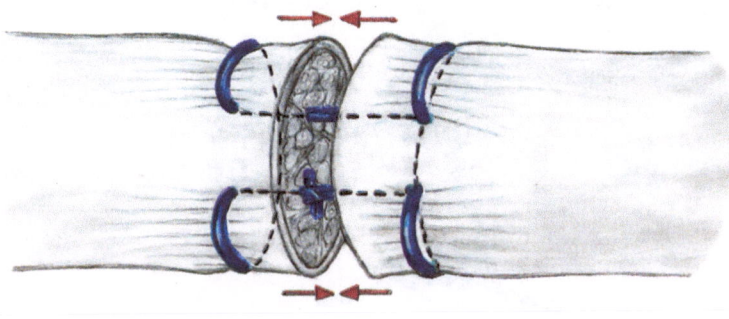

Modified Kessler: One or two sutures (two-strand) with intratendinous knots. Cross section demonstrates optimal position of core sutures

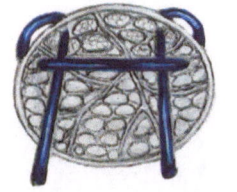
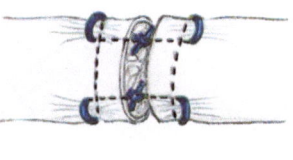

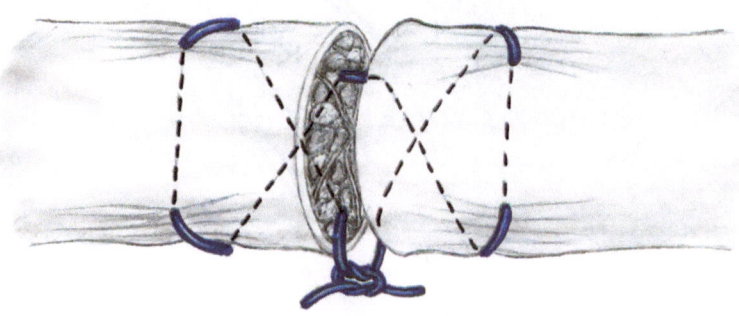

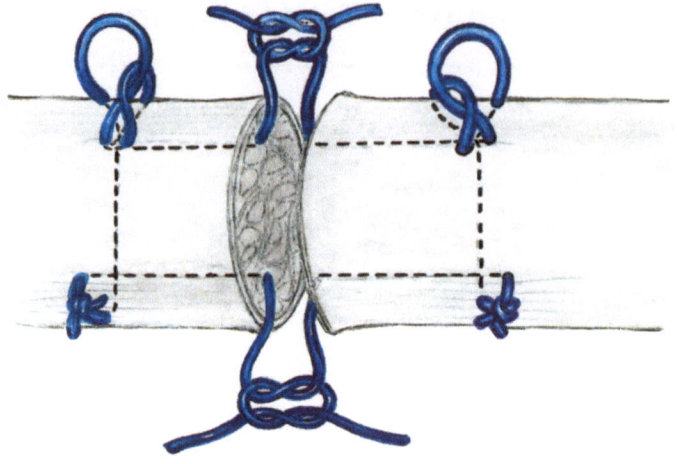

Strickland's "double grasp" modification of the Kirchmaier-Kessler technique (two-strand)

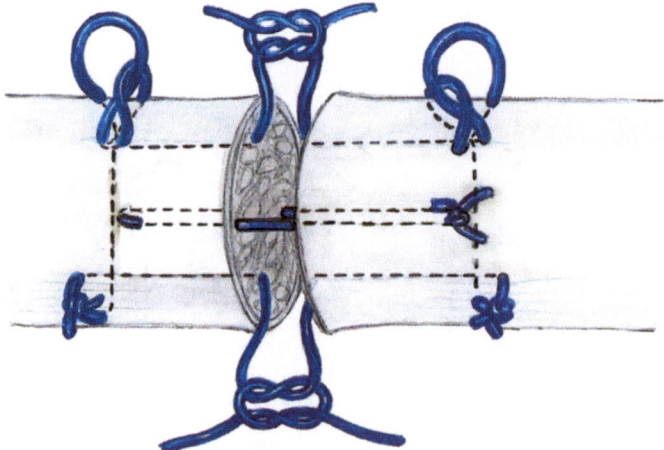

„Double grasp" technique with an additional rectangular mattress suture (four-strand)

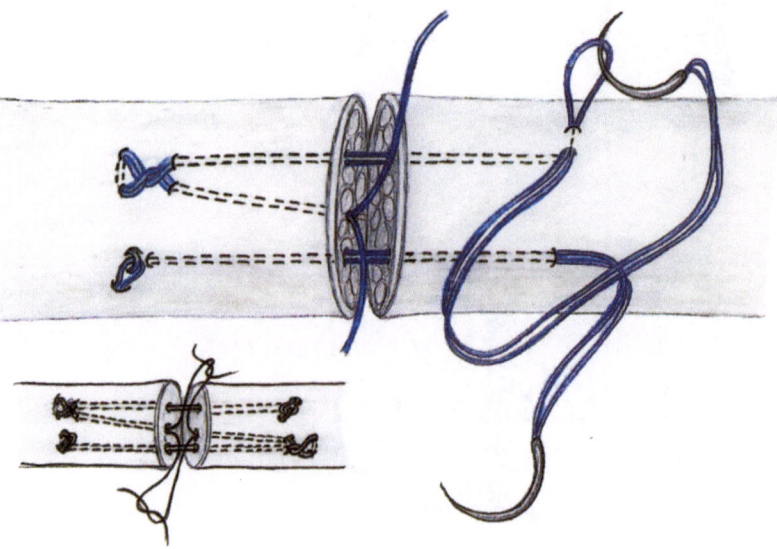

Recent modification of Tsuge's loop technique: Double loop (six-strand)

Pulvertaft technique: The tendon stumps are connected in a braided pattern – excellent tensile strength, allows early active mobilization

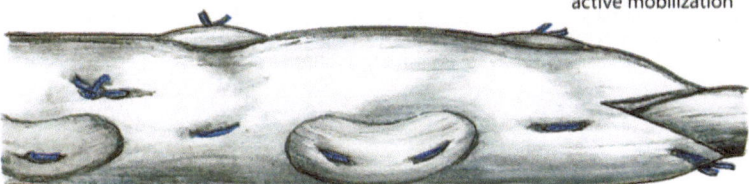

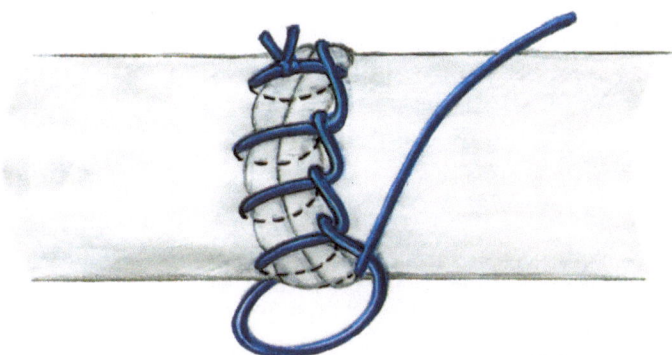

Epitenon sutures:
Epitenon sutures add considerable tensile strength to the tendon repair. They also smoothe the contour of the tendon repair, thereby improving gliding properties. The two most commonly used patterns are running stitches (5–0) or interlocking sutures (5–0). The most recent modification is a criss-cross pattern that may increase tensile strength

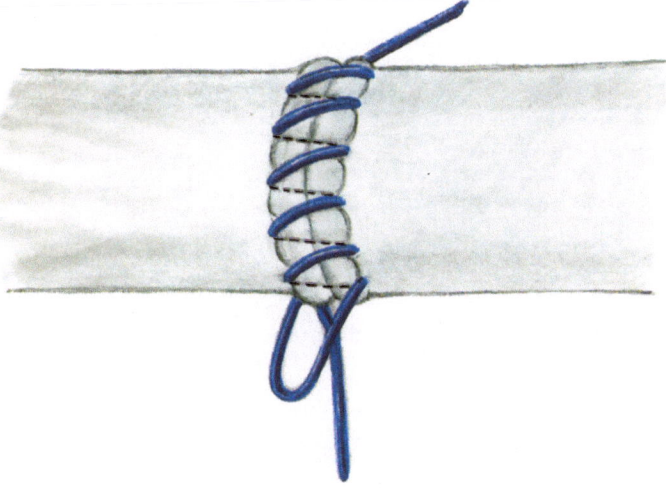

Techniques of Vascular Repair

Several techniques of vascular repair are frequently used. There is no preferred technique, since many techniques can give excellent results and patency rates. Best results are usually achieved with familiar techniques

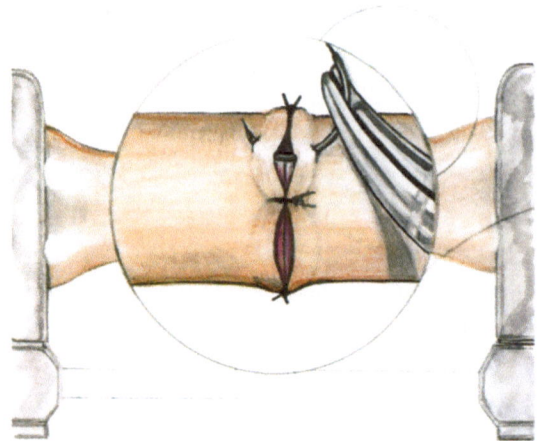

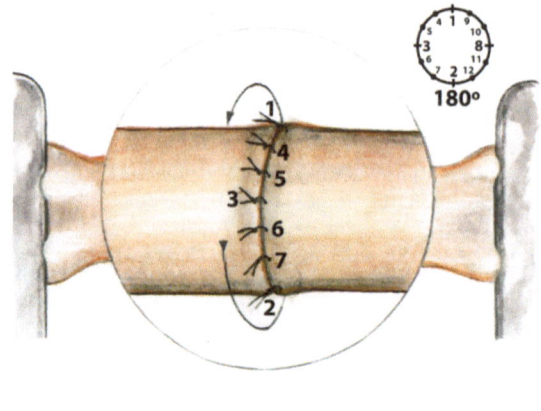

End-to-end anastomosis, 180° Technique:
Two corner sutures are placed at a 180° position (*1, 2*); third stitch in position *3* of the front wall; completion of front wall. Vessel is then flipped over; stitch in position *8*, completion of backwall

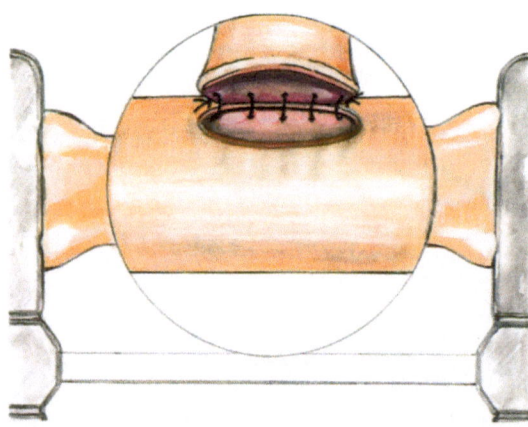

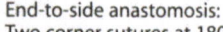

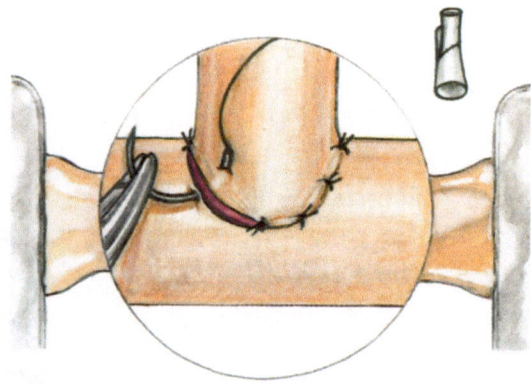

End-to-side anastomosis:
Two corner sutures at 180° Interrupted stitches (in larger vessels, running suture) for the vessel wall, with the more difficult access to complete the most difficult part first. Rinsing of the vessel lumen. Inspection of correct placement of stitches; completion of anterior wall

Trick: Place two sutures closely at either side of the corner sutures to prevent leakage from the angles. Take great care to grasp the intima of the recipient vessel

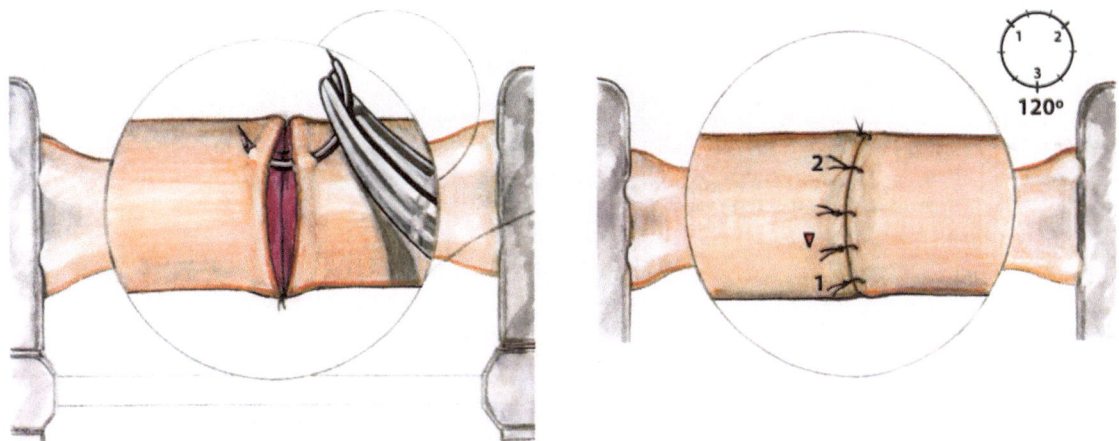

End-to-end anastomosis, 120° technique:
Two corner sutures at a 120° position on the front wall. Vessel is flipped over. Third
stitch at a 120° position. Segmental completion of backwall. Vessel is flipped over.
Completion of front wall

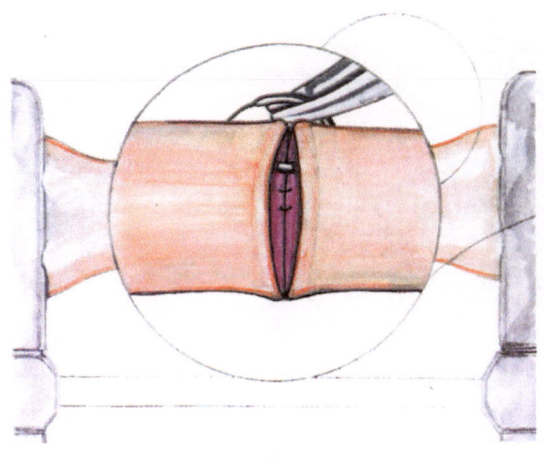

End-to-end anastomosis, "Backwall-first technique":
One everting suture is placed in the center of the back of the
back wall. Back wall is subsequently completed under vision.
Completion of the anastomoses is achieved by working from
both sides towards the center of the vessel; vessel is not flipped
over during the anastomoses

Techniques of Nerve Repair

Epi-perineural suture

Indicated in oligo fascicular nerves

Allows fascicle matching techniques (visual/staining)

Stronger suture in the epineurium of the back wall may reduce the tension on the suture line. The same goal can be achieved by using a strip of facia/tendon that is anchored to the back wall of both nerve stumps

Perfect alignment of nerve stumps and simultaneous sealing of the epineurial envelope

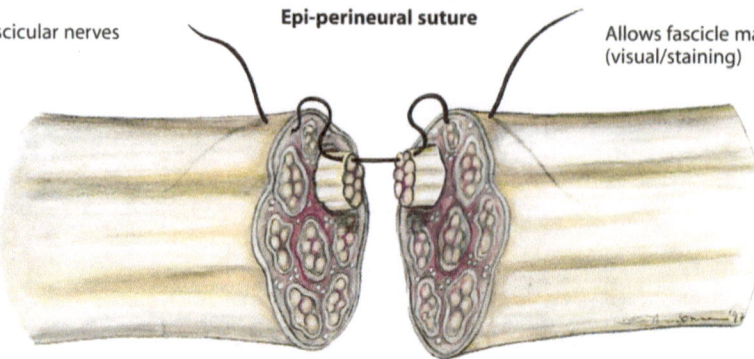

Avoid focal increase of pressure on the suture line to prevent bulging and/or poor alignment of the fascicles

Epineural suture:

Trim edges perpendicular to long axis of the nerve

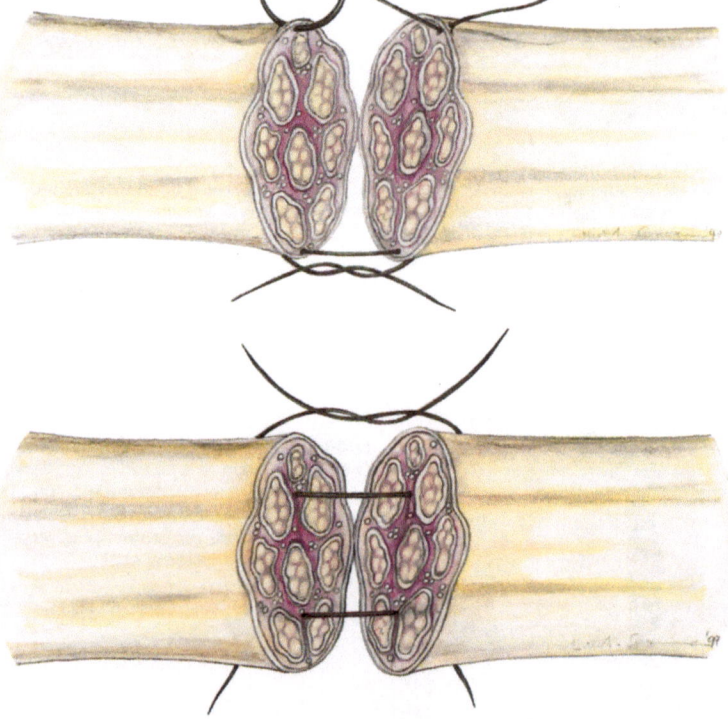

Use 180° technique to guarantee perfect coaptation

Rarely indicated in single fascicle nerves, when no "fascicle mapping" is required

Avoid focal increase of pressure on the suture line to prevent bulging and poor alignment of the fascicles

Individual fascicular suture:

Indicated only in nerve grafting; otherwise, too much suture material is brought into the nerve

Secure well-perfused soft tissue envelope in case of nerve grafting

Use 10/0 or maximum 9/0 for exact adaptation

Nerve graft donor sites:
Sural nerve
Medial ante-brachial cutaneous nerve
Lateral ante-brachial cutaneous nerve

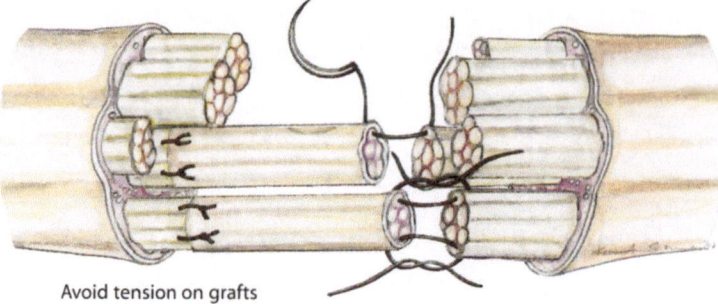

Avoid tension on grafts

Fibrin glue may be used in place of sutures in selected cases

Choice of Procedure

After a clear injury pattern has been established and documented, the next step is operative reconstruction. The following algorithms will be useful to direct this part of treatment.

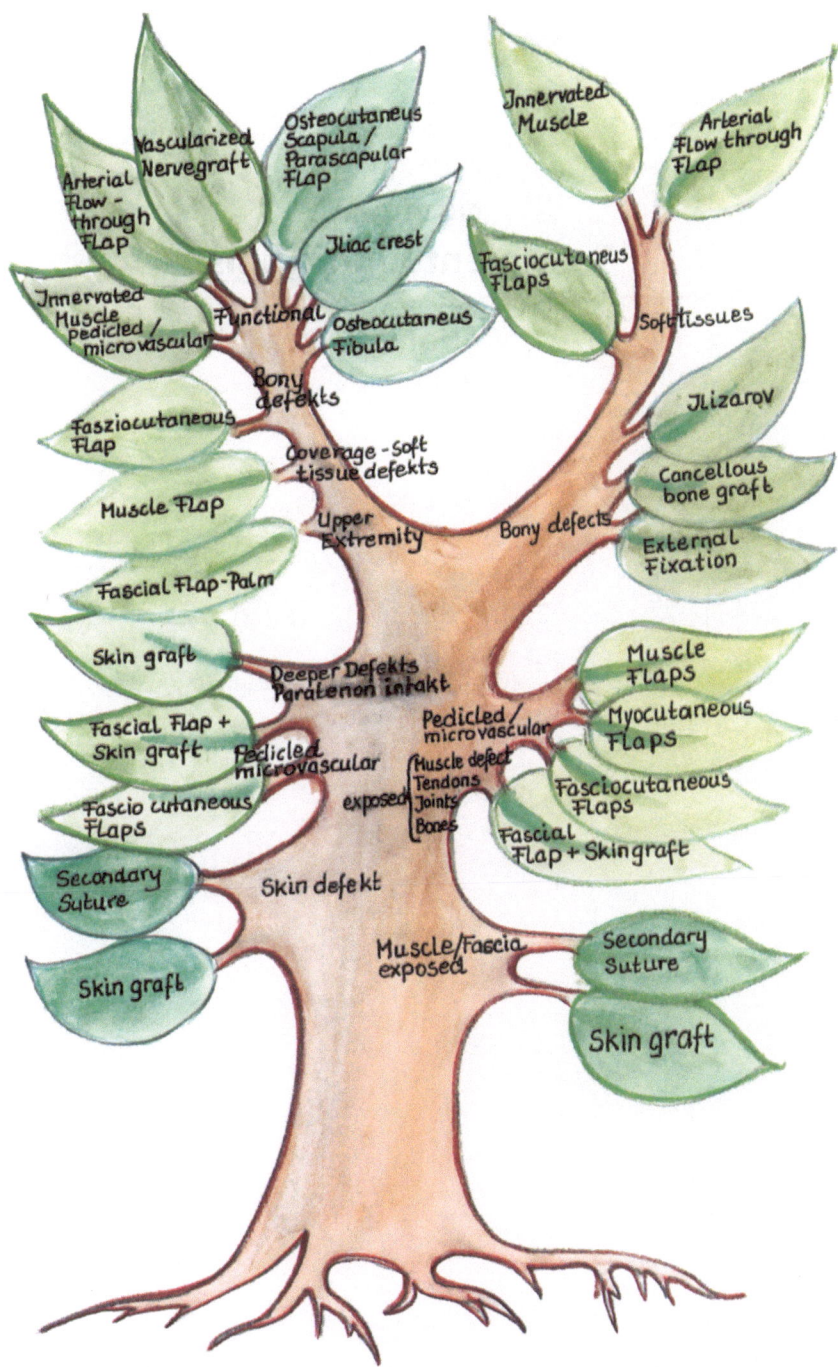

The reconstructive tree illustrates the treatment options in soft tissue defects. The surgeon's decision is based on his/her experience and abilities to realiably perform procedures in the acute setting. The following treatment algorithms will outline the particular decision making processes pertinent to anatomical structures and the types of injury.

CHAPTER III
Treatment Algorithms

Bones

Distal Phalanx

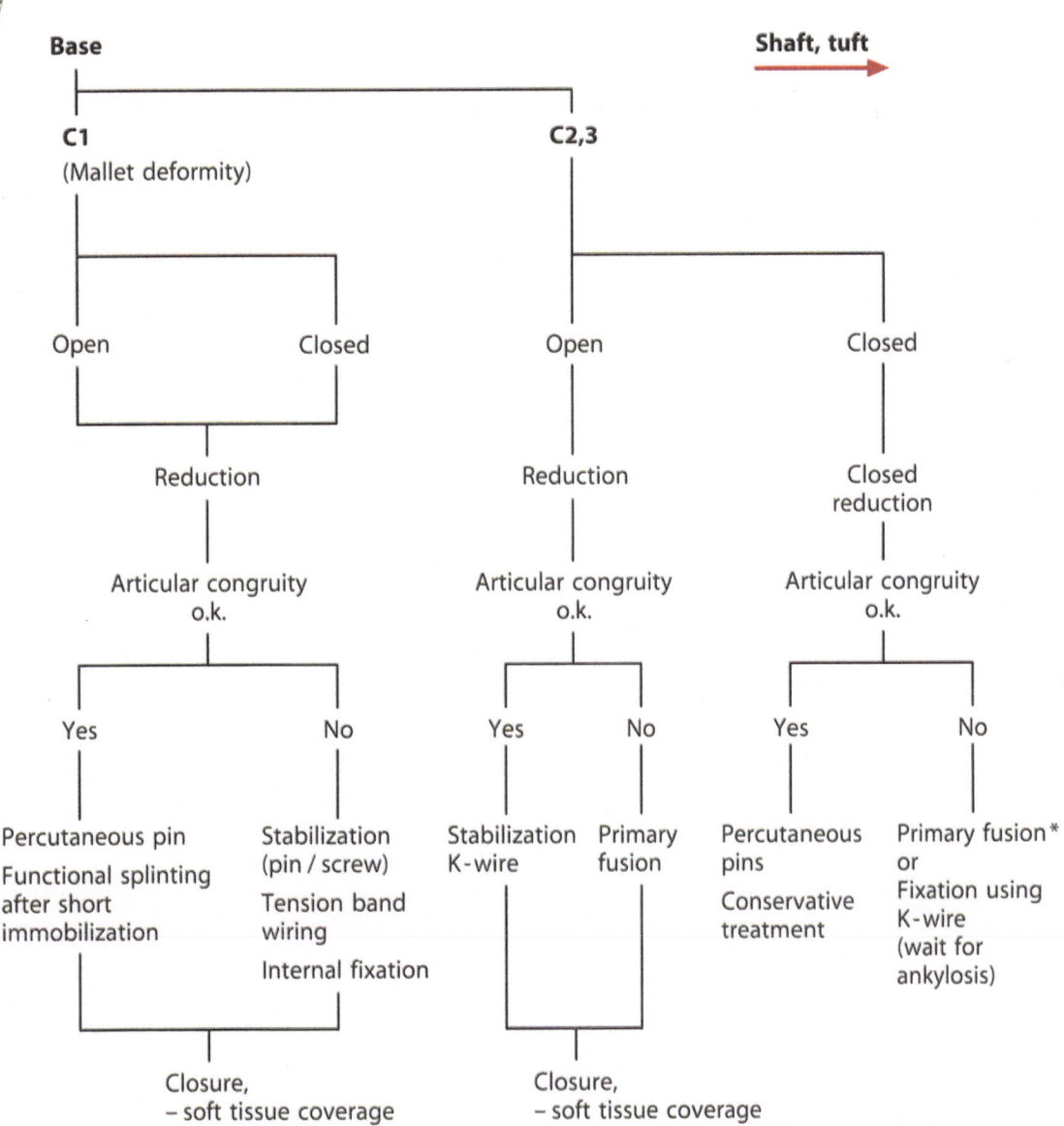

Base   **Shaft, tuft** →

C1   **C2,3**
(Mallet deformity)

Open   Closed   Open   Closed

Reduction   Reduction   Closed
                                                            reduction

Articular congruity   Articular congruity   Articular congruity
        o.k.   o.k.   o.k.

Yes   No   Yes   No   Yes   No

Percutaneous pin   Stabilization   Stabilization   Primary   Percutaneous   Primary fusion*
                        (pin / screw)   K-wire   fusion   pins   or
Functional splinting   Fixation using
after short   Tension band   Conservative   K-wire
immobilization   wiring   treatment   (wait for
                                                                                         ankylosis)
                        Internal fixation

        Closure,   Closure,
        – soft tissue coverage   – soft tissue coverage

* Primary fusion if
  joint reconstruction
  does not seem
  to allow painfree
  motion or patient desires
  definitive solution

Distal Phalanx

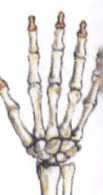

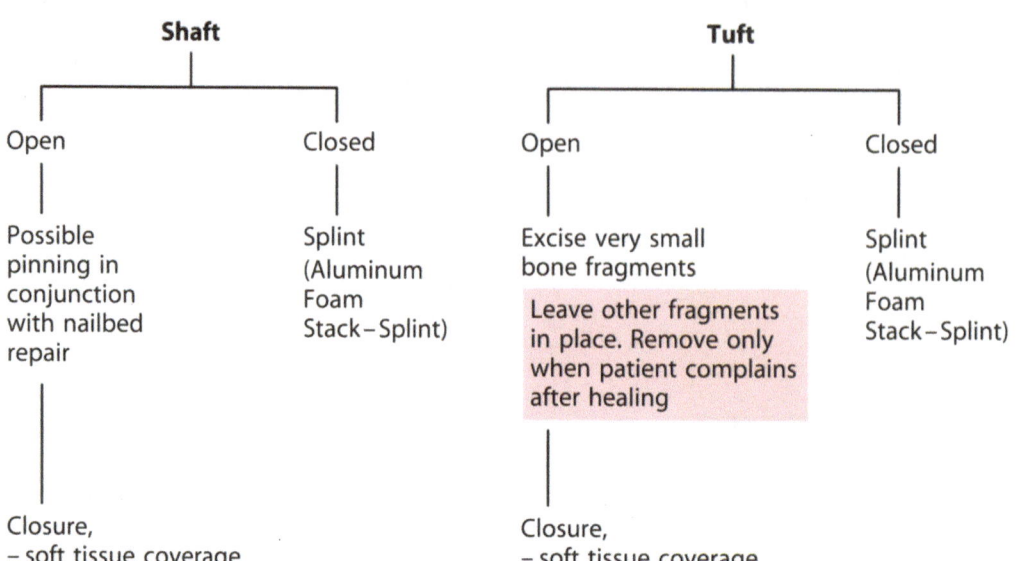

Shaft

Open

Possible
pinning in
conjunction
with nailbed
repair

Closure,
– soft tissue coverage

Closed

Splint
(Aluminum
Foam
Stack – Splint)

Tuft

Open

Excise very small
bone fragments

Leave other fragments
in place. Remove only
when patient complains
after healing

Closure,
– soft tissue coverage

Closed

Splint
(Aluminum
Foam
Stack – Splint)

Metacarpals, Proximal and Middle Phalanges

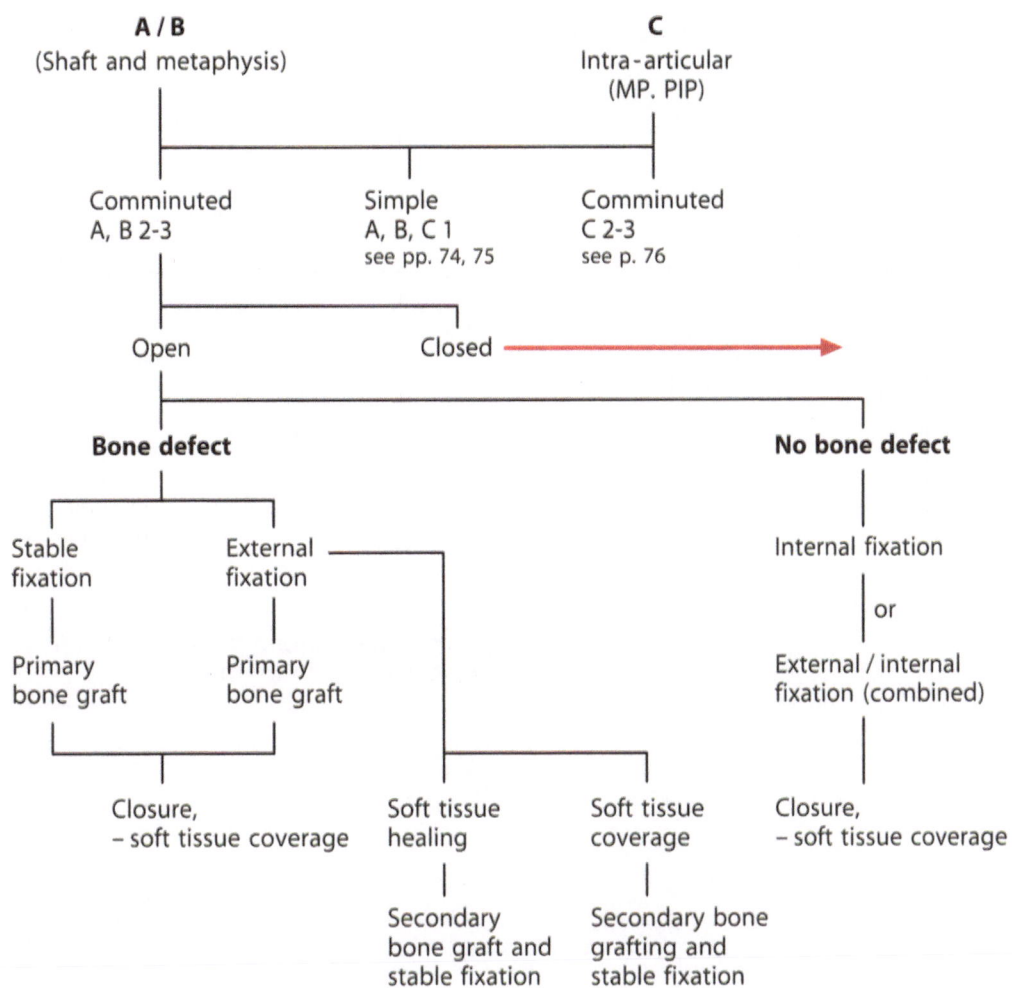

A / B
(Shaft and metaphysis)

C
Intra-articular
(MP. PIP)

Comminuted
A, B 2-3

Simple
A, B, C 1
see pp. 74, 75

Comminuted
C 2-3
see p. 76

Open   Closed

Bone defect   **No bone defect**

Stable
fixation

External
fixation

Internal fixation

or

Primary
bone graft

Primary
bone graft

External / internal
fixation (combined)

Closure,
– soft tissue coverage

Soft tissue
healing

Soft tissue
coverage

Closure,
– soft tissue coverage

Secondary
bone graft and
stable fixation

Secondary bone
grafting and
stable fixation

Metacarpals, Proximal and Middle Phalanges

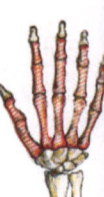

**Closed comminuted fractures
A, B 2-3**

Soft tissue
intact

Soft tissue
compromised

Internal fixation*

Percutaneous
K-wire
External fixation

Conservative
treatment

Percutaneous
K-wires

Functional brace
(Splint)

Functional
brace
(Splint)

Immobilization
(children)

External
fixation

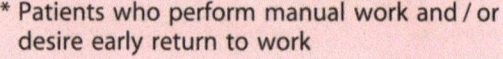

* Patients who perform manual work and / or
desire early return to work

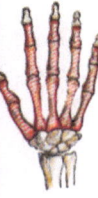

Metacarpals, Proximal and Middle Phalanges

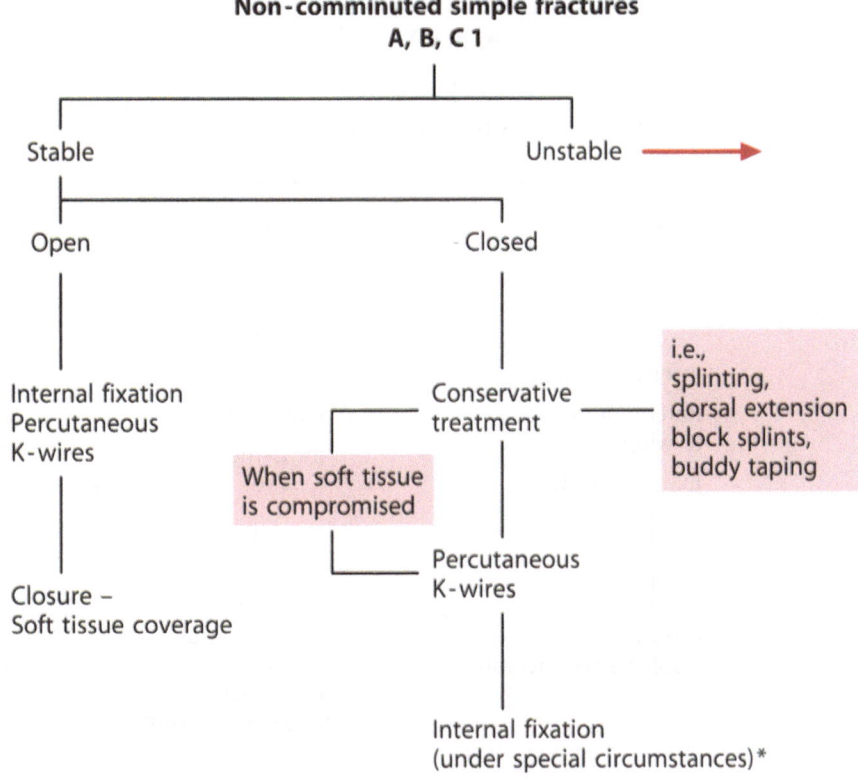

Non-comminuted simple fractures
A, B, C 1

Stable   Unstable →

Open   Closed

Internal fixation   Conservative   i.e.,
Percutaneous   treatment   splinting,
K-wires   dorsal extension
                                                   block splints,
                  When soft tissue   buddy taping
                  is compromised

                          Percutaneous
                          K-wires

Closure –
Soft tissue coverage

                          Internal fixation
                          (under special circumstances)*

* Patients who perform manual work and / or
  desire early return to work

Metacarpals, Proximal and Middle Phalanges

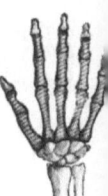

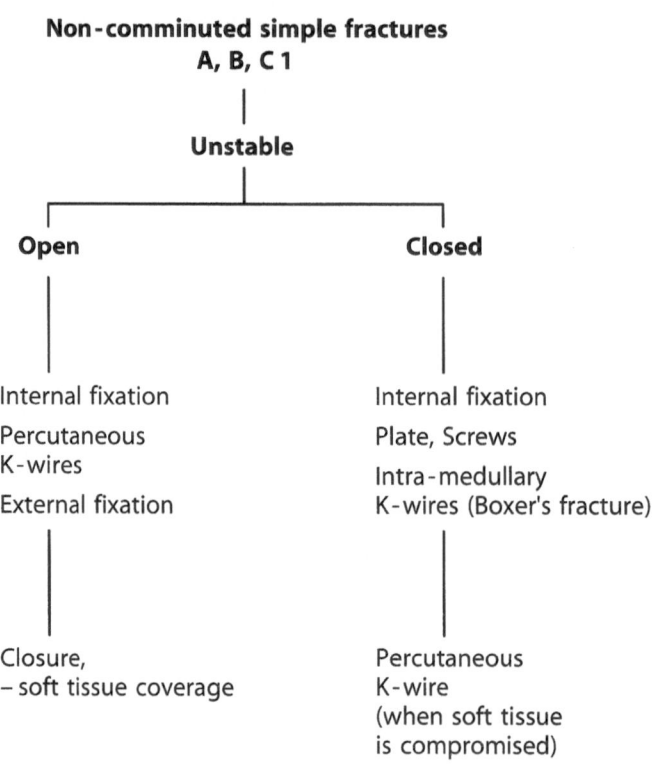

Non-comminuted simple fractures
A, B, C 1

|
Unstable

Open   **Closed**

Internal fixation   Internal fixation

Percutaneous   Plate, Screws
K-wires
                                                    Intra-medullary
External fixation   K-wires (Boxer's fracture)

Closure,   Percutaneous
– soft tissue coverage   K-wire
                                                    (when soft tissue
                                                    is compromised)

Metacarpals, Proximal and Middle Phalanges

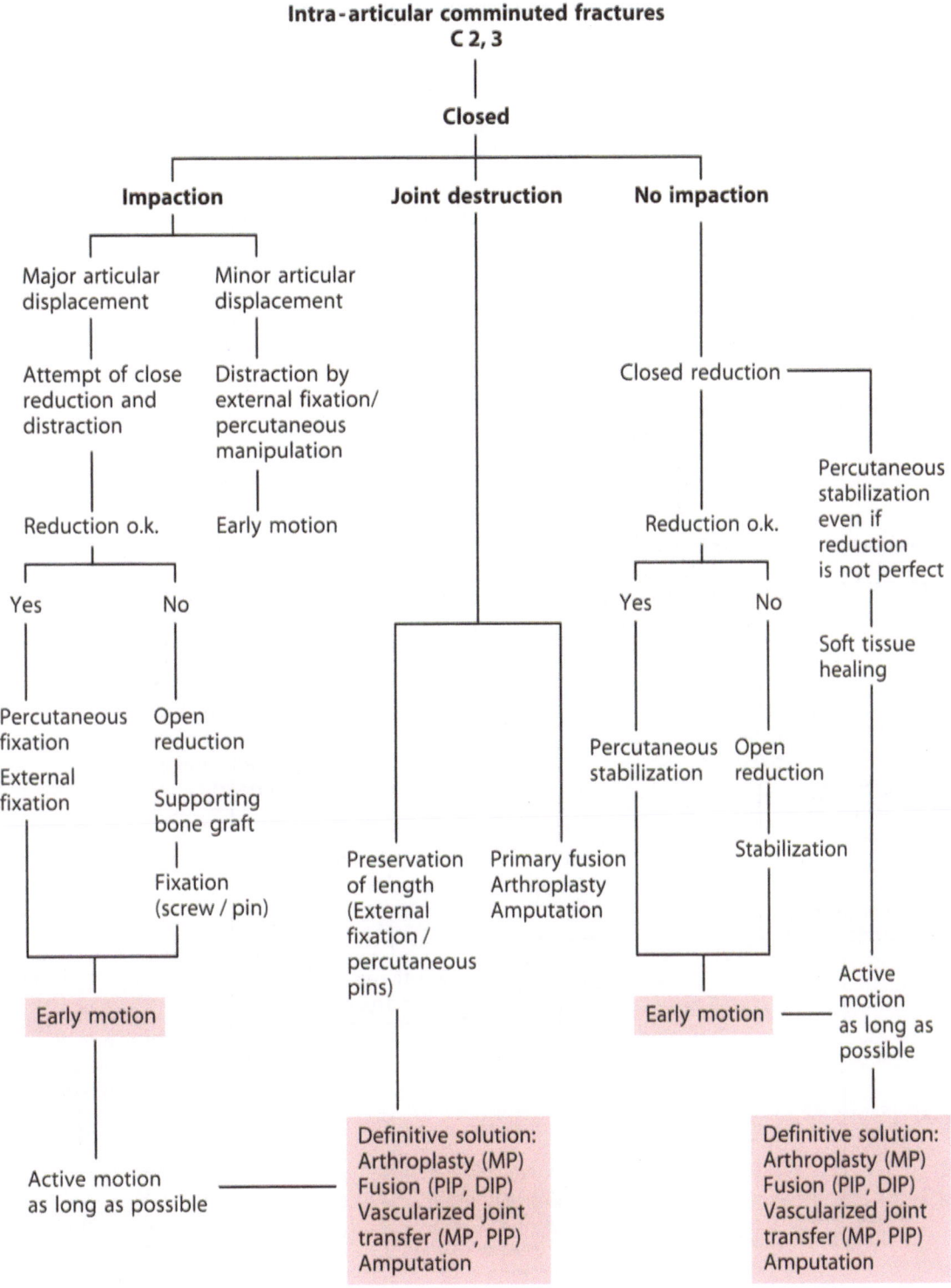

Intra-articular comminuted fractures
C 2, 3

Closed

Impaction   **Joint destruction**   **No impaction**

Major articular displacement   Minor articular displacement

Attempt of close reduction and distraction   Distraction by external fixation/ percutaneous manipulation

Closed reduction

Reduction o.k.   Early motion

Percutaneous stabilization even if reduction is not perfect

Yes   No   Reduction o.k.

Soft tissue healing

Percutaneous fixation   Open reduction   Yes   No

External fixation   Supporting bone graft   Percutaneous stabilization   Open reduction

Fixation (screw / pin)   Stabilization

Preservation of length (External fixation / percutaneous pins)   Primary fusion Arthroplasty Amputation

Active motion as long as possible

Early motion   Early motion

Active motion as long as possible

Definitive solution: Arthroplasty (MP) Fusion (PIP, DIP) Vascularized joint transfer (MP, PIP) Amputation   Definitive solution: Arthroplasty (MP) Fusion (PIP, DIP) Vascularized joint transfer (MP, PIP) Amputation

Metacarpals, Proximal and Middle Phalanges

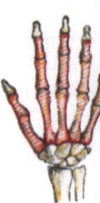

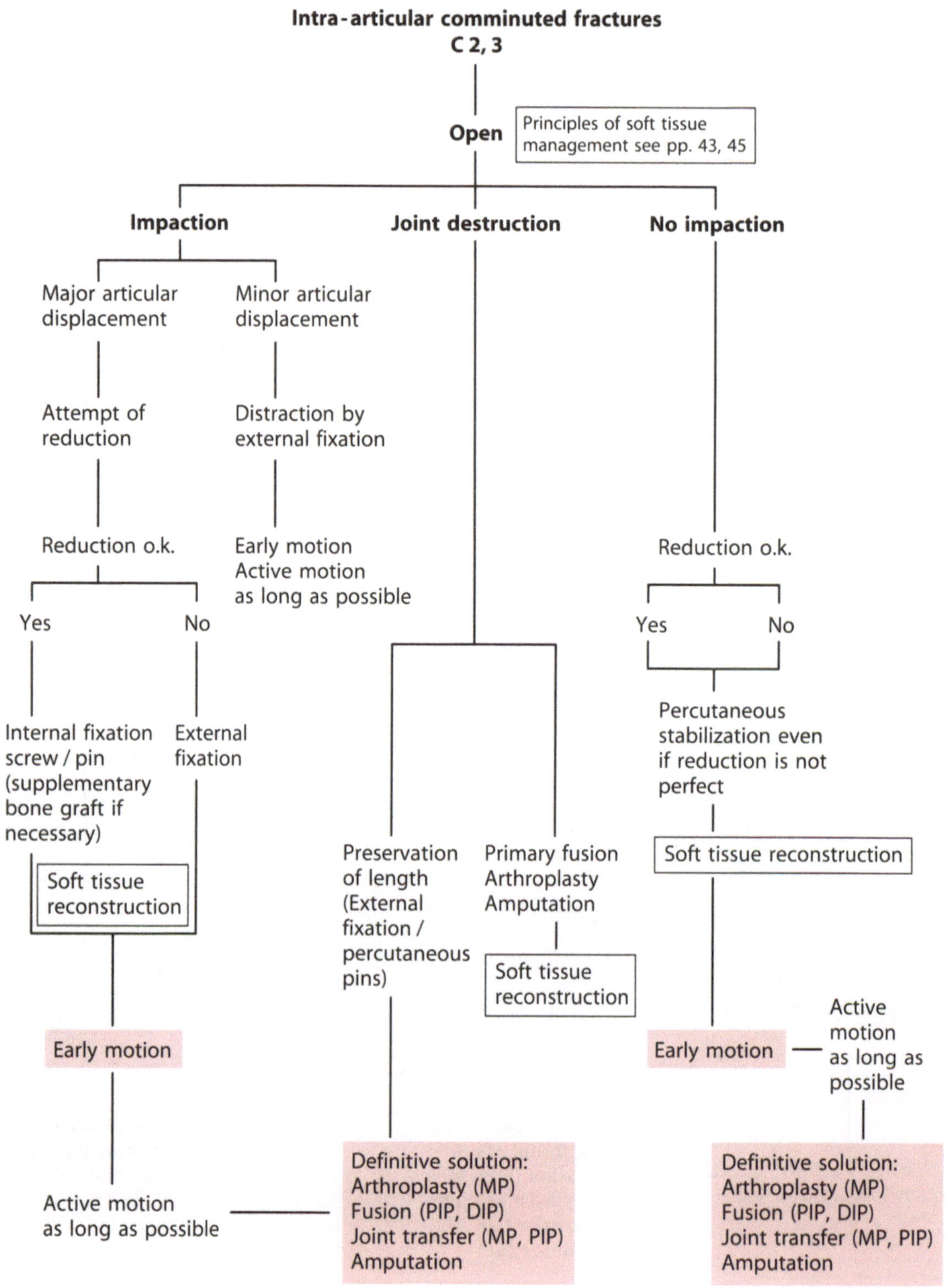

Intra-articular comminuted fractures
C 2, 3

Open | Principles of soft tissue management see pp. 43, 45

Impaction   **Joint destruction**   **No impaction**

Major articular displacement   Minor articular displacement

Attempt of reduction   Distraction by external fixation

Reduction o.k.   Early motion Active motion as long as possible   Reduction o.k.

Yes   No   Yes   No

Internal fixation screw / pin (supplementary bone graft if necessary)   External fixation

Percutaneous stabilization even if reduction is not perfect

Soft tissue reconstruction   Preservation of length (External fixation / percutaneous pins)   Primary fusion Arthroplasty Amputation   Soft tissue reconstruction

Soft tissue reconstruction

Early motion   **Early motion**   Active motion as long as possible

Active motion as long as possible   Definitive solution: Arthroplasty (MP) Fusion (PIP, DIP) Joint transfer (MP, PIP) Amputation   Definitive solution: Arthroplasty (MP) Fusion (PIP, DIP) Joint transfer (MP, PIP) Amputation

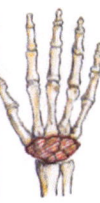

Carpus

Open	**Closed**

Open

Same treatment
as closed

Proceed with soft
tissue algorithms
for corresponding
areas

Closed

Scaphoid, lunate, trapezium, trapezoidem,
capitate, hamate, pisiform, triquetrum

CT-scan / spiral CT
special views / scaphoid series

Displaced

Consider ORIF
for lunate, capitate,
hook of hamate if
gap is >1 mm

Non-displaced

Casting –
see below for scaphoid
(short arm cast for 6 weeks)

Scaphoid

Proximal
B3
B3
(Unstable)

Displaced

ORIF
(dorsal
approach,
mini-Herbert
screw)

Non-displaced

ORIF
dorsal
approach,
mini-Herbert
screw

Cast 6 weeks

(Long arm or
short arm – no
definitive data
in literature.
Confirm union
with CT-scan!/
tomography)

Waist
B1/2
B2/3, C1-3
(Unstable)

Displaced

ORIF
Herbert screw
Cannulated AO
screw
Accutrac screw

Non-displaced

ORIF

* Cast 1 day – 2 weeks

(Long arm or
short arm – no
definitive data
in literature.
Confirm union
with CT-scan!/
tomography)

Distal
A1/2
A1-3, B1
(Stable)

Displaced

ORIF

Non-displaced

Cast 4-6 weeks

(Long arm or
short arm – no
definitive data
in literature.
Confirm union
with CT-scan!/
tomography)

Herbert
AO/ASIF

| A… = AO/ASIF classification |
| A… = *Herbert* classification |

* Length of casting depends
on quality of fixation

Beware:
Trans-scaphoid dislocation fractures
TFCC lesions
S-L dissociation, L-T lesions
Peri-lunate dislocation
Arthroscopy

Radius

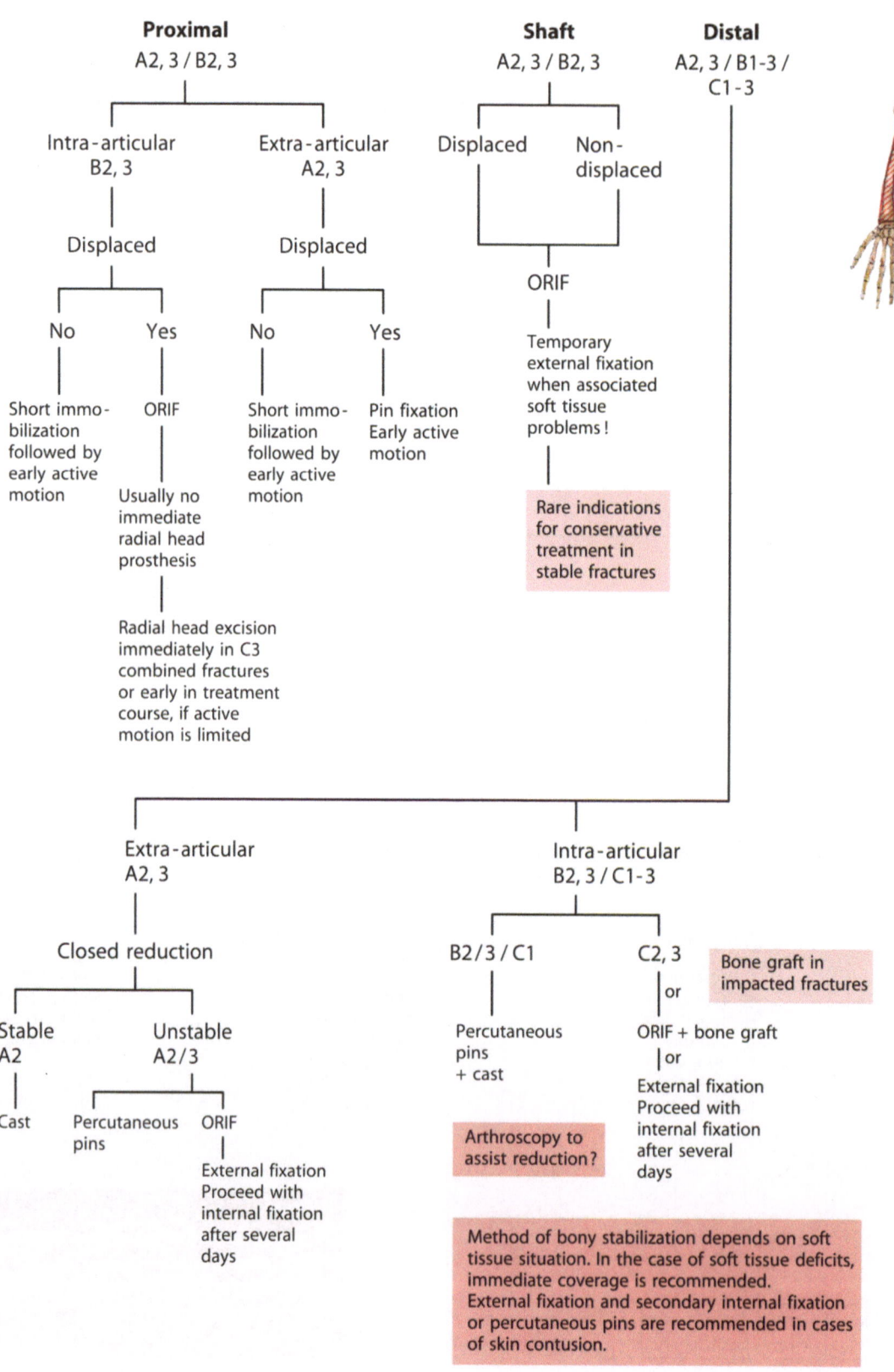

Proximal
A2, 3 / B2, 3

Shaft
A2, 3 / B2, 3

Distal
A2, 3 / B1-3 /
C1-3

Intra-articular
B2, 3

Extra-articular
A2, 3

Displaced

Non-displaced

Displaced

Displaced

ORIF

No

Yes

No

Yes

Temporary
external fixation
when associated
soft tissue
problems!

Short immo-
bilization
followed by
early active
motion

ORIF

Short immo-
bilization
followed by
early active
motion

Pin fixation
Early active
motion

Rare indications
for conservative
treatment in
stable fractures

Usually no
immediate
radial head
prosthesis

Radial head excision
immediately in C3
combined fractures
or early in treatment
course, if active
motion is limited

Extra-articular
A2, 3

Intra-articular
B2, 3 / C1-3

Closed reduction

B2/3 / C1

C2, 3

Bone graft in
impacted fractures

Stable
A2

Unstable
A2/3

Percutaneous
pins
+ cast

ORIF + bone graft

or

Cast

Percutaneous
pins

ORIF

External fixation
Proceed with
internal fixation
after several
days

External fixation
Proceed with
internal fixation
after several
days

Arthroscopy to
assist reduction?

Method of bony stabilization depends on soft
tissue situation. In the case of soft tissue deficits,
immediate coverage is recommended.
External fixation and secondary internal fixation
or percutaneous pins are recommended in cases
of skin contusion.

Ulna

Proximal
A1/B1/C1-3

Shaft
A1/B1/C1-2

Distal
A1/B1/C1-3

Intra-articular
B1

Extra-articular
A1

Displaced

Non-
displaced

Displaced

Displaced

ORIF

No   Yes No   Yes

ORIF

Short immo-
bilization
followed by
early active
motion

Pin fixation
Early active
motion

Temporary
external fixation
when associated
soft tissue
problems!

Bone graft
in case of
bone loss
in C3
comminuted
fractures

Tension band
wiring

Rare indications
for conservative
treatment in
stable fractures

Extra-articular
A1

Intra-articular
Styloid
C1-3

Watch out for
TFCC lesions!
Arthroscopy!

Closed reduction

C1-3   Styloid

Stable   Unstable

ORIF
Percutaneous
pins + cast

ORIF +
external fixation
and proceed with
internal fixation

Fixation of
styloid
to re-insert
ligaments

Cast   ORIF

Method of bony stabilization depends on soft
tissue situation. In the case of soft tissue deficits,
immediate coverage is recommended.
External fixation and secondary internal fixation
is recommended in cases of skin contusion.

Both Forearm Fractures

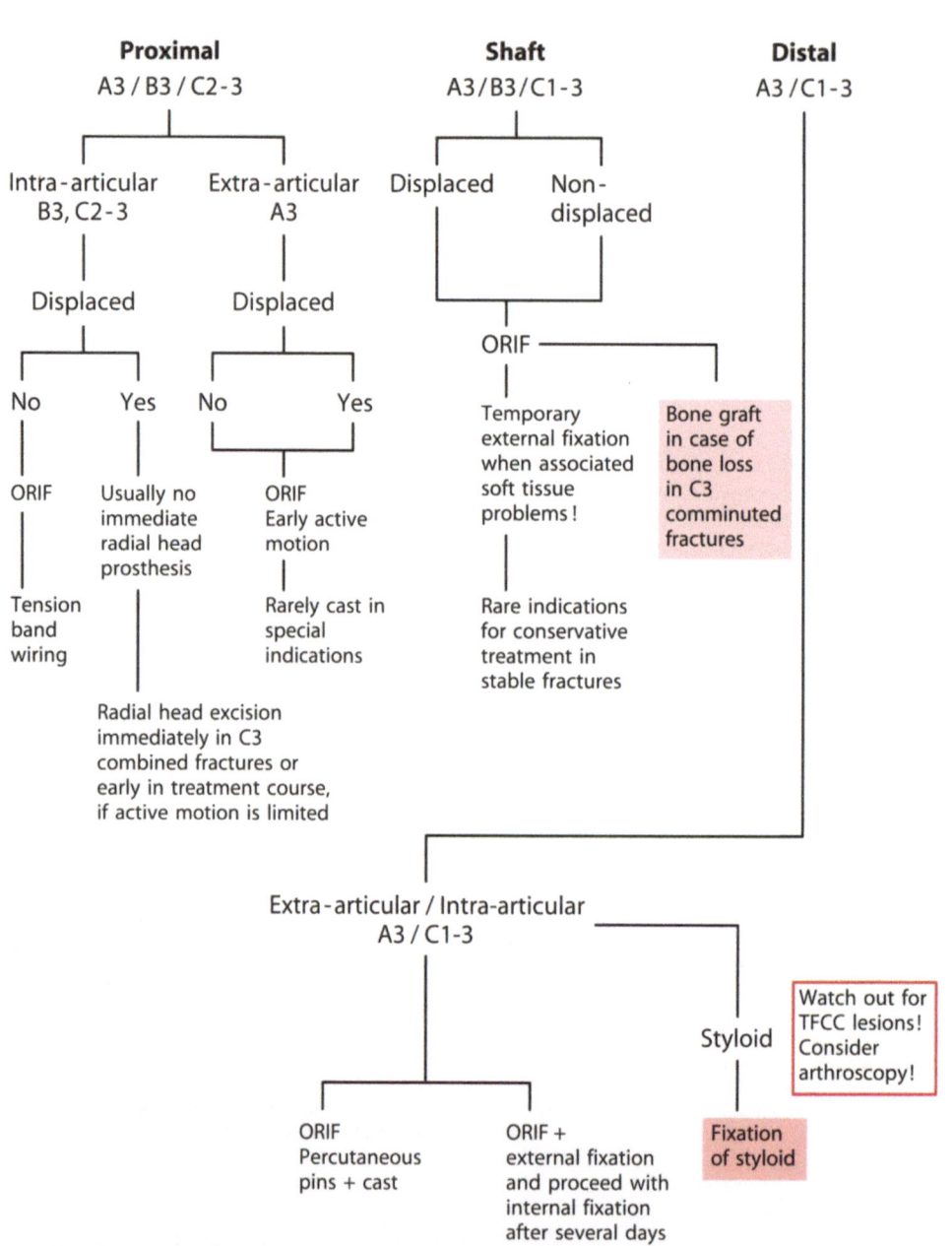

Proximal
A3 / B3 / C2-3

Shaft
A3 / B3 / C1-3

Distal
A3 / C1-3

Intra-articular
B3, C2-3

Extra-articular
A3

Displaced

Non-displaced

Displaced

Displaced

ORIF

No

Yes

No

Yes

ORIF

Usually no immediate radial head prosthesis

ORIF
Early active motion

Temporary external fixation when associated soft tissue problems!

Bone graft in case of bone loss in C3 comminuted fractures

Tension band wiring

Rarely cast in special indications

Rare indications for conservative treatment in stable fractures

Radial head excision immediately in C3 combined fractures or early in treatment course, if active motion is limited

Extra-articular / Intra-articular
A3 / C1-3

Styloid

Watch out for TFCC lesions! Consider arthroscopy!

ORIF
Percutaneous pins + cast

ORIF + external fixation and proceed with internal fixation after several days

Fixation of styloid

Method of bony stabilization depends on soft tissue situation. In the case of soft tissue deficits, immediate coverage is recommended. External fixation and secondary internal fixation is recommended in cases of skin contusion.

Humerus

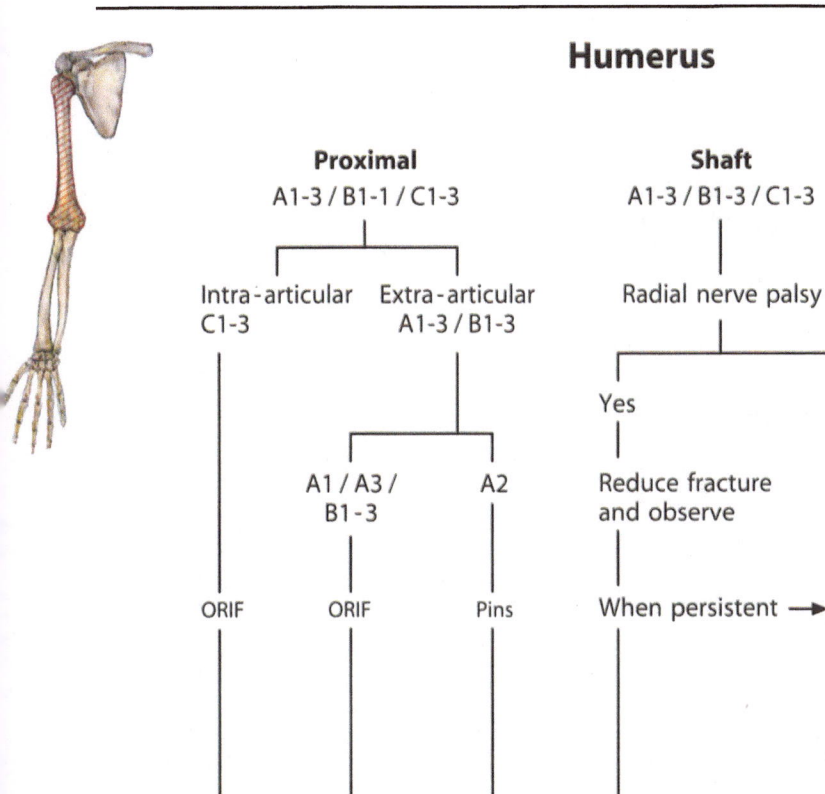

Proximal	Shaft	Distal
A1-3 / B1-1 / C1-3	A1-3 / B1-3 / C1-3	A1-3 / B1-3 / C1-3

Proximal

Intra-articular C1-3 → ORIF → Consider head prosthesis in case of severe destruction

Extra-articular A1-3 / B1-3
- A1 / A3 / B1-3 → ORIF → Percutaneous pins → Consider head prosthesis in B2/B3 cases
- A2 → Pins → Cast/brace Functional treatment

Shaft

Radial nerve palsy

Yes → Reduce fracture and observe → When persistent →

Or occurs after reduction

Consider nerve exploration

Consider early tendon transfer in the case of nerve laceration to accelerate rehabilitation

No

- A1 / B1 → ORIF Cast/brace Functional treatment
- A2-3 → ORIF (i.m. nailing) → Cast/brace Functional treatment
- B2-3 / C1-3 → ORIF (Plate) → External fixation if soft tissue is inadequate

Cast brace
or

Distal

Intra-articular
- Partial B1-B3 → ORIF Pins Screws
- Complete C1-C3 → ORIF Plate (bilateral) Screws

Extra-articular A1-A3
- A1-2 → ORIF Pins Screws
- A3 → ORIF Plate Screws

Scapula

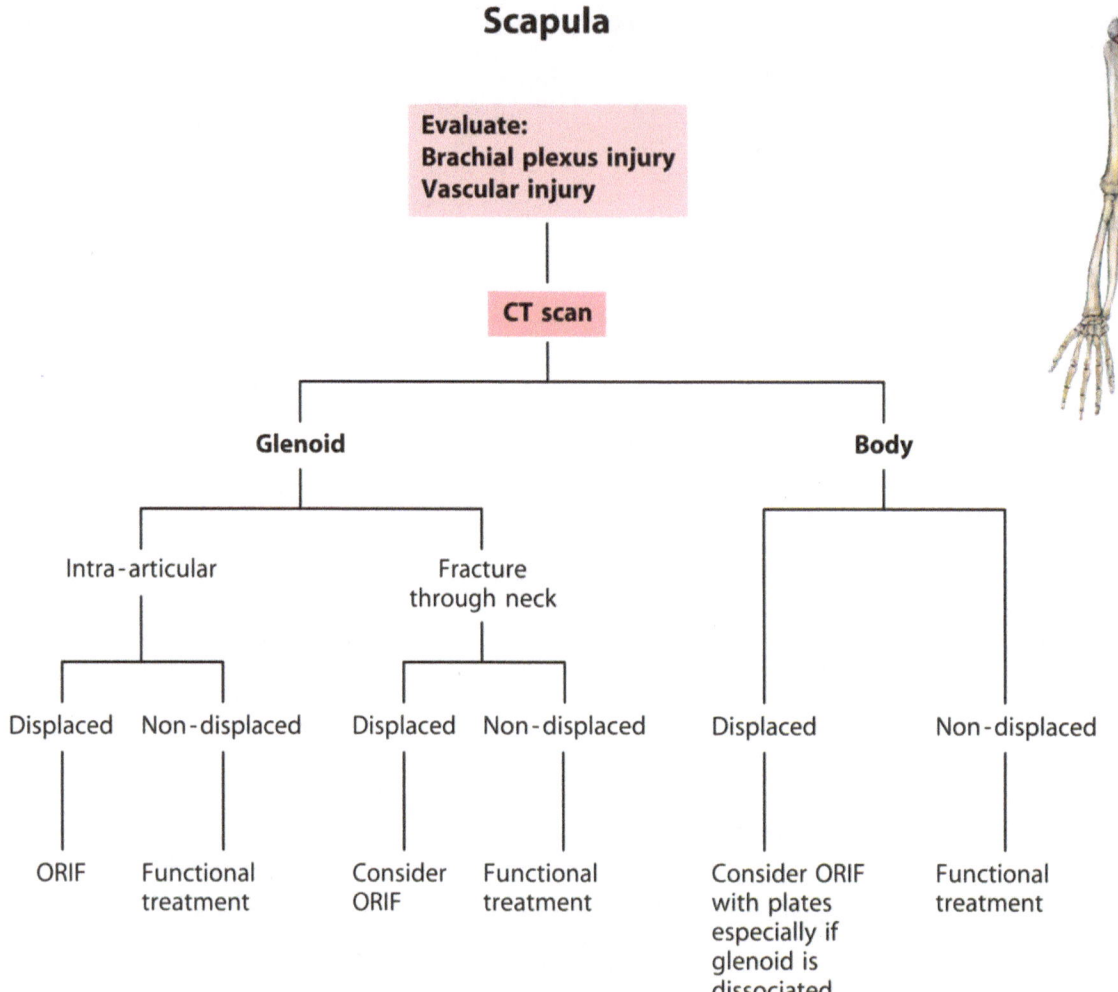

Evaluate:
Brachial plexus injury
Vascular injury

CT scan

Glenoid

Body

Intra-articular

Fracture
through neck

Displaced

Non-displaced

Displaced

Non-displaced

Displaced

Non-displaced

ORIF

Functional
treatment

Consider
ORIF

Functional
treatment

Consider ORIF
with plates
especially if
glenoid is
dissociated

Functional
treatment

Ligamentous Injuries

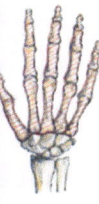

Digits
(PIP, MP)

Collateral ligament

Stress exam
X-ray deviation (> 35°) or
compare with opposite
side under fluoroscopy

Joint stable

Yes | No

Functional treatment | Functional treatment

Surgical repair in MP injury
of the radial aspect of the
index finger and the ulnar
aspect of the little finger

4 weeks | 6 weeks

Re-examination

If still symptomatic
Consider:

Surgical ligament reconstruction/ repair | Fusion (PIP joints in older patients)

Volar plate

Exam (instability, tendency of
dislocation, pain in flexion or
extension)
X-ray of PIP to exclude fracture

Bone involvement?

Yes | No

Small fragment | Large/displaced fragment | Immobilization for one week

Immobilization for 1 week | | Followed by

Followed by

Limited increasing
flexion with extension
block (5-6 weeks) when
fragment reduces! | | Limited increasing flexion with extension block for 5-6 weeks

(see Appendix:
Rehabilitation
protocols) | Open or closed reduction Fixation Screw / K-wires | (see Appendix: Rehabilitation protocols)

Thumb

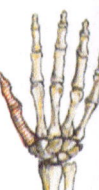

Ulnar and radial collateral ligament

|

Examination
(Instability, pain,
loss of grip strength)

X-ray — >35°-40° indicates rupture
>10° side difference
digital block to assess
deviation in acute situation

Bone fragment

Yes
- **Displaced**
  - Large fragment
  - Small fragment
    - Excise fragment
      Re-insertion of ligament
      (transosseous bone anchor)
  - Closed reduction
    Percutaneous pins
  - ORIF
    Lag screw
    K-wire
- **Non-displaced**
  - Casting for 6 weeks
    Thumb spica

No
- Stress test >40°
  - **No**
    Indicates partial tear
    Thumb spica
  - **Yes**
    Indicates complete tear
    Stener lesion
    Open repair
    (Re-insertion with bone anchor if stump is not appropriate for suture)
    Transosseous suture
    Trial cast
    Ligament reconstruction if chronic instability results (PL tendon graft)

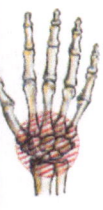

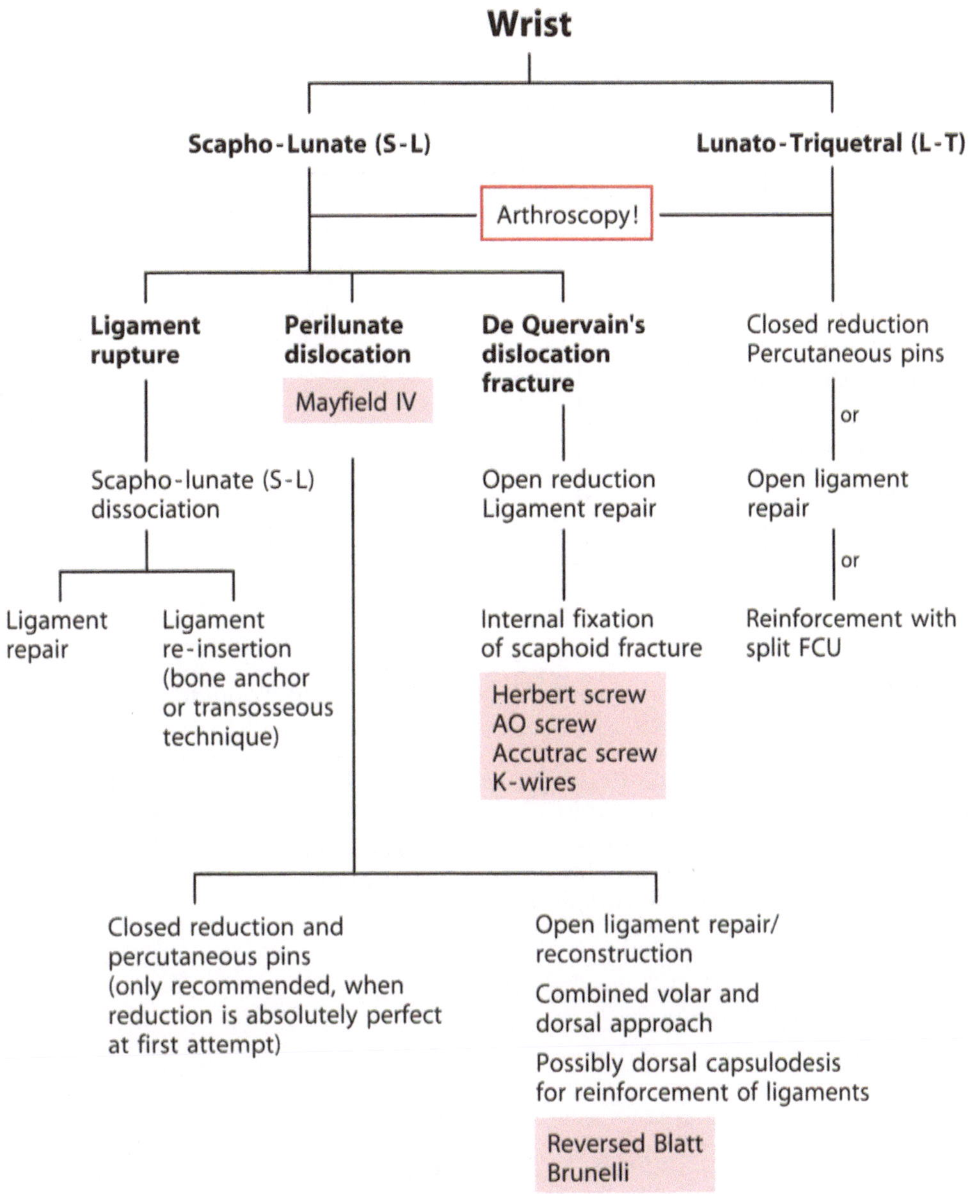

Wrist

Scapho-Lunate (S-L)   **Lunato-Triquetral (L-T)**

Arthroscopy!

Ligament rupture   **Perilunate dislocation**   **De Quervain's dislocation fracture**   Closed reduction Percutaneous pins

Mayfield IV

Scapho-lunate (S-L) dissociation   Open reduction Ligament repair   or

                                                                                                Open ligament repair

Ligament repair   Ligament re-insertion (bone anchor or transosseous technique)   Internal fixation of scaphoid fracture   or

                                                                                                Reinforcement with split FCU

Herbert screw
AO screw
Accutrac screw
K-wires

Closed reduction and percutaneous pins (only recommended, when reduction is absolutely perfect at first attempt)

Open ligament repair/ reconstruction

Combined volar and dorsal approach

Possibly dorsal capsulodesis for reinforcement of ligaments

Reversed Blatt
Brunelli

Arthroscopy has to be considered the gold standard for the diagnosis of ligamentous injuries. The predictive power of MRI is approximately 50 %, except high-powered gadolinium sequence MRI. CT scan only shows bony ligament avulsions and is only the third choice in imaging procedures.

Wrist

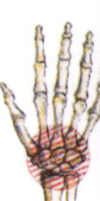

Chronic instability

Diagnosis

Clinical signs (pain, instability, loss of motion, loss of strength)

Plain X-ray (p.a., lateral, 20 % ulnar elevated)

Kinematic investigation with amplification (Fluoroscopy)

Arthroscopy

Classification

Mayo
Taleisnik
Viegas

Therapy

Scapho-Lunate (S-L)

Static – CID
(Symptomatic: carpal instability dissociative)

Scapho-trapzio-trapezoidal (STT) fusion

Ligament reconstruction capsulodesis

Dynamic – CIND
(Symptomatic: carpal instability non-dissociative)

Dorsal capsulodesis

Lunato-Triquetral (L-T)

L-T fusion

Ligament reconstruction

Midcarpal fusion

SLAC wrist

Stage I + II

Midcarpal fusion
(4 corner fusion)
(radial stylectomy)

Proximal row carpectomy
(if more residual motion is desired)

Stage III

Midcarpal fusion

Wrist fusion
+ denervation

Flexor Systems

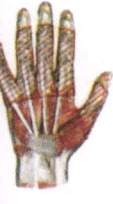

Zone 1 and 2

**Laceration
FDP, FDS**

Complete   **Incomplete**

Cross-section

Tendon repair —————— **> 50%**   **< 50%**

Simple suture

FDP   **FDS**   **FDP/FDS**

Zone I   **Zone II**

Tendon repair   Primary repair   Repair FDP and FDS

Transosseous   Repair tendon sheath   Repair FDP
fixation   Repair pulley   Single slip FDS and
(Bunnell)   excision of other slip

Bone anchor   Excise FDS

Dynamic follow-up protocol
except in children under 10-12 years
See p. 225

Insertion   **Single slip**   **Common tendon**

Repair   Excise/repair   Repair
(Do not create   (Depending on
chiasma stenosis)   local situation)

Tendon Loss, Rupture, Avulsion

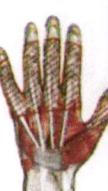

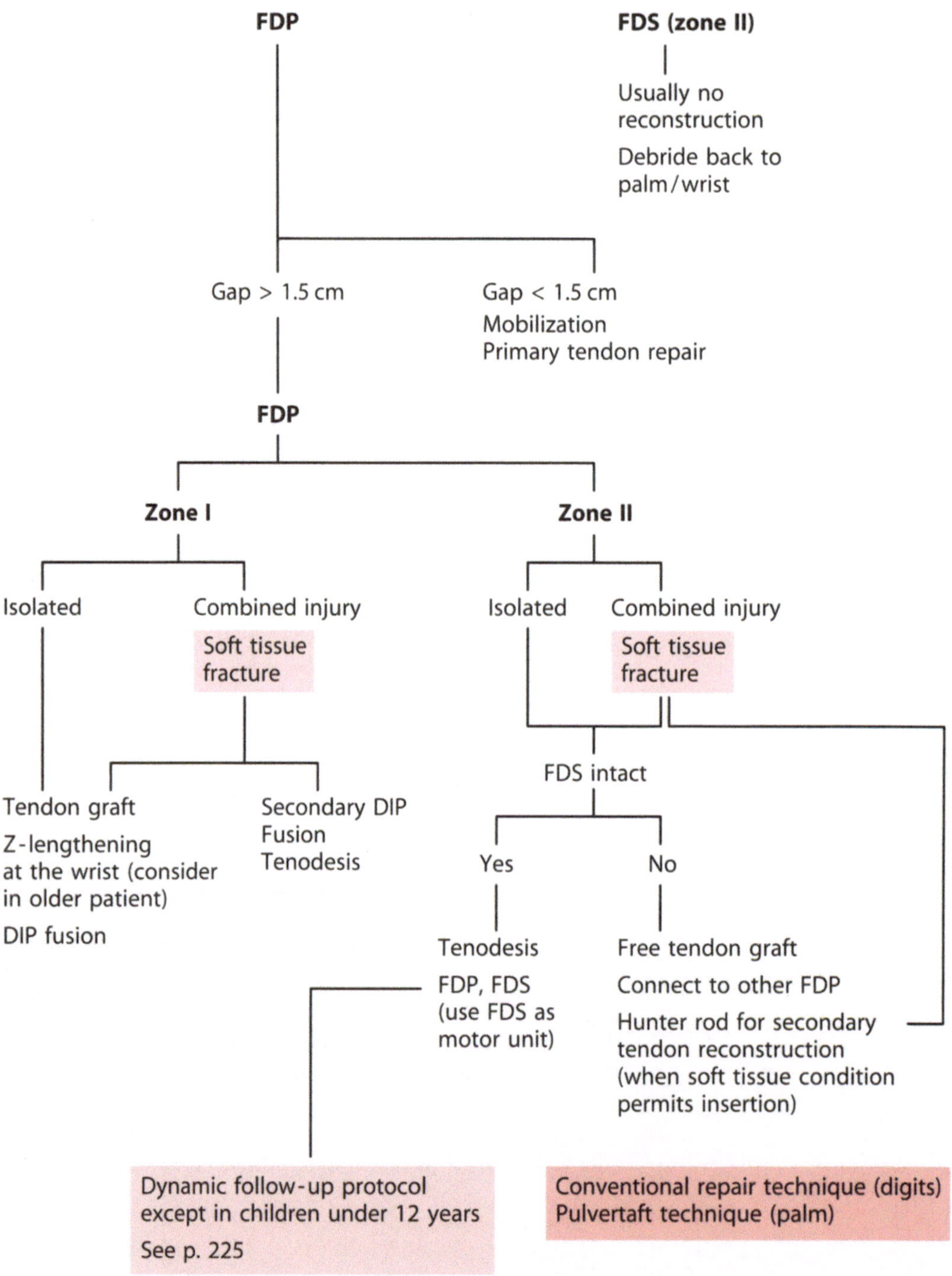

FDP   **FDS (zone II)**

Usually no
reconstruction

Debride back to
palm / wrist

Gap > 1.5 cm   Gap < 1.5 cm
                      Mobilization
                      Primary tendon repair

FDP

Zone I   **Zone II**

Isolated   Combined injury   Isolated   Combined injury
            Soft tissue   Soft tissue
            fracture   fracture

                                    FDS intact

Tendon graft   Secondary DIP   Yes   No
                Fusion
Z-lengthening   Tenodesis
at the wrist (consider   Tenodesis   Free tendon graft
in older patient)   FDP, FDS   Connect to other FDP
                                    (use FDS as
DIP fusion   motor unit) Hunter rod for secondary
                                                 tendon reconstruction
                                                 (when soft tissue condition
                                                 permits insertion)

Dynamic follow-up protocol   Conventional repair technique (digits)
except in children under 12 years   Pulvertaft technique (palm)

See p. 225

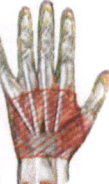

Zone 3 and 4

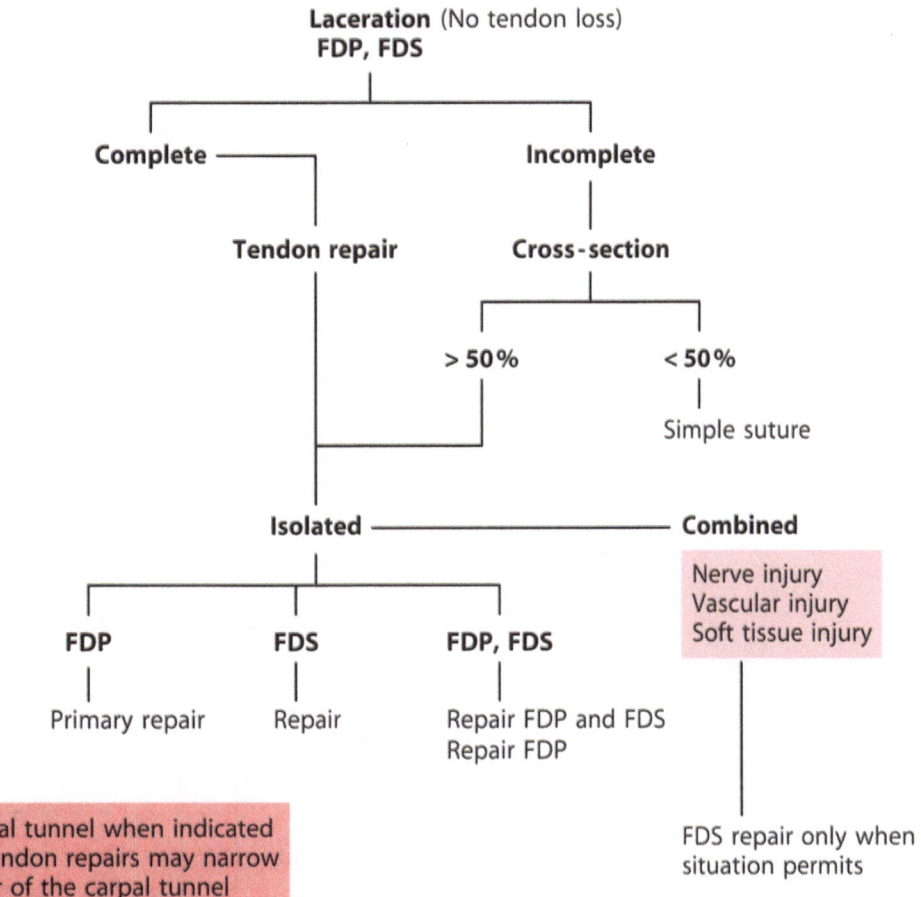

Laceration (No tendon loss)
FDP, FDS

Complete ──────── **Incomplete**

Tendon repair   **Cross-section**

> 50 %   **< 50 %**

Simple suture

Isolated ─────────────────── **Combined**

FDP   **FDS**   **FDP, FDS**

Primary repair   Repair   Repair FDP and FDS
Repair FDP

Nerve injury
Vascular injury
Soft tissue injury

FDS repair only when
situation permits

Release carpal tunnel when indicated
Too many tendon repairs may narrow
the diameter of the carpal tunnel

Dynamic follow-up protocol
except in children under 12 years
See p. 225

Zone 3 and 4

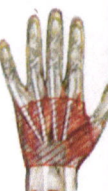

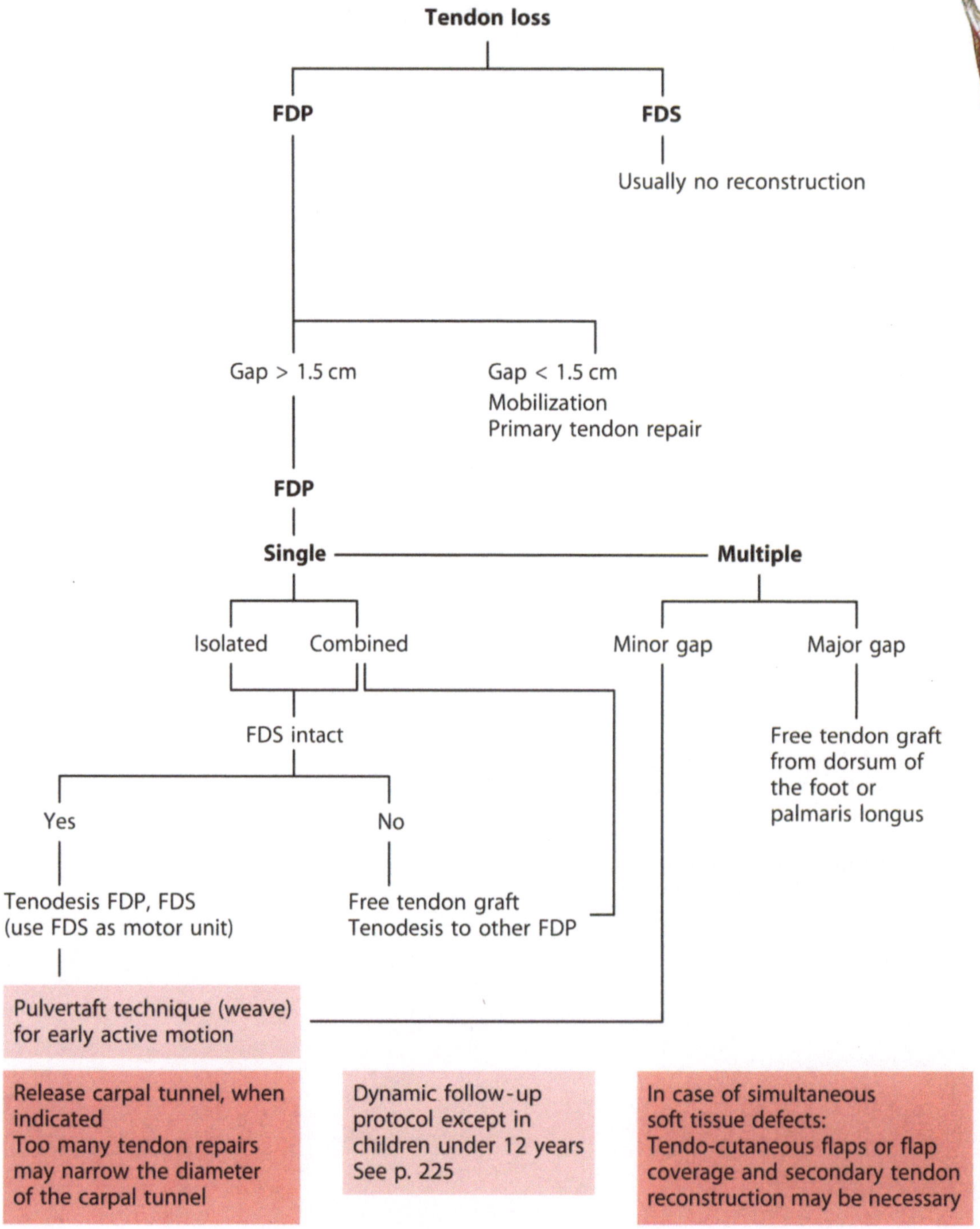

Tendon loss

FDP

FDS

Usually no reconstruction

Gap > 1.5 cm

Gap < 1.5 cm
Mobilization
Primary tendon repair

FDP

Single ———————————————————————— **Multiple**

Isolated   Combined

Minor gap   Major gap

FDS intact

Free tendon graft
from dorsum of
the foot or
palmaris longus

Yes

No

Tenodesis FDP, FDS
(use FDS as motor unit)

Free tendon graft
Tenodesis to other FDP

Pulvertaft technique (weave)
for early active motion

Release carpal tunnel, when
indicated
Too many tendon repairs
may narrow the diameter
of the carpal tunnel

Dynamic follow-up
protocol except in
children under 12 years
See p. 225

In case of simultaneous
soft tissue defects:
Tendo-cutaneous flaps or flap
coverage and secondary tendon
reconstruction may be necessary

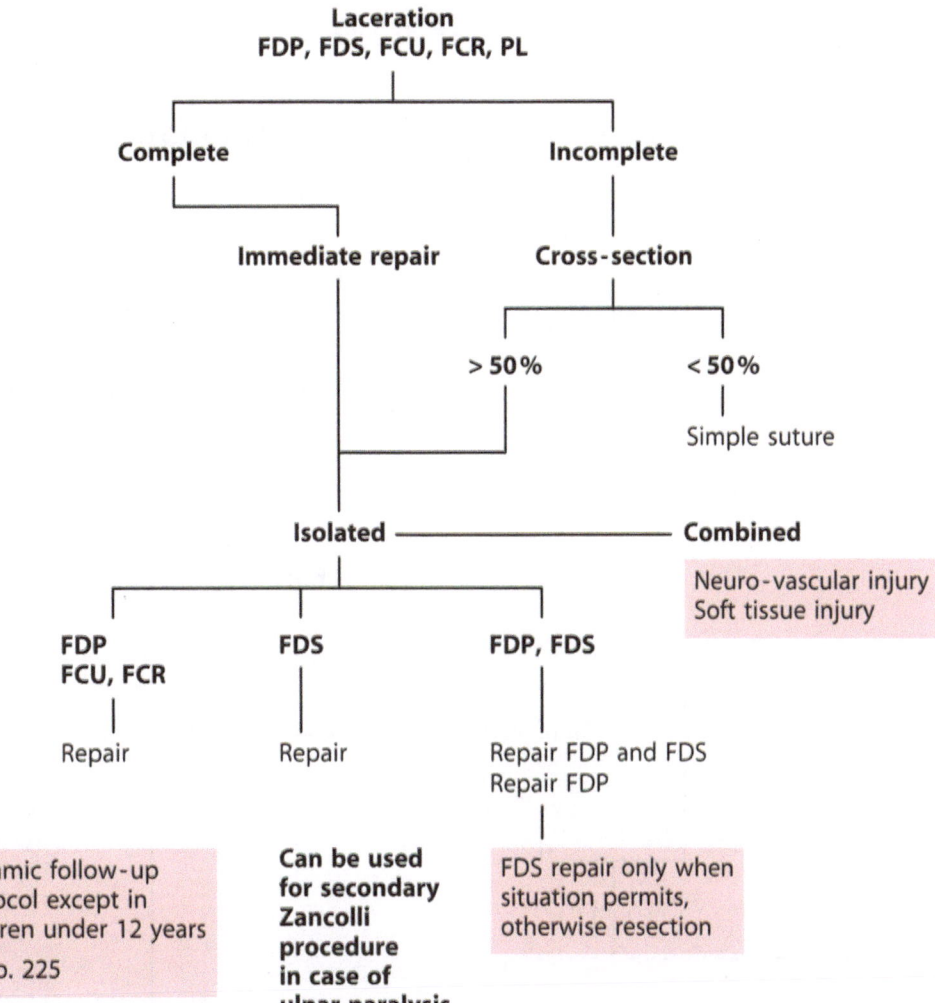

Zone 5 and 6 (Wrist/Forearm)

Laceration
FDP, FDS, FCU, FCR, PL

Complete

Incomplete

Immediate repair

Cross-section

> 50%

< 50%

Simple suture

Isolated ──────────── **Combined**

Neuro-vascular injury
Soft tissue injury

FDP
FCU, FCR

FDS

FDP, FDS

Repair

Repair

Repair FDP and FDS
Repair FDP

Dynamic follow-up
protocol except in
children under 12 years
See p. 225

**Can be used
for secondary
Zancolli
procedure
in case of
ulnar paralysis**

FDS repair only when
situation permits,
otherwise resection

Zone 5 and 6 (Wrist/Forearm)

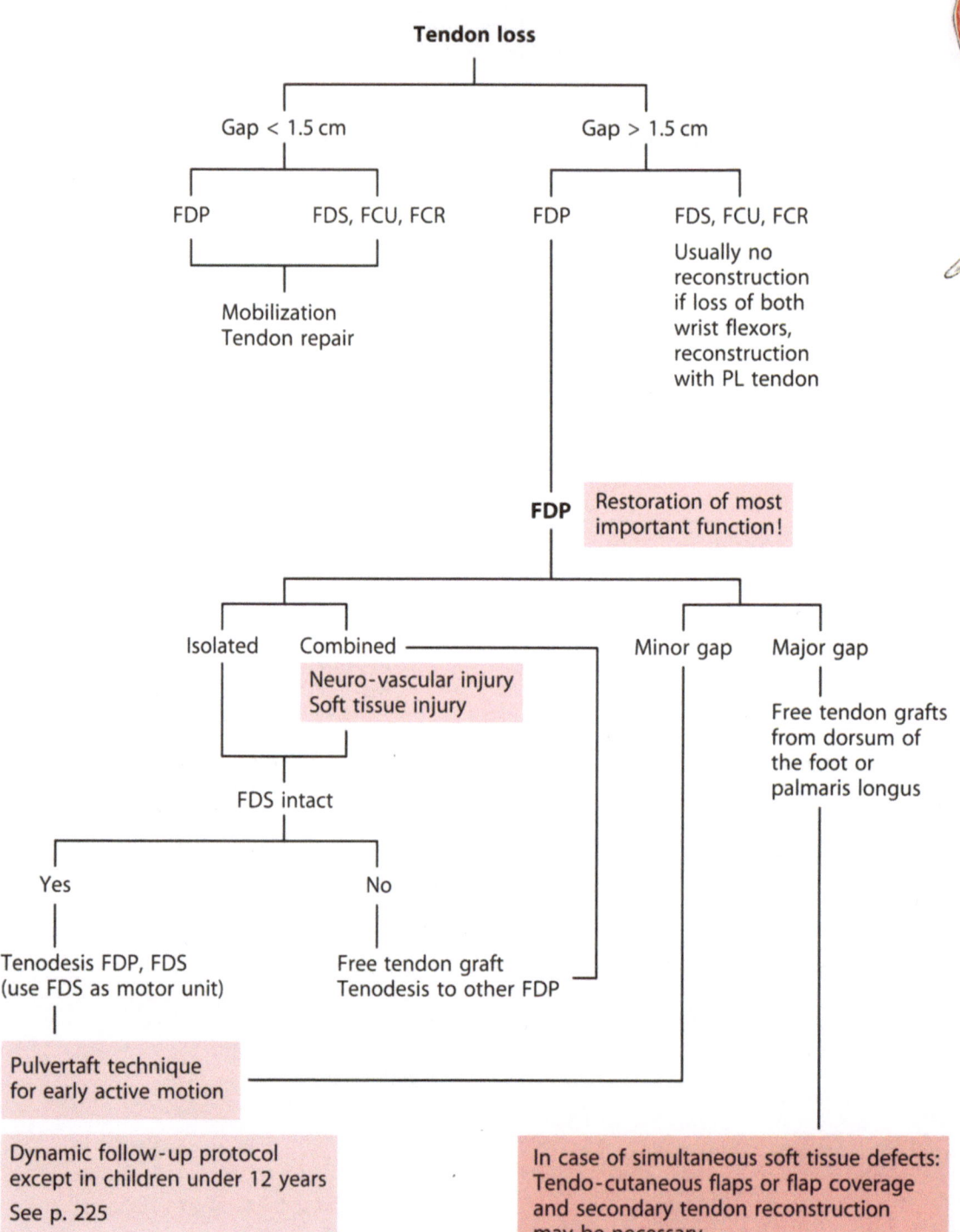

Tendon loss

Gap < 1.5 cm

FDP   FDS, FCU, FCR

Mobilization
Tendon repair

Gap > 1.5 cm

FDP   FDS, FCU, FCR

Usually no
reconstruction
if loss of both
wrist flexors,
reconstruction
with PL tendon

FDP Restoration of most
important function!

Isolated   Combined

Neuro-vascular injury
Soft tissue injury

FDS intact

Yes   No

Tenodesis FDP, FDS   Free tendon graft
(use FDS as motor unit)   Tenodesis to other FDP

Pulvertaft technique
for early active motion

Dynamic follow-up protocol
except in children under 12 years
See p. 225

Minor gap   Major gap

Free tendon grafts
from dorsum of
the foot or
palmaris longus

In case of simultaneous soft tissue defects:
Tendo-cutaneous flaps or flap coverage
and secondary tendon reconstruction
may be necessary

Zone 6 (Musculotendinous Junction)

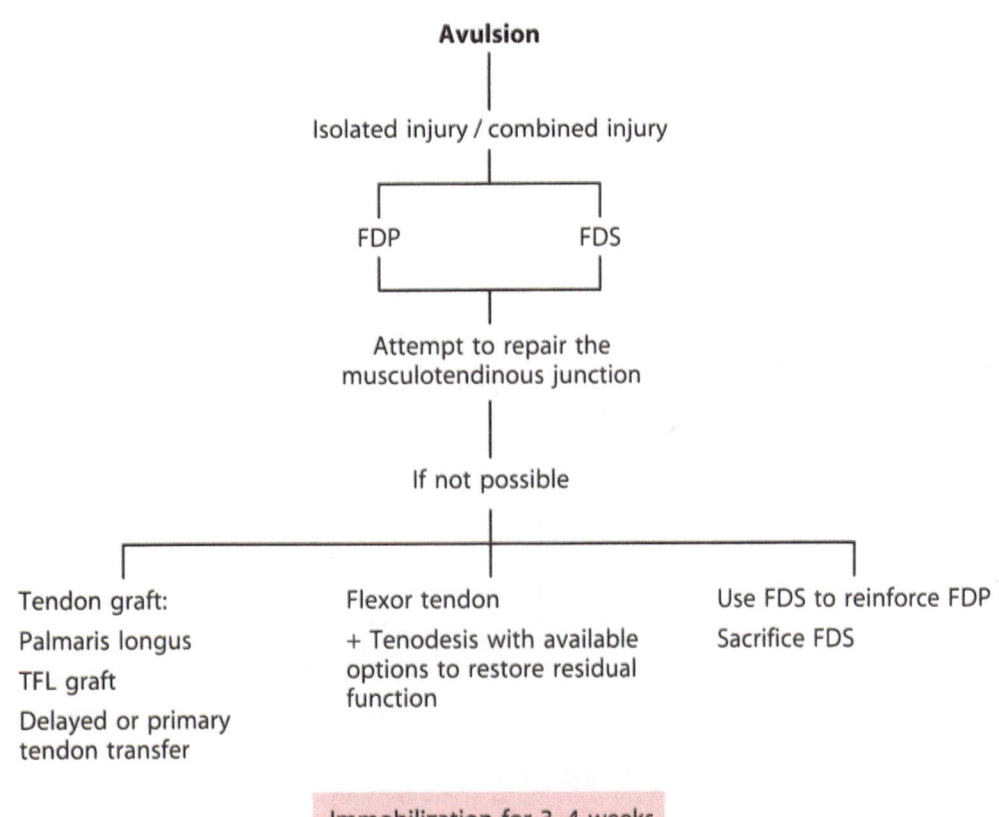

Avulsion

Isolated injury / combined injury

FDP   FDS

Attempt to repair the
musculotendinous junction

If not possible

Tendon graft:

Palmaris longus

TFL graft

Delayed or primary
tendon transfer

Flexor tendon

+ Tenodesis with available
options to restore residual
function

Use FDS to reinforce FDP

Sacrifice FDS

Immobilization for 3-4 weeks

Forearm

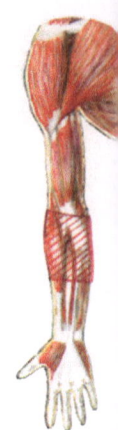

Laceration
FDP, FDS, Muscular portions
FCU, FCR, PT

Complete ——————— Incomplete

Muscular repair
(Approximation of
epimysium and
deep fascia)

Isolated ——————— Combined
or

Neurovascular
Soft tissue

Immobilization for 4-5 weeks (if no tension) – on repair
Immobilization for 5 weeks (if slight tension) – on repair

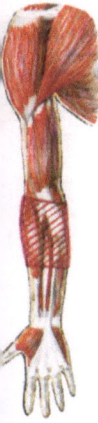

Forearm

Muscle loss

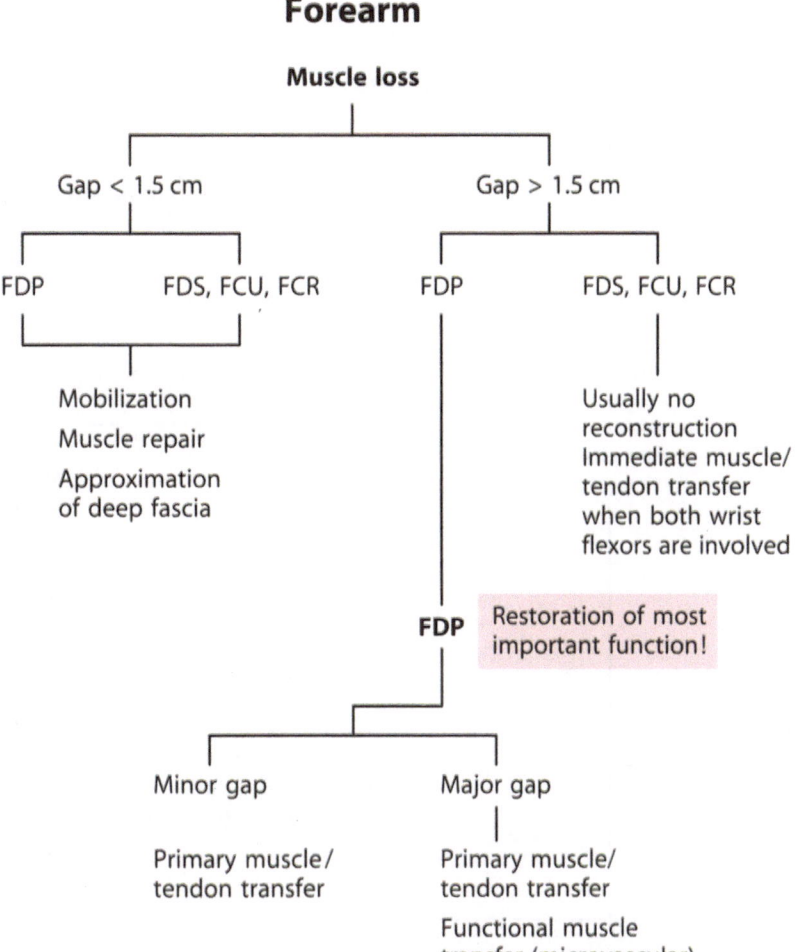

Gap < 1.5 cm   Gap > 1.5 cm

FDP   FDS, FCU, FCR   FDP   FDS, FCU, FCR

Mobilization

Muscle repair

Approximation
of deep fascia

Usually no
reconstruction
Immediate muscle/
tendon transfer
when both wrist
flexors are involved

FDP   Restoration of most
important function!

Minor gap   Major gap

Primary muscle/
tendon transfer

Primary muscle/
tendon transfer

Functional muscle
transfer (microvascular)

Immobilization for 4 weeks

Forearm

Avulsion

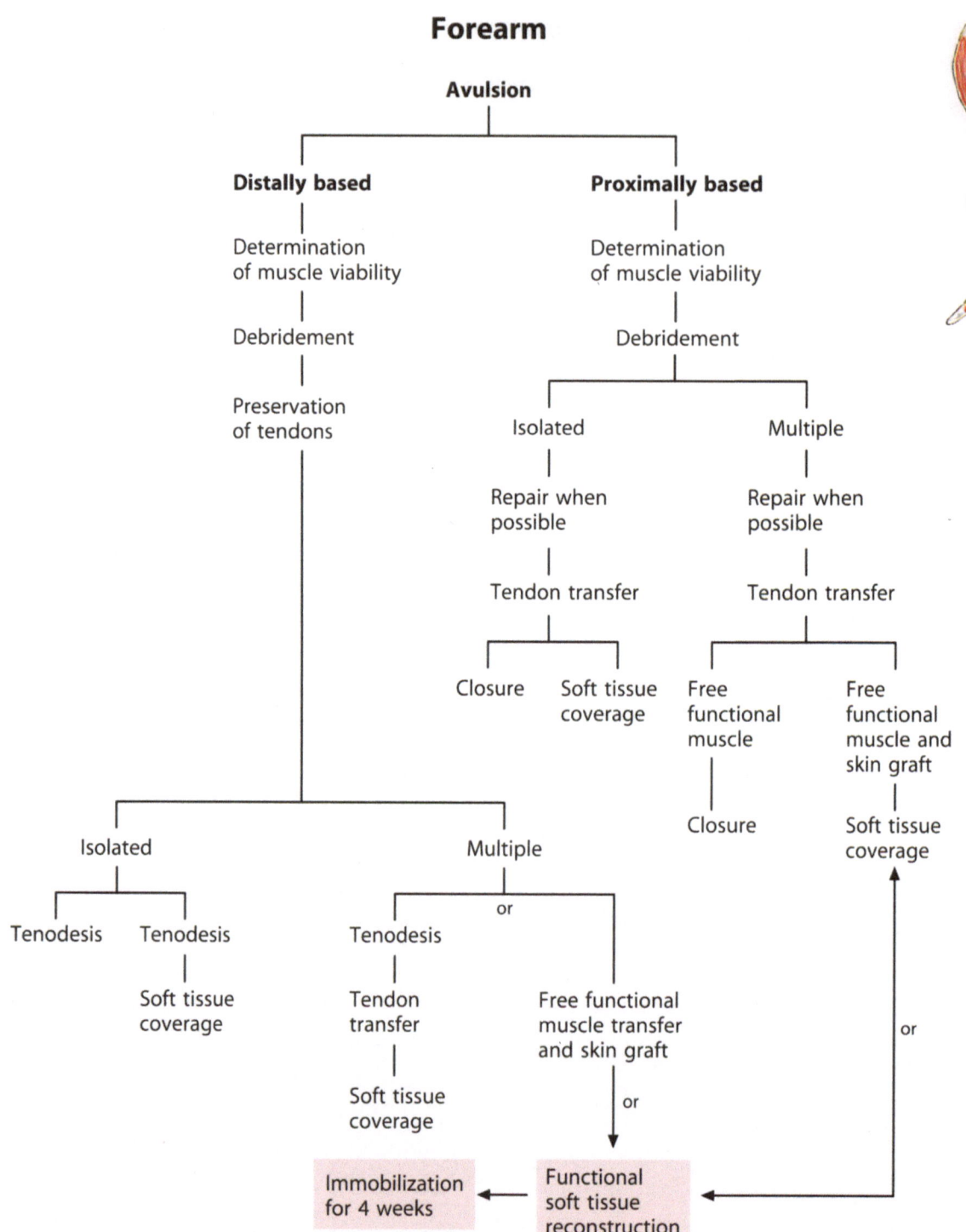

Distally based

Determination
of muscle viability

Debridement

Preservation
of tendons

Proximally based

Determination
of muscle viability

Debridement

Isolated

Repair when
possible

Tendon transfer

Closure   Soft tissue
coverage

Multiple

Repair when
possible

Tendon transfer

Free
functional
muscle

Closure

Free
functional
muscle and
skin graft

Soft tissue
coverage

Isolated

Tenodesis   Tenodesis

Soft tissue
coverage

Multiple

or

Tenodesis

Tendon
transfer

Soft tissue
coverage

Free functional
muscle transfer
and skin graft

or

Immobilization
for 4 weeks

Functional
soft tissue
reconstruction

or

Brachium and Elbow

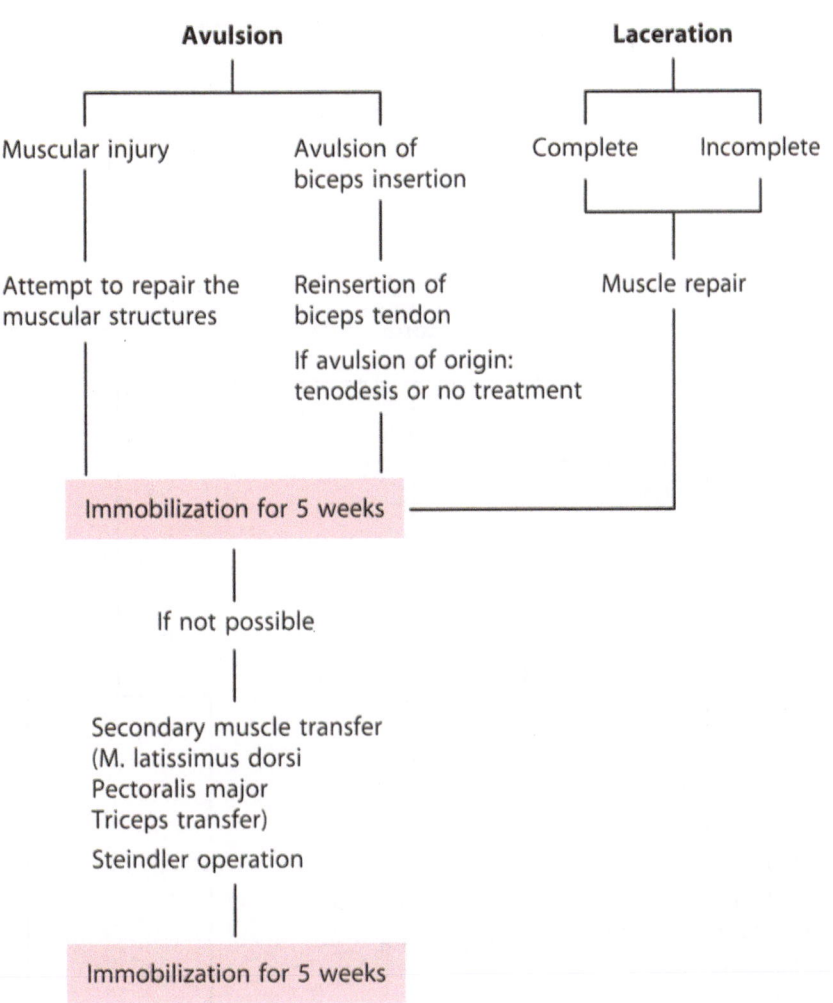

Avulsion   **Laceration**

Muscular injury   Avulsion of   Complete   Incomplete
                         biceps insertion

Attempt to repair the   Reinsertion of   Muscle repair
muscular structures   biceps tendon

                         If avulsion of origin:
                         tenodesis or no treatment

Immobilization for 5 weeks

If not possible

Secondary muscle transfer
(M. latissimus dorsi
Pectoralis major
Triceps transfer)

Steindler operation

Immobilization for 5 weeks

Flexor Tendon Reconstruction

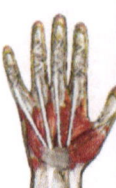

FDP

FDS

Full passive ROM for
all digital joints is
absolutely mandatory

Usually no secondary
reconstruction

Zone

1

2

3-6

Two stage
reconstruction

Stage one

Hunter rod
Pulley reconstruction

Hunter rod +
pulley reconstruction

FDS intact

Stage two
(wait 12-16 weeks)

Free tendon graft

PL, plantaris, FDS slip
(transosseous fixation)

Z-lengthening
(thumb)

FDS transfer

Free tendon graft

PL, plantaris

Yes

No

Motor transfer

FDS, FDP
(side-to-side
tenoraphy)

Free tendon graft

PL, plantaris

Tendon transfer

Free muscle
transplant if no
flexors are available

Dynamic follow-up protocol

Extensor Systems

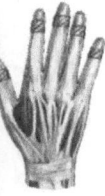

Zone 1

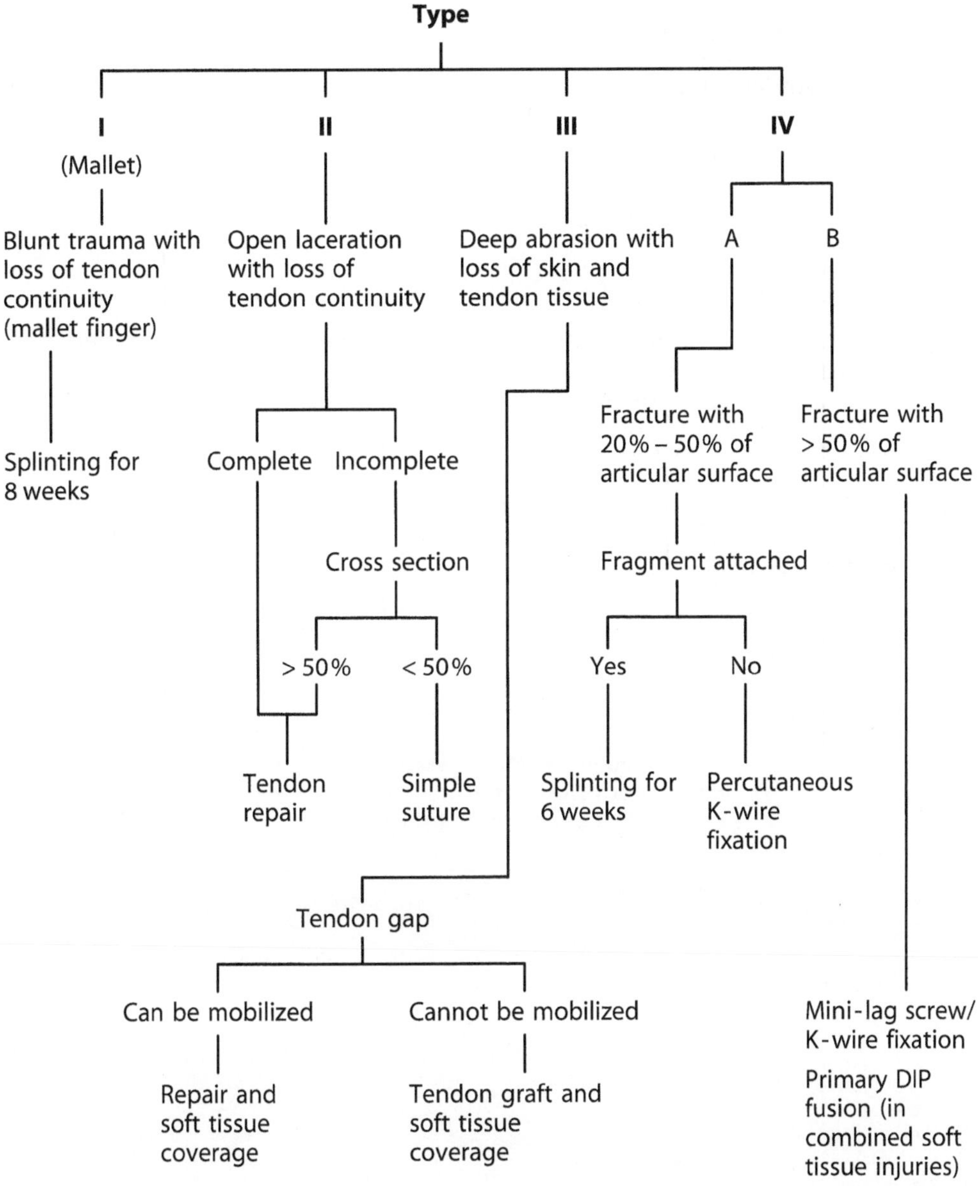

Type

I
(Mallet)

Blunt trauma with loss of tendon continuity (mallet finger)

Splinting for 8 weeks

II

Open laceration with loss of tendon continuity

Complete   Incomplete

Cross section

> 50%   < 50%

Tendon repair   Simple suture

III

Deep abrasion with loss of skin and tendon tissue

Tendon gap

Can be mobilized   Cannot be mobilized

Repair and soft tissue coverage

Tendon graft and soft tissue coverage

IV

A   B

Fracture with 20% – 50% of articular surface

Fracture with > 50% of articular surface

Fragment attached

Yes   No

Splinting for 6 weeks   Percutaneous K-wire fixation

Mini-lag screw/ K-wire fixation

Primary DIP fusion (in combined soft tissue injuries)

Zone 2 and 4 – Thumb

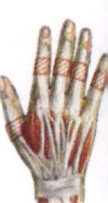

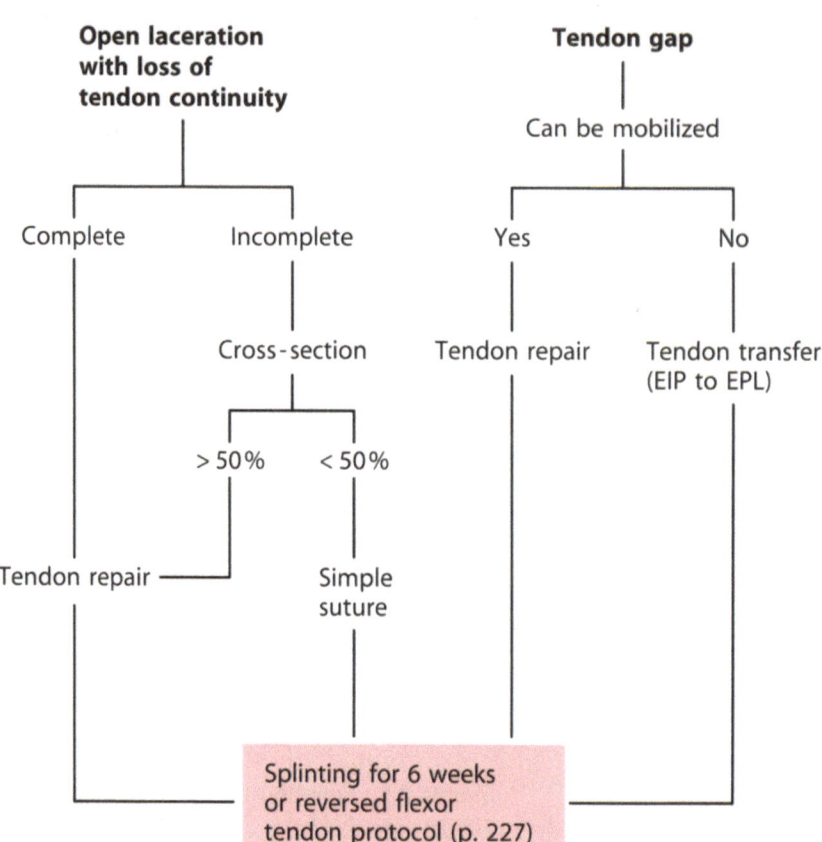

Open laceration with loss of tendon continuity

- Complete
- Incomplete
  - Cross-section
    - > 50 %
    - < 50 %

Tendon repair

Simple suture

Tendon gap

Can be mobilized

- Yes → Tendon repair
- No → Tendon transfer (EIP to EPL)

Splinting for 6 weeks or reversed flexor tendon protocol (p. 227)

Zone 3 and 4 – Central Slip

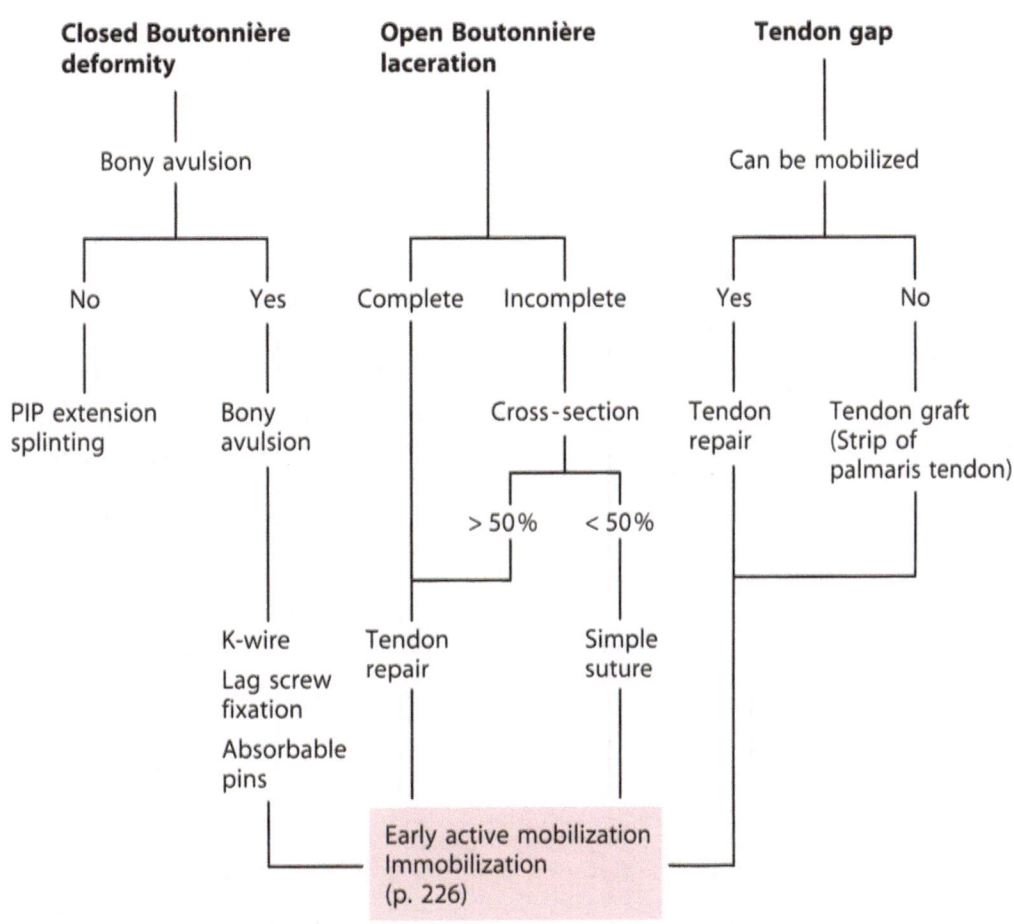

Closed Boutonnière deformity

|
Bony avulsion
|
No / Yes

No → PIP extension splinting

Yes → Bony avulsion → K-wire / Lag screw fixation / Absorbable pins

Open Boutonnière laceration

|
Bony avulsion
|
Complete / Incomplete

Complete → Tendon repair

Incomplete → Cross-section → > 50% / < 50%

> 50% → Tendon repair

< 50% → Simple suture

Tendon gap

|
Can be mobilized
|
Yes / No

Yes → Tendon repair

No → Tendon graft (Strip of palmaris tendon)

Early active mobilization
Immobilization
(p. 226)

Zone 5 and 6 – Thumb

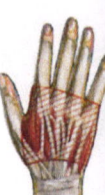

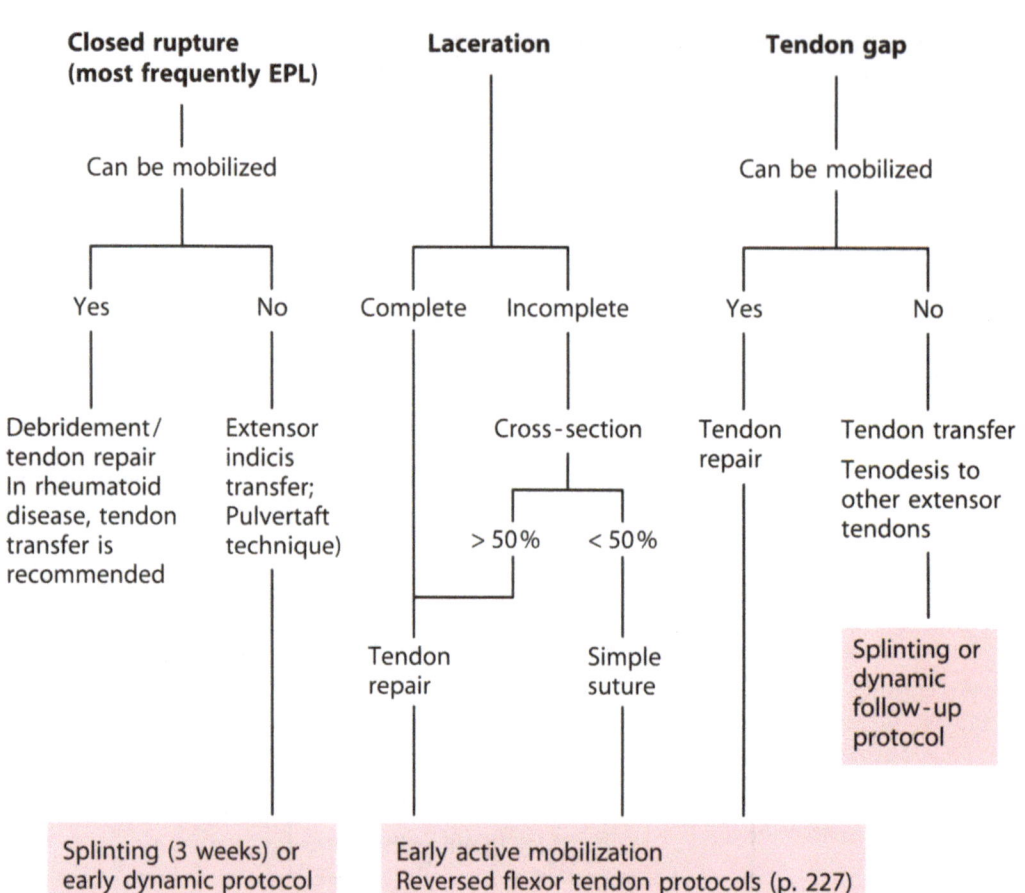

Closed rupture (most frequently EPL)

Can be mobilized

Yes → Debridement/ tendon repair In rheumatoid disease, tendon transfer is recommended

No → Extensor indicis transfer; Pulvertaft technique)

Laceration

Complete → Tendon repair

Incomplete → Cross-section → > 50% → Tendon repair / < 50% → Simple suture

Tendon gap

Can be mobilized

Yes → Tendon repair

No → Tendon transfer Tenodesis to other extensor tendons

Splinting (3 weeks) or early dynamic protocol

Early active mobilization Reversed flexor tendon protocols (p. 227)

Splinting or dynamic follow-up protocol

Zone 7

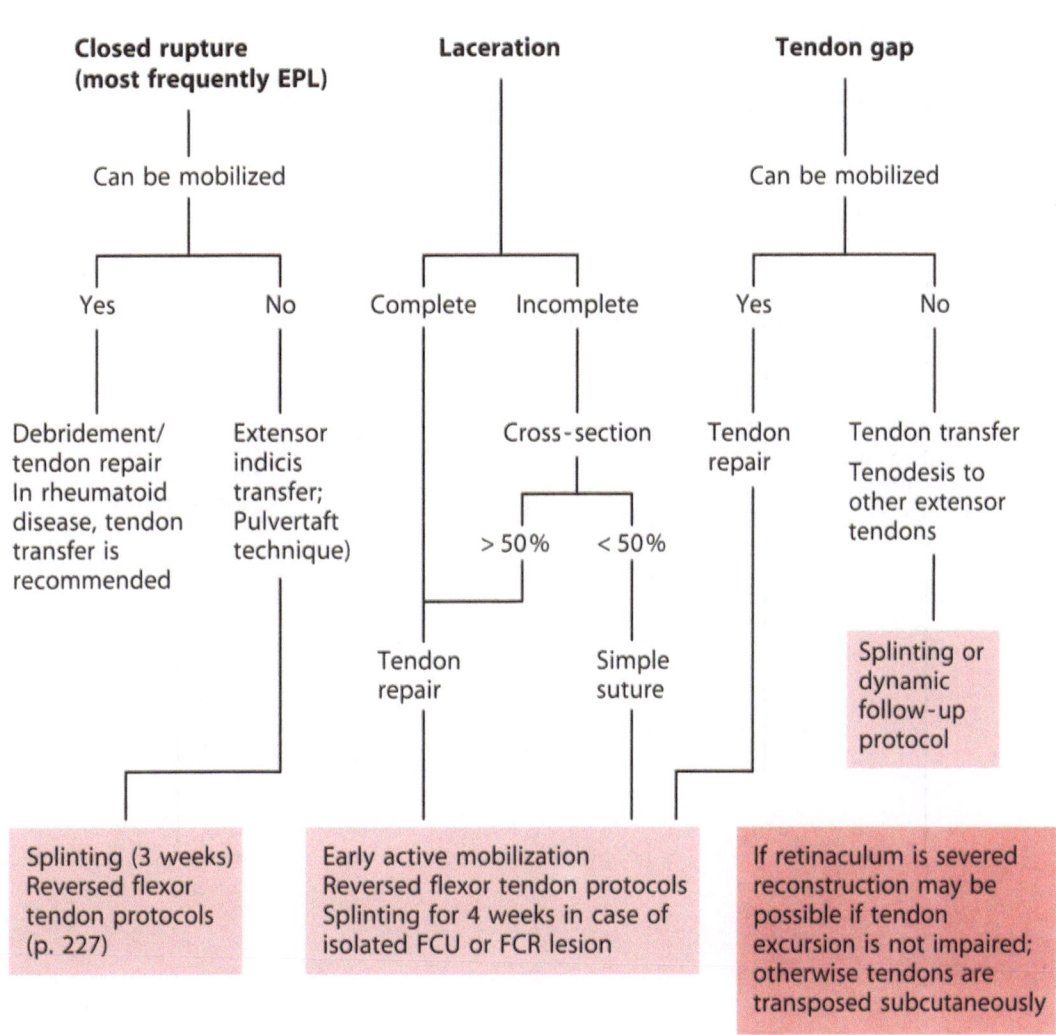

Closed rupture (most frequently EPL)

Can be mobilized

Yes — No

Yes: Debridement/ tendon repair In rheumatoid disease, tendon transfer is recommended

No: Extensor indicis transfer; Pulvertaft technique)

Splinting (3 weeks) Reversed flexor tendon protocols (p. 227)

Laceration

Complete — Incomplete

Cross-section

> 50%   < 50%

Tendon repair

Simple suture

Early active mobilization Reversed flexor tendon protocols Splinting for 4 weeks in case of isolated FCU or FCR lesion

Tendon gap

Can be mobilized

Yes — No

Yes: Tendon repair

No: Tendon transfer Tenodesis to other extensor tendons

Splinting or dynamic follow-up protocol

If retinaculum is severed reconstruction may be possible if tendon excursion is not impaired; otherwise tendons are transposed subcutaneously

Zone 8

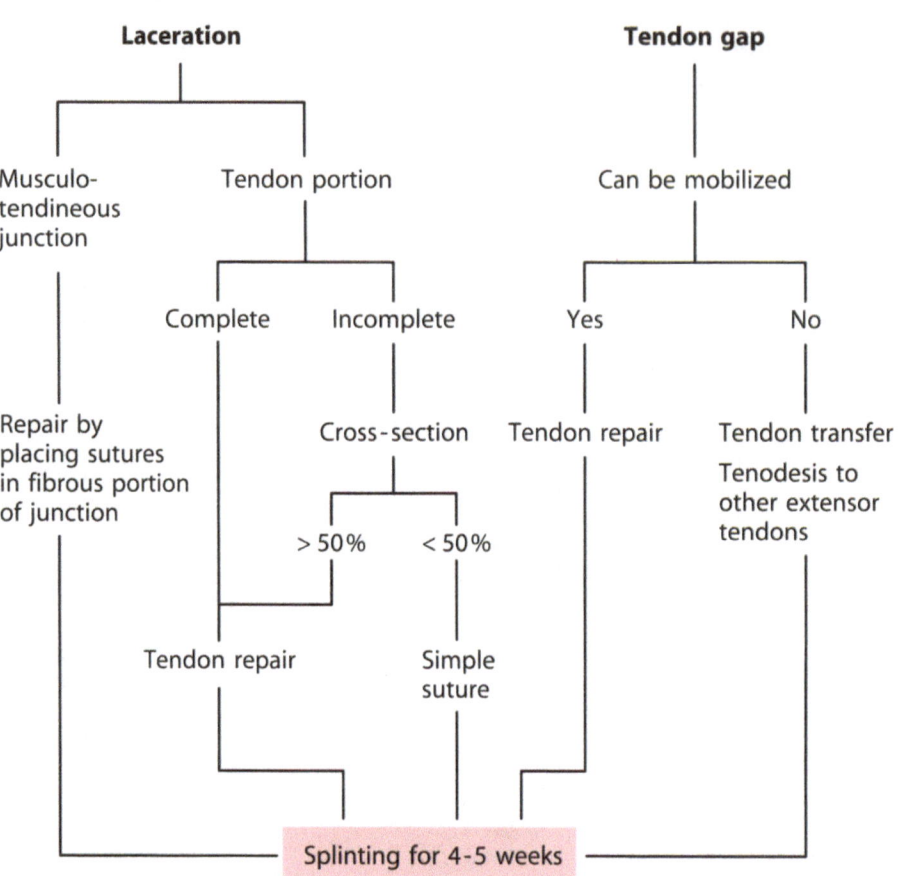
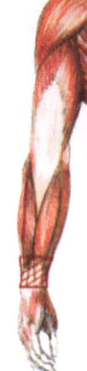

Laceration

Tendon gap

Musculo-
tendineous
junction

Tendon portion

Can be mobilized

Complete   Incomplete

Yes   No

Repair by
placing sutures
in fibrous portion
of junction

Cross-section

Tendon repair

Tendon transfer

Tenodesis to
other extensor
tendons

> 50 %   < 50 %

Tendon repair   Simple
suture

Splinting for 4-5 weeks

Zone 8 – Forearm

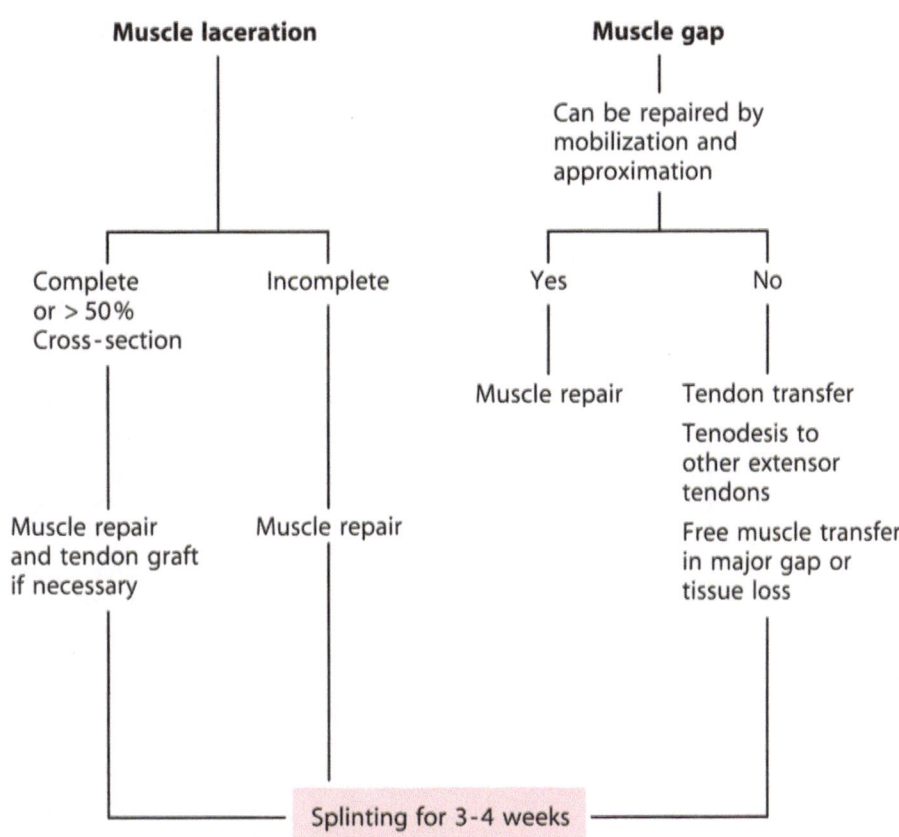

Muscle laceration

Muscle gap

Can be repaired by
mobilization and
approximation

Complete
or > 50 %
Cross-section

Incomplete

Yes

No

Muscle repair

Tendon transfer

Tenodesis to
other extensor
tendons

Muscle repair
and tendon graft
if necessary

Muscle repair

Free muscle transfer
in major gap or
tissue loss

Splinting for 3-4 weeks

Forearm

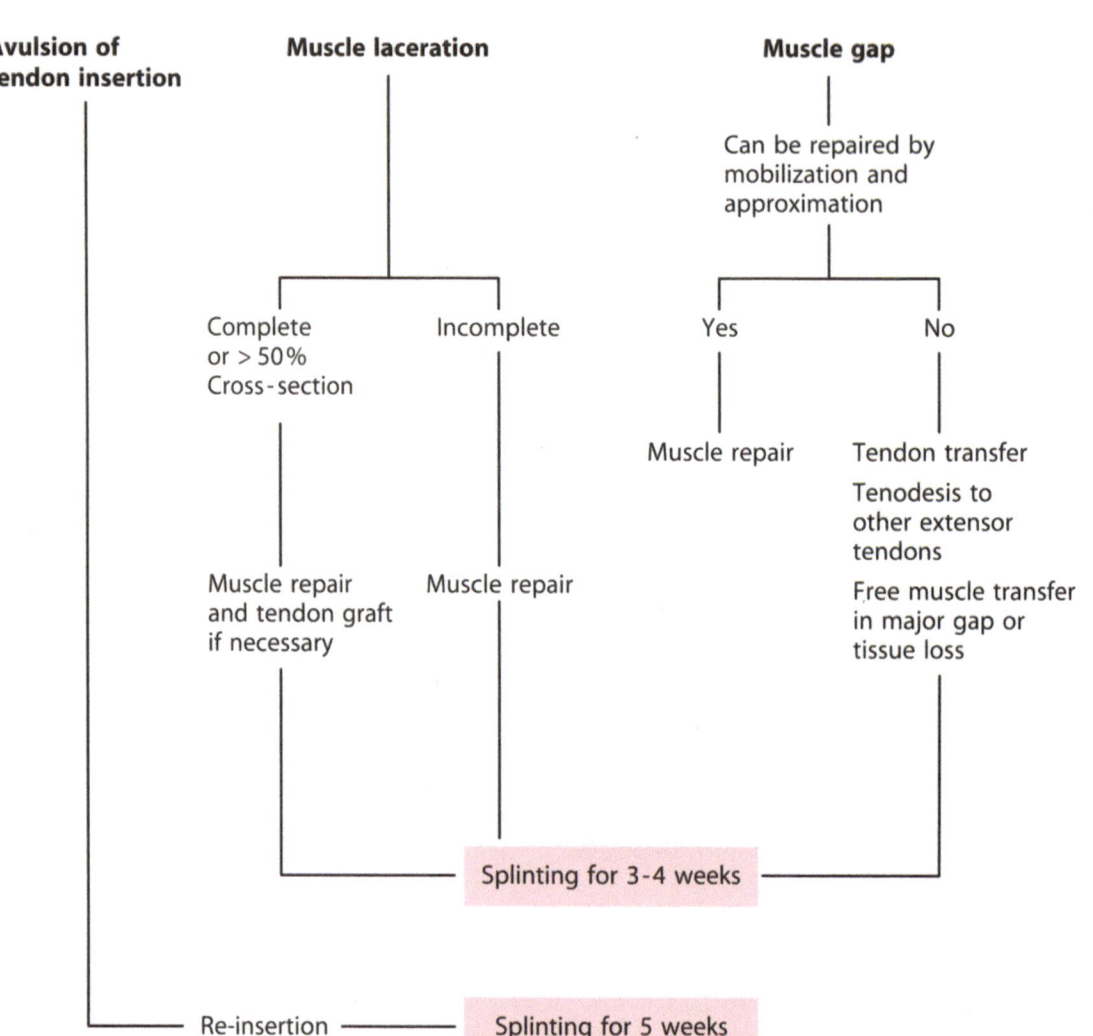

**Avulsion of
tendon insertion**

Muscle laceration

Muscle gap

Can be repaired by
mobilization and
approximation

Complete
or > 50 %
Cross-section

Incomplete

Yes

No

Muscle repair

Tendon transfer

Tenodesis to
other extensor
tendons

Free muscle transfer
in major gap or
tissue loss

Muscle repair
and tendon graft
if necessary

Muscle repair

Splinting for 3-4 weeks

Re-insertion ———— Splinting for 5 weeks

Brachium

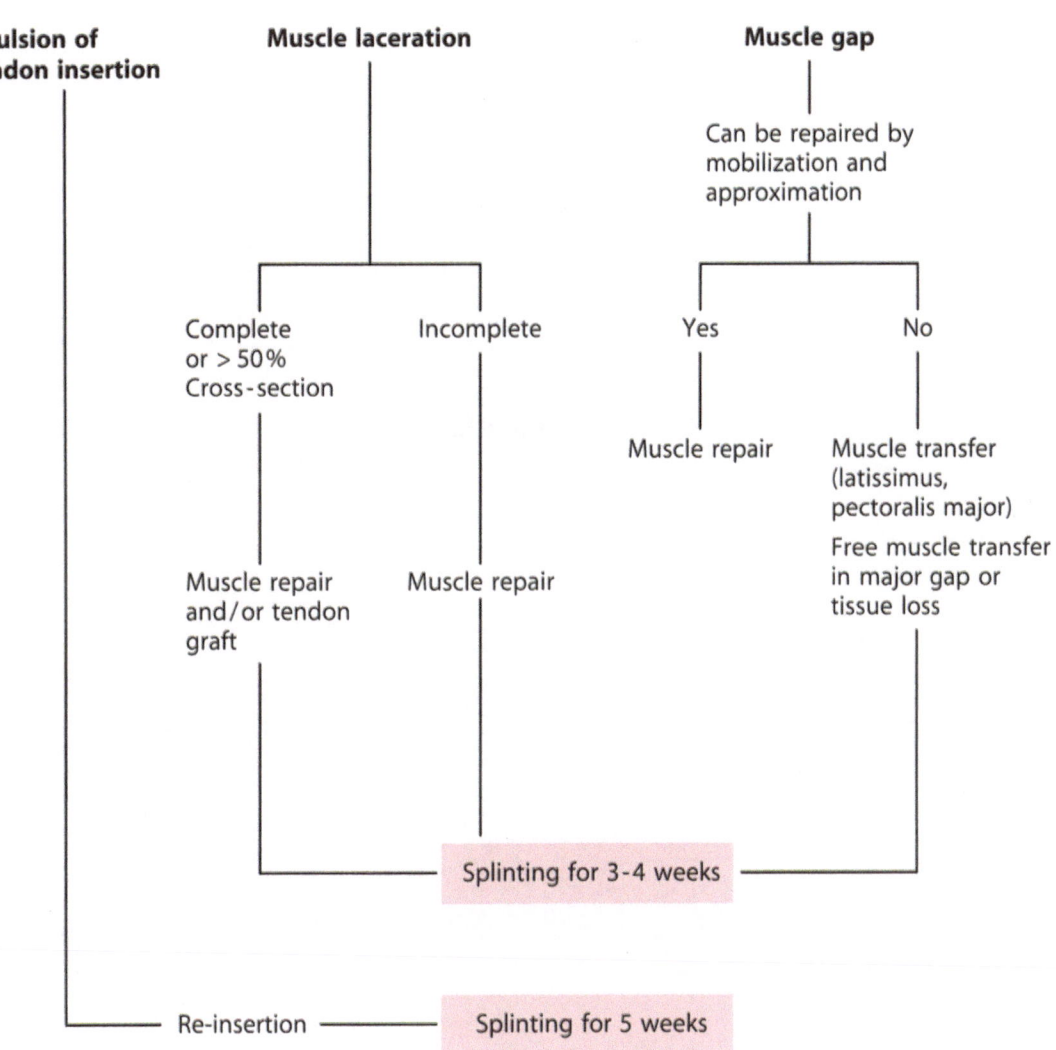

Avulsion of tendon insertion	Muscle laceration		Muscle gap	
			Can be repaired by mobilization and approximation	
	Complete or > 50 % Cross-section	Incomplete	Yes	No
			Muscle repair	Muscle transfer (latissimus, pectoralis major)
				Free muscle transfer in major gap or tissue loss
	Muscle repair and/or tendon graft	Muscle repair		

Splinting for 3-4 weeks

Re-insertion ——— Splinting for 5 weeks

Vessels

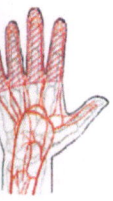

Digits

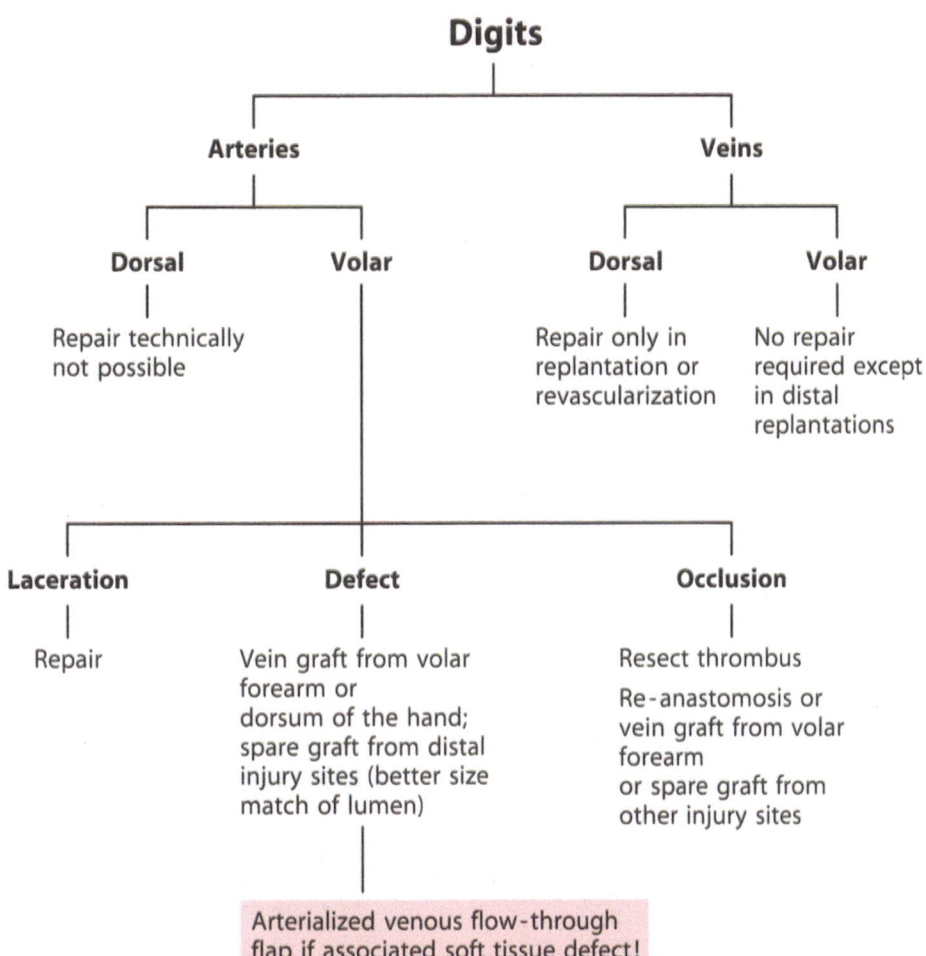

Arteries

    Dorsal

Repair technically
not possible

    Volar

Veins

    Dorsal

Repair only in
replantation or
revascularization

    Volar

No repair
required except
in distal
replantations

Laceration

Repair

Defect

Vein graft from volar
forearm or
dorsum of the hand;
spare graft from distal
injury sites (better size
match of lumen)

Occlusion

Resect thrombus

Re-anastomosis or
vein graft from volar
forearm
or spare graft from
other injury sites

Arterialized venous flow-through
flap if associated soft tissue defect!

Palm and Dorsum of the Hand

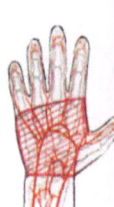

Arteries

Veins

Dorsal

Volar

Dorsal

Volar

Repair A. princeps
pollicis

Repair only in
replantation or
revascularization

No repair
required
(unless
distally
based skin
avulsion)

Superficial arch

Deep arch

Deep arch usually
not repaired

Laceration

Defect

Occlusion

Repair

Vein graft from
dorsum of the hand,
volar forearm,
or spare graft from distal
injury sites

Resect thrombus

Re-anastomosis or vein graft from
dorsum of the hand (caliber!),
volar forearm
or spare graft

Arterial graft from sub-
scapular system possible when
arterial arch is destroyed?

Arterial graft from sub-
scapular system possible when
entire arterial arch is occluded?

Controversial in the literature

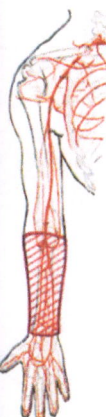

Forearm

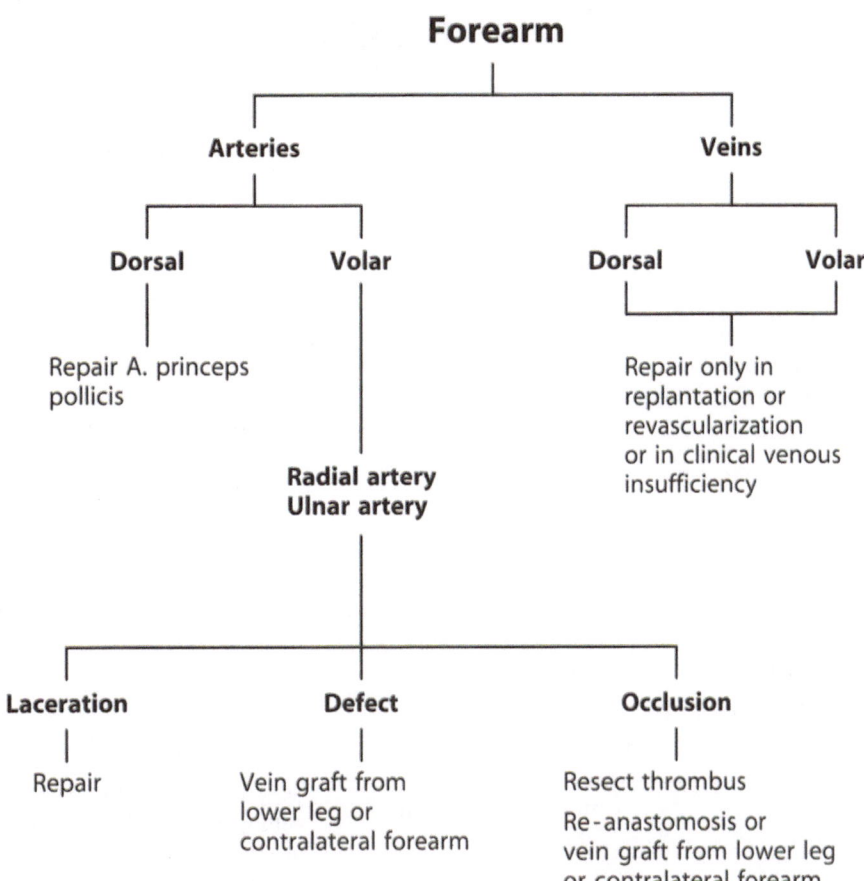

Arteries

Dorsal

Repair A. princeps
pollicis

Volar

Radial artery
Ulnar artery

Veins

Dorsal

Repair only in
replantation or
revascularization
or in clinical venous
insufficiency

Volar

Laceration

Repair

Defect

Vein graft from
lower leg or
contralateral forearm

Occlusion

Resect thrombus

Re-anastomosis or
vein graft from lower leg
or contralateral forearm

Always repair both arteries
for the following reasons:
1. Reserve capacity
2. Possible secondary occlusion
   due to sequelae of trauma
3. Reinjury later in life

Brachium

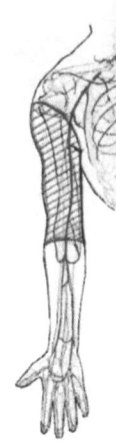

Arteries

Dorsal

No repair of
recurrent arteries

Volar

Brachial artery

Laceration

Repair

Defect

Vein graft from
lower leg or
contralateral forearm

Occlusion

Resect thrombus

Re-anastomosis or
vein graft from lower leg
or contralateral forearm

Veins

Dorsal

Volar

Repair only in
replantation or
revascularization
or clinical venous
insufficiency

Nerves

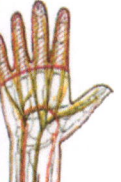

Digits

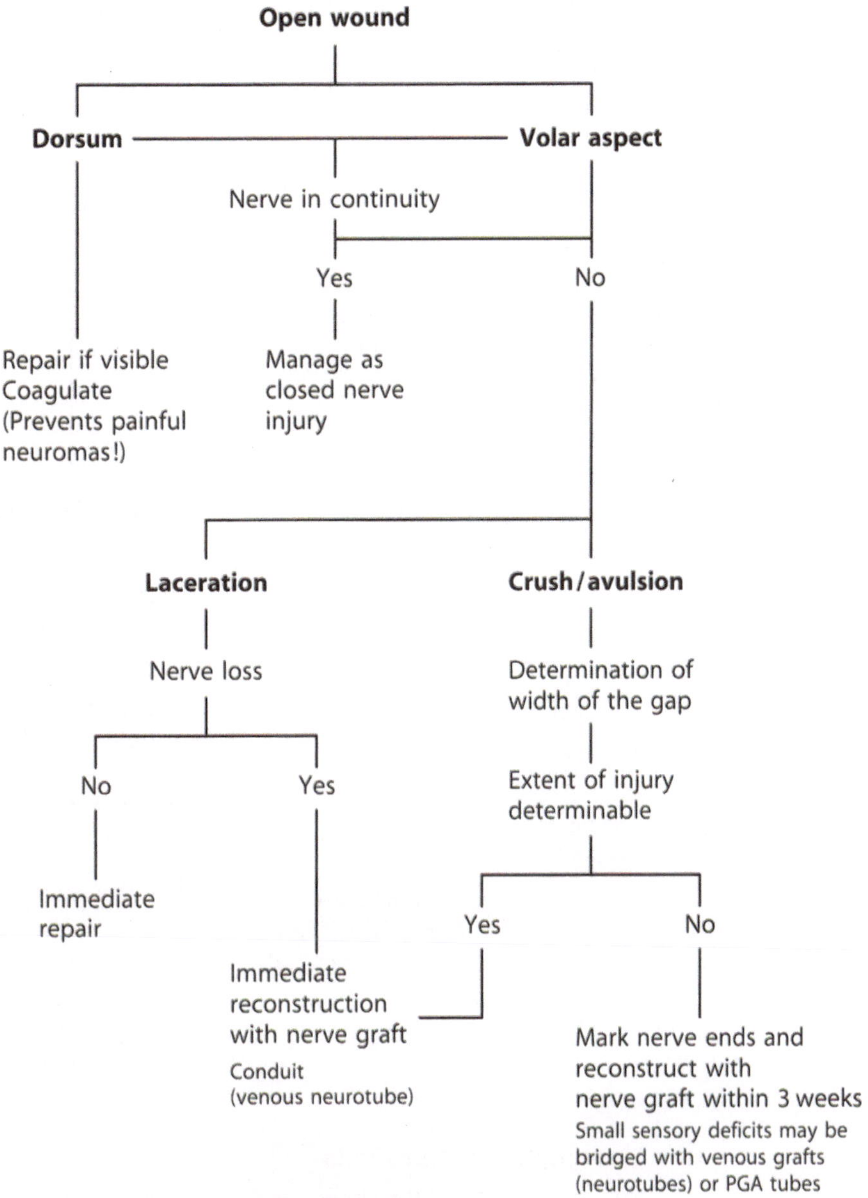

Open wound

Dorsum ——————————————————— **Volar aspect**

Nerve in continuity

Yes   No

Repair if visible   Manage as
Coagulate   closed nerve
(Prevents painful   injury
neuromas!)

Laceration   **Crush/avulsion**

Nerve loss   Determination of
                                     width of the gap

No   Yes   Extent of injury
                                     determinable

Immediate   Yes   No
repair

          Immediate   Mark nerve ends and
          reconstruction   reconstruct with
          with nerve graft   nerve graft within 3 weeks
          Conduit   Small sensory deficits may be
          (venous neurotube)   bridged with venous grafts
                                             (neurotubes) or PGA tubes

Spare parts for nerve grafts

Medial or lateral antebrachial
cutaneous nerve

Posterior interosseous nerve (distal)

Small defects with venous conduit

Palm / Dorsum

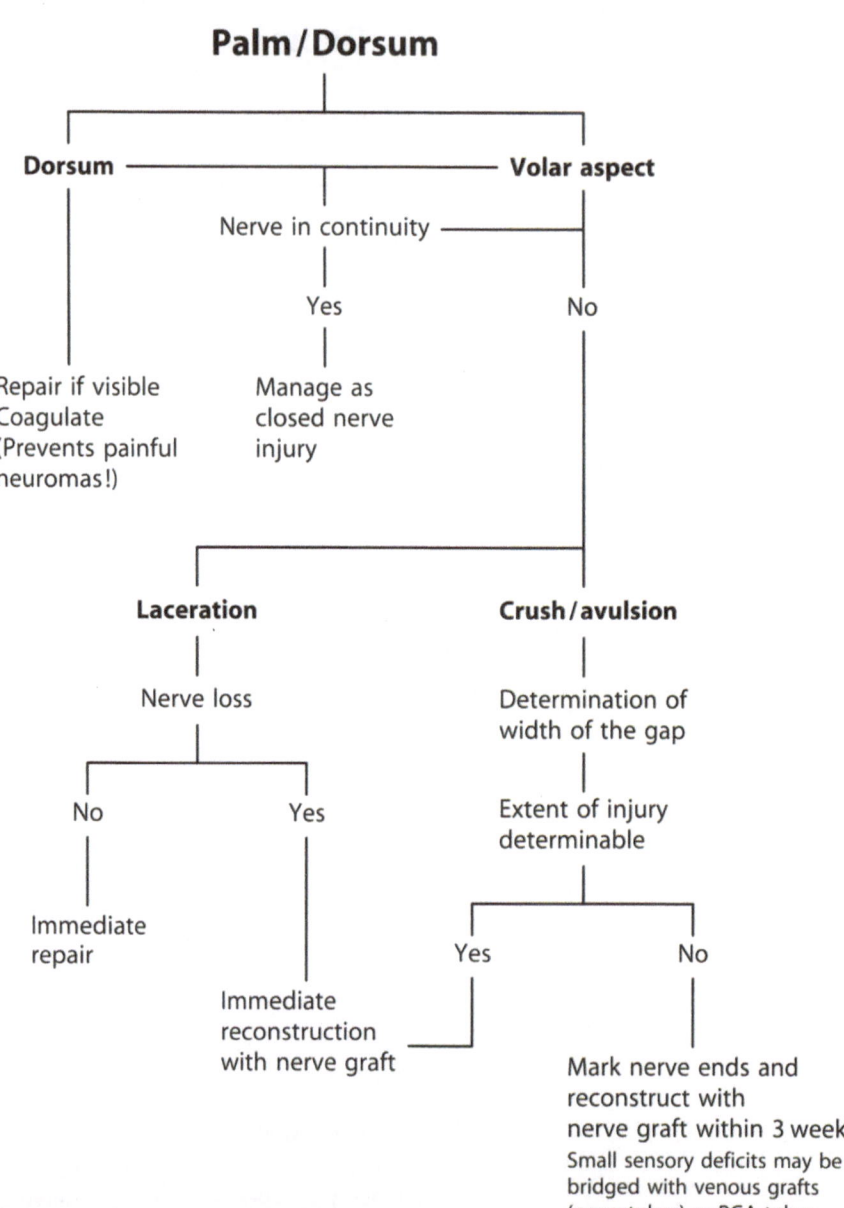

Dorsum ———————————————— **Volar aspect**

Nerve in continuity ————————

Yes   No

Repair if visible   Manage as
Coagulate   closed nerve
(Prevents painful   injury
neuromas!)

Laceration   **Crush / avulsion**

Nerve loss   Determination of
                             width of the gap

No   Yes   Extent of injury
                             determinable

Immediate   Yes   No
repair

            Immediate   Mark nerve ends and
            reconstruction   reconstruct with
            with nerve graft   nerve graft within 3 weeks
                                           Small sensory deficits may be
                                           bridged with venous grafts
                                           (neurotubes) or PGA tubes

Spare parts for nerve grafts

Medial or lateral antebrachial
cutaneous nerve

Posterior interosseous nerve (distal)

Sural nerve

Small defects with venous conduit

Wrist / Distal Forearm

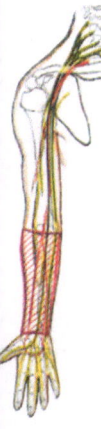

- **Dorsum**
  - Repair all branches of radial nerve! (Prevents painful neuromas!) Determine level and extent of motor deficit! Consider immediate tendon transfer in patients over 30 years or aimed at early rehabilitation
- **Volar aspect**
  - Nerve in continuity
    - Yes
      - Manage as closed nerve injury
    - No
      - **Laceration**
        - Nerve loss
          - No
            - Immediate repair
              - **Median nerve**
                - Consider post-primary opponens plasty in patients over 20 years EIP, FDS 4, Abductor digiti minimi
          - Yes
            - Immediate reconstruction with nerve graft
              - **Ulnar nerve**
                - Consider immediate tendon transfer in patients over 30 years or aimed at early rehabilitation Wait with Zancolli plasty or similar procedure until extent of ulnar palsy (claw hand) can be determined
      - **Crush / avulsion**
        - Determination of width of the gap
          - Extent of injury determinable
            - Yes
              - Immediate reconstruction with nerve graft
            - No
              - Mark nerve ends and reconstruct with nerve graft within 3 weeks
              - Small sensory deficits may be bridged with venous neurotubes

Spare parts
Sural nerve

Brachium

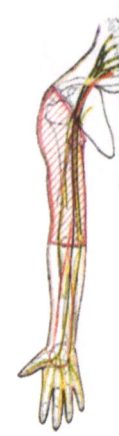

Nerve in continuity

Yes — No

Yes:
Manage as
closed nerve injury

No:

Laceration | **Crush/avulsion**

Laceration → Nerve loss

No — Yes

No: Immediate repair

Yes: Immediate reconstruction with nerve graft

Crush/avulsion:
Determination of width of the gap

Extent of injury determinable

No

Mark nerve ends and reconstruct with nerve graft within 3 weeks

Spare parts
Sural nerve grafts

Median nerve

Consider post-primary opponens plasty in patients over 20 years

EIP, FDS 4,
Abductor digiti minimi

Ulnar nerve

Consider immediate tendon transfer (FDS, FDP) in patients > 30 years or aimed for early rehabilitation

Wait with Zancolli plasty or similar procedure until extent of ulnar palsy is determined

Radial nerve

Consider immediate tendon transfer in patients > 30 years or aimed for early rehabilitation

FCU, EDC,
FDS 4, EPL,
PT, ECRL/ECRB

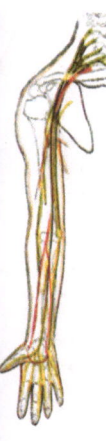

Closed Nerve Injury

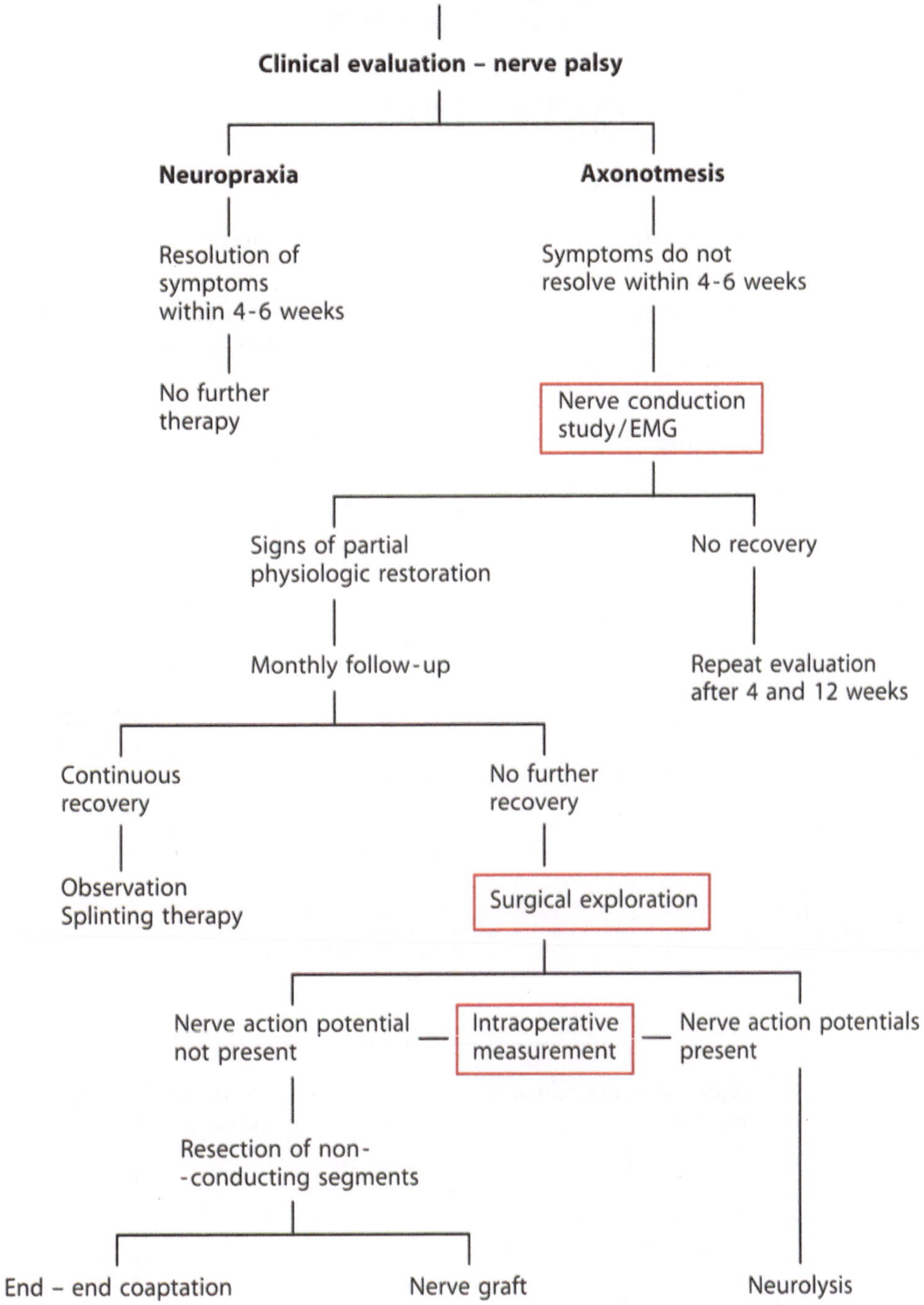

Clinical evaluation – nerve palsy

Neuropraxia   **Axonotmesis**

Resolution of   Symptoms do not
symptoms   resolve within 4-6 weeks
within 4-6 weeks

No further   Nerve conduction
therapy   study / EMG

                Signs of partial   No recovery
                physiologic restoration

                Monthly follow-up   Repeat evaluation
                                                          after 4 and 12 weeks

Continuous   No further
recovery   recovery

Observation   Surgical exploration
Splinting therapy

        Nerve action potential ___ Intraoperative ___ Nerve action potentials
        not present   measurement   present

        Resection of non-
        -conducting segments

End – end coaptation   Nerve graft   Neurolysis

Closed Brachial Plexus Injury
with Complete Palsy

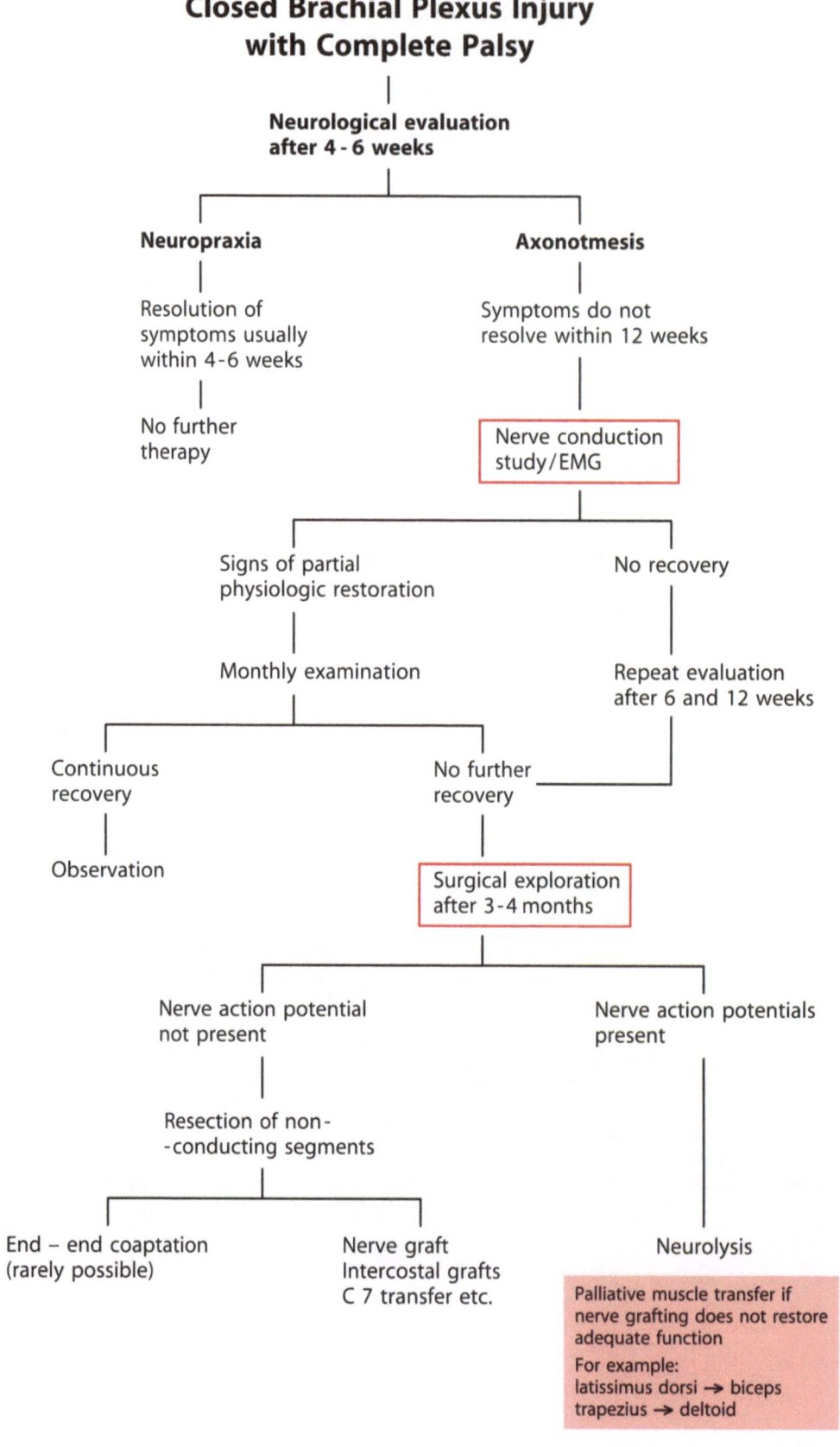

**Neurological evaluation
after 4 - 6 weeks**

Neuropraxia

Resolution of
symptoms usually
within 4-6 weeks

No further
therapy

Axonotmesis

Symptoms do not
resolve within 12 weeks

Nerve conduction
study/EMG

Signs of partial
physiologic restoration

Monthly examination

No recovery

Repeat evaluation
after 6 and 12 weeks

Continuous
recovery

Observation

No further
recovery

Surgical exploration
after 3-4 months

Nerve action potential
not present

Nerve action potentials
present

Resection of non-
-conducting segments

End – end coaptation
(rarely possible)

Nerve graft
Intercostal grafts
C 7 transfer etc.

Neurolysis

Palliative muscle transfer if
nerve grafting does not restore
adequate function

For example:
latissimus dorsi ➔ biceps
trapezius ➔ deltoid

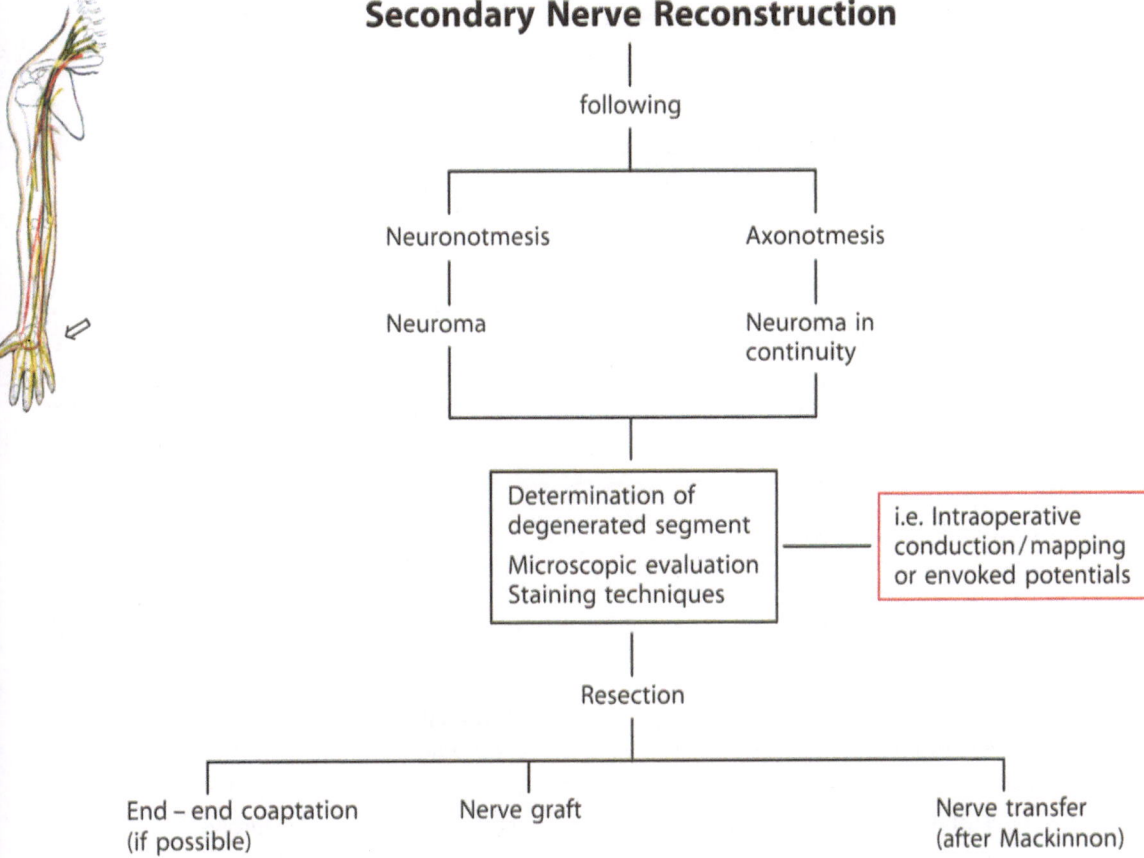

Secondary Nerve Reconstruction

following

Neuronotmesis   Axonotmesis

Neuroma   Neuroma in
                                       continuity

Determination of   i.e. Intraoperative
degenerated segment   conduction/mapping
                          or envoked potentials
Microscopic evaluation
Staining techniques

Resection

End – end coaptation   Nerve graft   Nerve transfer
(if possible)   (after Mackinnon)

Medial or lateral antebrachial nerve

Cutaneous antebrachial nerves

Posterior interosseous nerve

Sural nerve

Consider vascularized nerve graft in
large defects

Neuroma

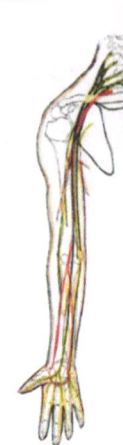

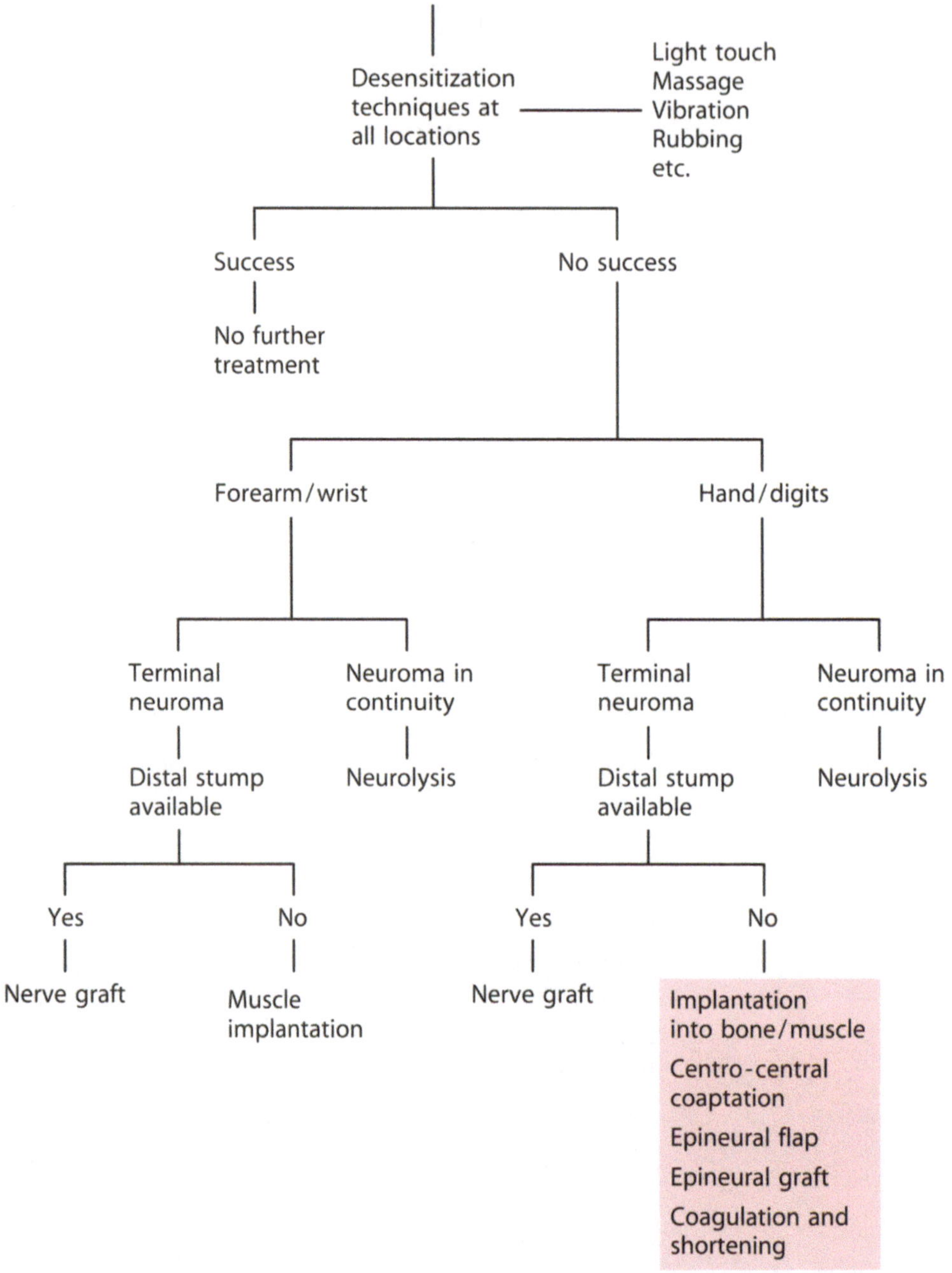

Desensitization techniques at all locations ——— Light touch
Massage
Vibration
Rubbing
etc.

Success

No further treatment

No success

Forearm/wrist

Terminal neuroma

Distal stump available

Yes

Nerve graft

No

Muscle implantation

Neuroma in continuity

Neurolysis

Hand/digits

Terminal neuroma

Distal stump available

Yes

Nerve graft

No

Implantation into bone/muscle

Centro-central coaptation

Epineural flap

Epineural graft

Coagulation and shortening

Neuroma in continuity

Neurolysis

Skin and Soft Tissue

Skin and Soft Tissue

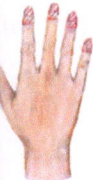

Injuries to the Nail Complex –
Nail Plate, Germinal, and Sterile Matrix

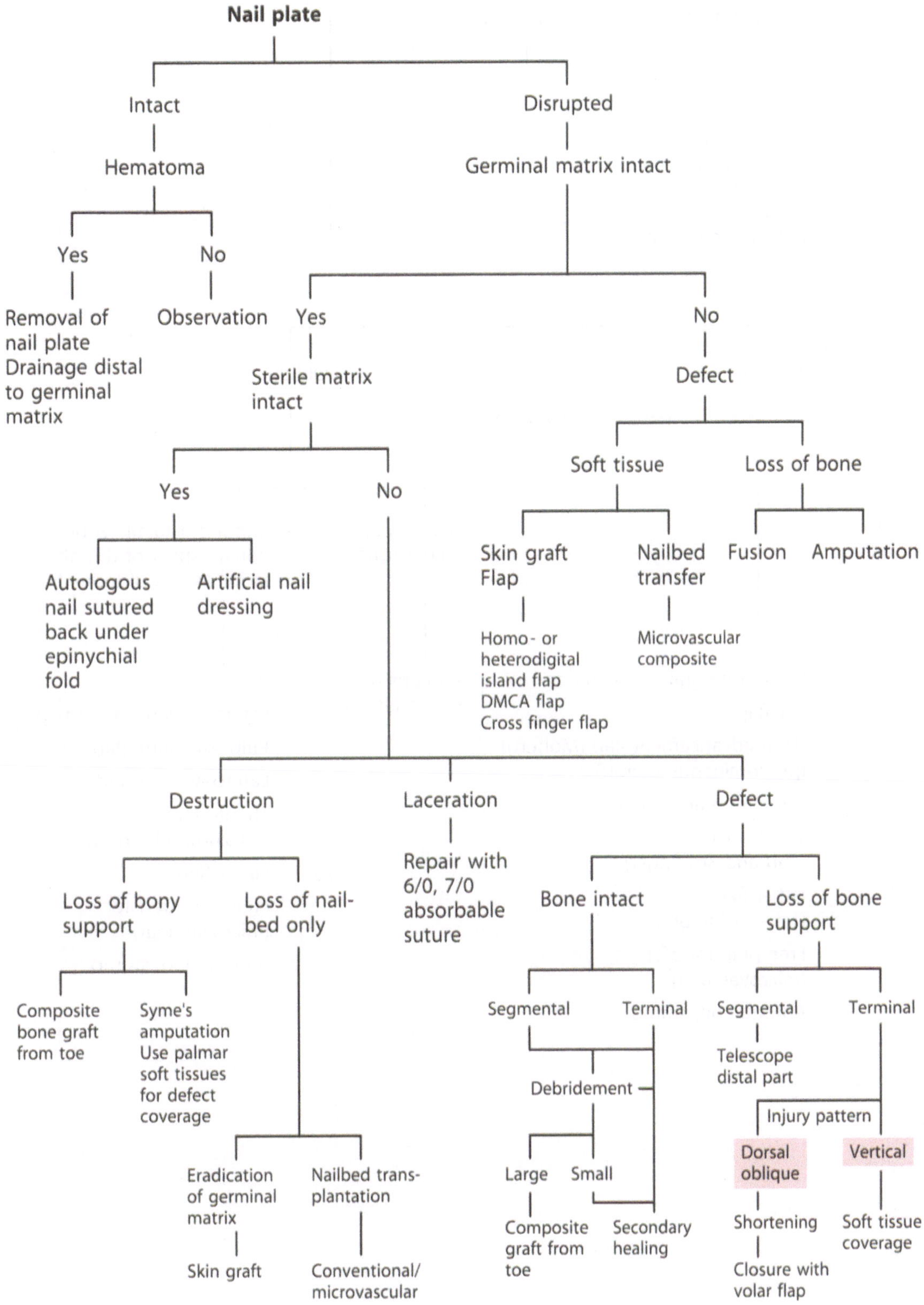

Nail plate

- **Intact**
  - **Hematoma**
    - **Yes** → Removal of nail plate Drainage distal to germinal matrix
    - **No** → Observation
- **Disrupted**
  - **Germinal matrix intact**
    - **Yes** → **Sterile matrix intact**
      - **Yes**
        - Autologous nail sutured back under epinychial fold
        - Artificial nail dressing
      - **No**
        - **Destruction**
          - **Loss of bony support**
            - Composite bone graft from toe
            - Syme's amputation Use palmar soft tissues for defect coverage
          - **Loss of nail-bed only**
            - Eradication of germinal matrix → Skin graft
            - Nailbed transplantation → Conventional/microvascular
        - **Laceration**
          - Repair with 6/0, 7/0 absorbable suture
        - **Defect**
          - **Bone intact**
            - **Segmental**
              - Debridement
                - **Large** → Composite graft from toe
                - **Small** → Secondary healing
            - **Terminal**
          - **Loss of bone support**
            - **Segmental** → Telescope distal part
            - **Terminal** → Injury pattern
              - **Dorsal oblique** → Shortening → Closure with volar flap
              - **Vertical** → Soft tissue coverage
    - **No**
      - **Defect**
        - **Soft tissue**
          - Skin graft Flap → Homo- or heterodigital island flap DMCA flap Cross finger flap
          - Nailbed transfer → Microvascular composite
        - **Loss of bone**
          - Fusion
          - Amputation

Fingertips

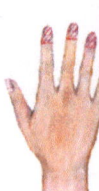

Superficial –	**Dorsal**	**Volar**
no bone exposed	Dorsal/oblique	

Secondary healing	Nail complex	Deep,
	see page 132	bone exposed

Dressing:
Silicone gauze
Artificial skin
Gauze
Polyurethan foil etc.

> If a very small bone segment is exposed, the bone can be trimmed and the wound may heal secondarily

Transverse   **Oblique**

——— Flap coverage ———

Less important tactile zone   **Important tactile zone (ulnar aspect of thumb; radial aspect of index finger)**

Transverse	Less important tactile zone	Important tactile zone
Composite graft replantation	All flaps or skin graft	V-Y flap
V-Y flap		Lateral advancement flap
Volar advancement flap (Moberg) (predominantly thumb)		Pulp exchange flap
Volar translation flap		Latero-volar island flap
Thenar flap (2nd and 3rd finger)		Thenar flap (for 2nd and 3rd finger)
Littler flap (1st – 3rd finger)		Littler flap
Free pulp transfer (microvascular)		Free pulp transfer (microvascular)
Amputation, stump		Amputation, stump

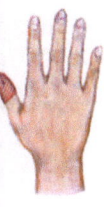

Thumb

Distal phalanx and fingertip

**Superficial –
no bone exposed**

Deep, bone exposed

> If a very small bone segment is exposed, the bone can be trimmed and the wound may heal secondarily

Secondary healing

Nailbed
see page 132

Dressing:
Silicone
Artificial skin
Gauze
Polyurethan foil etc.

Distal third

Middle/proximal
third

Transverse

V-Y flap

Volar advancement
flap (Moberg)

Volar translation flap

Lateral dorsal island
flap

**Oblique
(Dorsal or volar)**

V-Y

Lateral advancement
flap

Pulp exchange flap

Latero-volar island
flap

Transverse

Volar advancement
flap (Moberg)

Bipedicled
advancement flap
(O'Brien)

Volar translation flap

Lateral dorsal island
flap

Neuro-vascular island
flap

First DMCA flap

Mid-phalangeal island
flap

Free pulp transfer
(microvascular)

Oblique

V-Y flap

Lateral advancement
flap

Pulp exchange flap

Latero-volar island
flap

First DMCA flap

Free pulp transfer
(microvascular)

Free thenar flap
(microvascular)

Thumb

Proximal phalanx

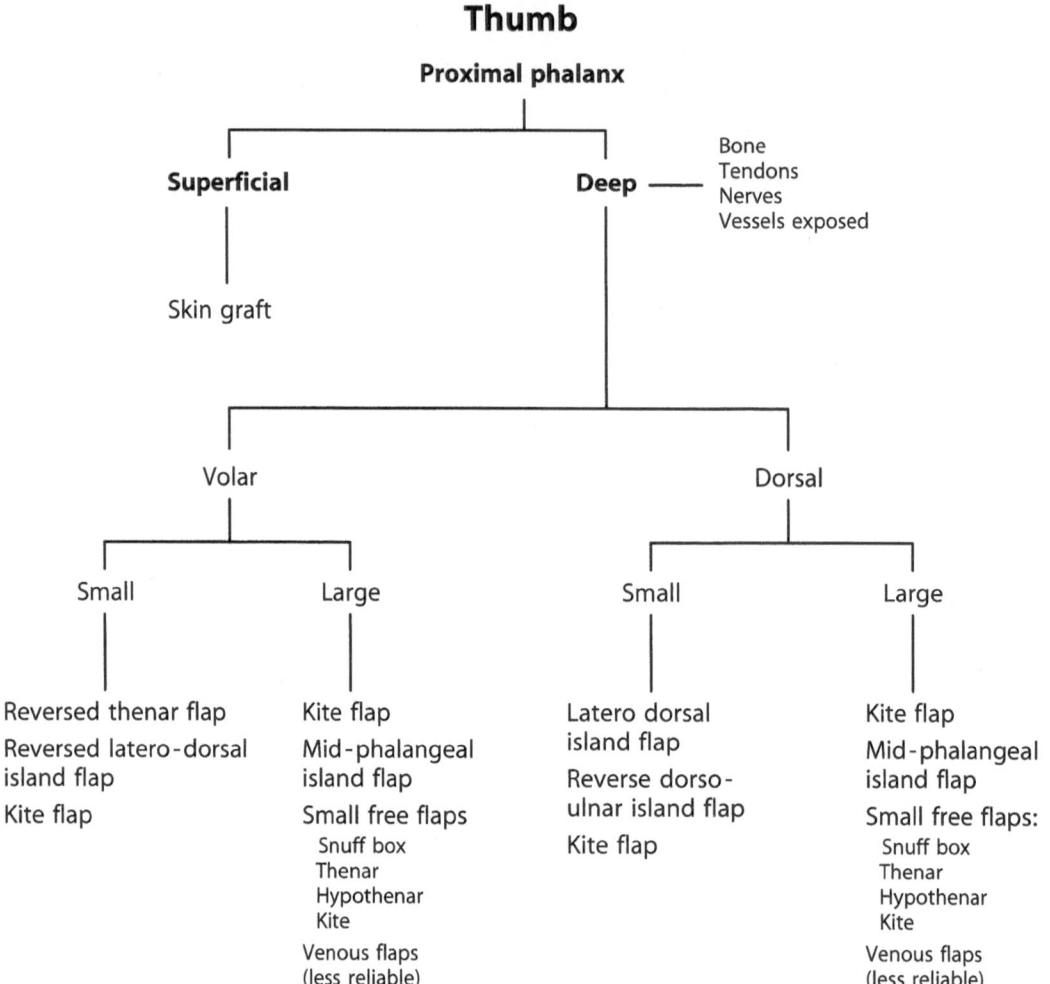

Superficial

Skin graft

Deep —— Bone
Tendons
Nerves
Vessels exposed

Volar

Dorsal

Small

Large

Small

Large

Reversed thenar flap

Reversed latero-dorsal
island flap

Kite flap

Kite flap

Mid-phalangeal
island flap

Small free flaps
  Snuff box
  Thenar
  Hypothenar
  Kite

Venous flaps
(less reliable)

Latero dorsal
island flap

Reverse dorso-
ulnar island flap

Kite flap

Kite flap

Mid-phalangeal
island flap

Small free flaps:
  Snuff box
  Thenar
  Hypothenar
  Kite

Venous flaps
(less reliable)

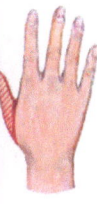

Thumb

Combined defects of proximal phalanx – palmar and dorsal

Superficial

Skin graft

Deep

Vessels, bones,
joints, tendons
exposed

In case of avulsion injury,
consider pedicle groin flap
for primary coverage to
provide the platform for
secondary reconstruction
with "wrap around flap" or
similar procedure

Pedicle flaps

Small/medium
size defects

Kite flap

Mid-phalangeal
island flap

Fillet flap or
pedicle flap from
injured adjacent
digit may be
necessary

Larger
defects

Posterior interosseous
island flap (cutaneous
and fascial)

Reverse radial forearm
flap (cutaneous and
fascial)

All forearm flaps need
coaptation to recipient
nerves to regain sensibility

Microvascular flaps

Small/medium
size defects

Kite flap

Fillet flap or
pedicle flap from
injured adjacent
digit may be
necessary

Venous flap
(less reliable)

Larger
defects

Lateral arm flap
(fascia)

Temporalis fascia flap

Free contralateral
forearm fascia flap

Compound Defects of Proximal and Distal Phalanx of Thumb

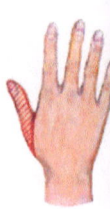

Injury assessment

Which functional structures are involved?

Is preservation/reconstruction possible?

Is preservation/reconstruction worthwhile?

Yes

Structure repair according to pertinent principles

Soft tissue reconstruction with all means available

In case of avulsion injury, consider pedicle groin flap for primary coverage to provide the platform for secondary reconstruction with "wrap around flap" or similar procedure

No

Amputation

Secondary reconstruction

(Depending on level of amputation)

Free great toe ⎫ microsurgical
Free 2nd toe ⎭ transfer
Pollicization
Web space deepening
Metacarpal lengthening

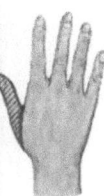

Thumb Reconstruction
(Mono and Compound Defects)

Level of amputation

	Metacarpal	Proximal phalanx	IP joint
Microvascular transfer of:	Great toe including metatarsal 2nd toe including metatarsal	Trimmed great toe Custom-tailored toe (1st and 2nd toes) 2nd toe	Wrap around toe Custom-tailored toe (1st and 2nd toe combined)
	Pollicization? Metacarpal distraction	Web space deepening Distraction	Web space deepening Distraction

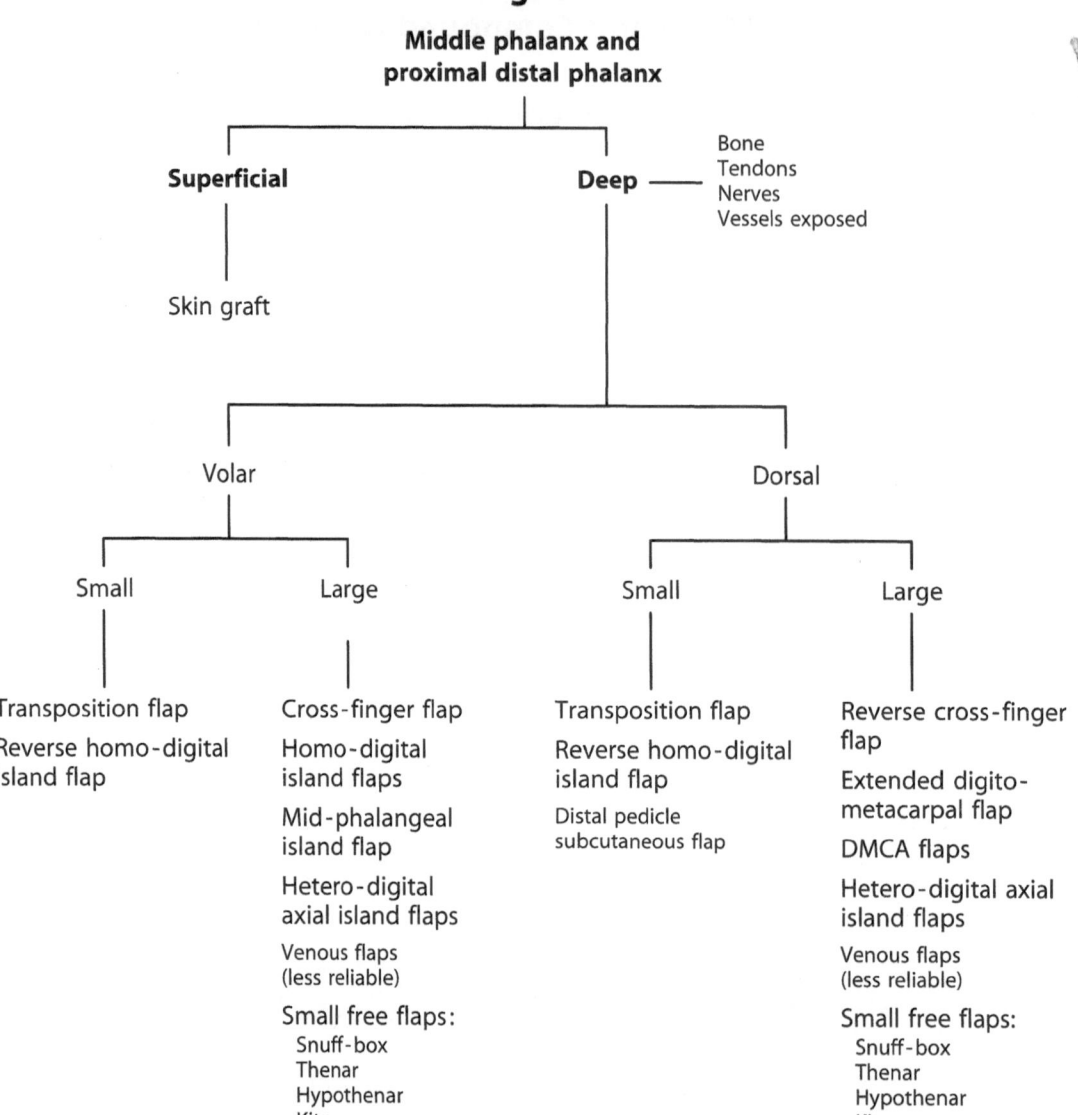

Digits

**Middle phalanx and
proximal distal phalanx**

Superficial   **Deep** ──── Bone
                                                                                    Tendons
                                                                                    Nerves
                                                                                    Vessels exposed

Skin graft

Volar   Dorsal

Small   Large   Small   Large

Transposition flap   Cross-finger flap   Transposition flap   Reverse cross-finger
                                                                               flap
Reverse homo-digital   Homo-digital   Reverse homo-digital
island flap   island flaps   island flap   Extended digito-
                                                                               metacarpal flap
                          Mid-phalangeal   Distal pedicle
                          island flap   subcutaneous flap   DMCA flaps

                          Hetero-digital   Hetero-digital axial
                          axial island flaps   island flaps

                          Venous flaps   Venous flaps
                          (less reliable)   (less reliable)

                          Small free flaps: Small free flaps:
                            Snuff-box   Snuff-box
                            Thenar   Thenar
                            Hypothenar   Hypothenar
                            Kite   Kite

Digits

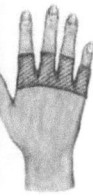

Proximal phalanx

Superficial	**Deep** —— Bone Tendons Nerves Vessels exposed

Superficial

Skin graft

Deep

Volar		Dorsal	
Small	Large	Small	Large

Small (Volar)

Transposition flap

Lateral transposition
flap (Bunnell)

Flag flap

Large (Volar)

Cross-finger flap

Homo-digital
island flaps

Extended digito-
metacarpal flaps

Venous flaps
(less reliable)

Small free flaps:
  Snuff-box
  Thenar
  Hypothenar
  Kite

Small (Dorsal)

Transposition flap

Lateral transposition
flap

Large (Dorsal)

Reverse cross-finger
flap

DMCA flaps

Hetero-digital axial
island flaps

Flag flap

Venous flaps
(less reliable)

Small free flaps:
  Snuff-box
  Thenar
  Hypothenar
  Kite

Digits

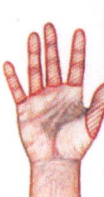

**Extended defects –
proximal / middle phalanx**

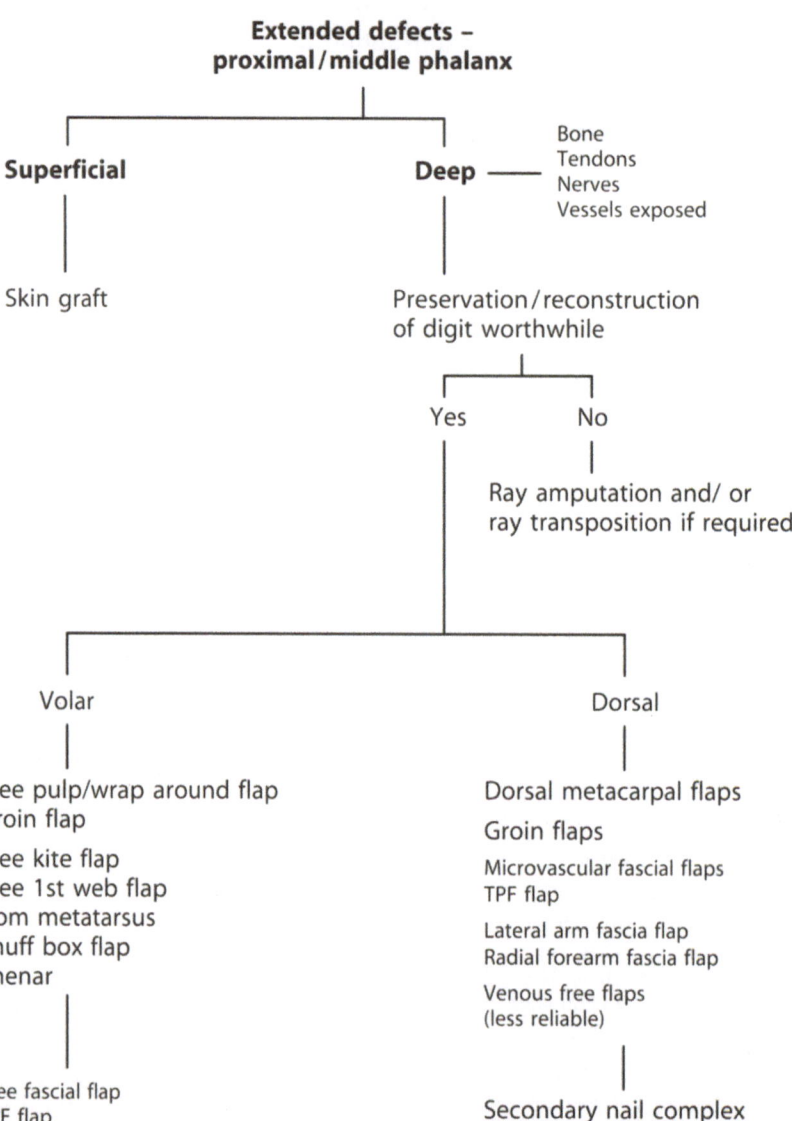

Superficial

Deep —— Bone
Tendons
Nerves
Vessels exposed

Skin graft

Preservation / reconstruction
of digit worthwhile

Yes   No

Ray amputation and/ or
ray transposition if required

Volar

Dorsal

Free pulp/wrap around flap
Groin flap

Free kite flap
Free 1st web flap
from metatarsus
Snuff box flap
Thenar

Free fascial flap
TPF flap
Lateral arm fascia
Distal pedicle,
Radial forearm fascia flap
Reverse DMCA flap

Dorsal metacarpal flaps

Groin flaps

Microvascular fascial flaps
TPF flap

Lateral arm fascia flap
Radial forearm fascia flap

Venous free flaps
(less reliable)

Secondary nail complex
reconstruction, if desired
by the patient

Secondary pulp reconstruction
if required / desired with:
  Littler flap
  Hetero-digital island flap
  Free pulp / wrap around flap

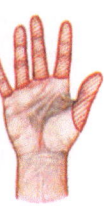

Multi-Digital Injuries

Assessment of the injury
Fracture classification

Which digits should be preserved?
Which position do they occupy?
Salvage of digit worthwhile?

Yes   No

Reconstruction   ◄────────────   Amputation –
                                 Consider tissue banking!

                                 Spare parts that can be
Compound flaps   used for reconstruction of
including functional   other digits:
tissues

Temporo-parietal fascia flap   Skin grafts
Radial forearm flap   Arterial grafts
Lateral arm flap   Nerve grafts
Posterior interosseous flap   Tendon grafts
Serratus fascia flap   Bone grafts
                                 Vascularized joints

Structure repair   Depending on   **Personal profile**
and flap coverage   ────────────────────►   **of the patient!**

                                                    Age, occupation,
                                                    personalitiy, motivation

Volar   Dorsal

Step by step single digital repair   Posterior interosseous flap
Multiple cross-finger flaps   Radial forearm flap
Hetero-digital island flaps   Dorsal-metacarpal flaps
Free fascial flaps and skin grafts   Free fascial flap and skin grafts
                                       Temporal fascia
                                       Serratus fascia

                                     Distant flaps:
                                     Groin flap
                                     Cross-arm flap

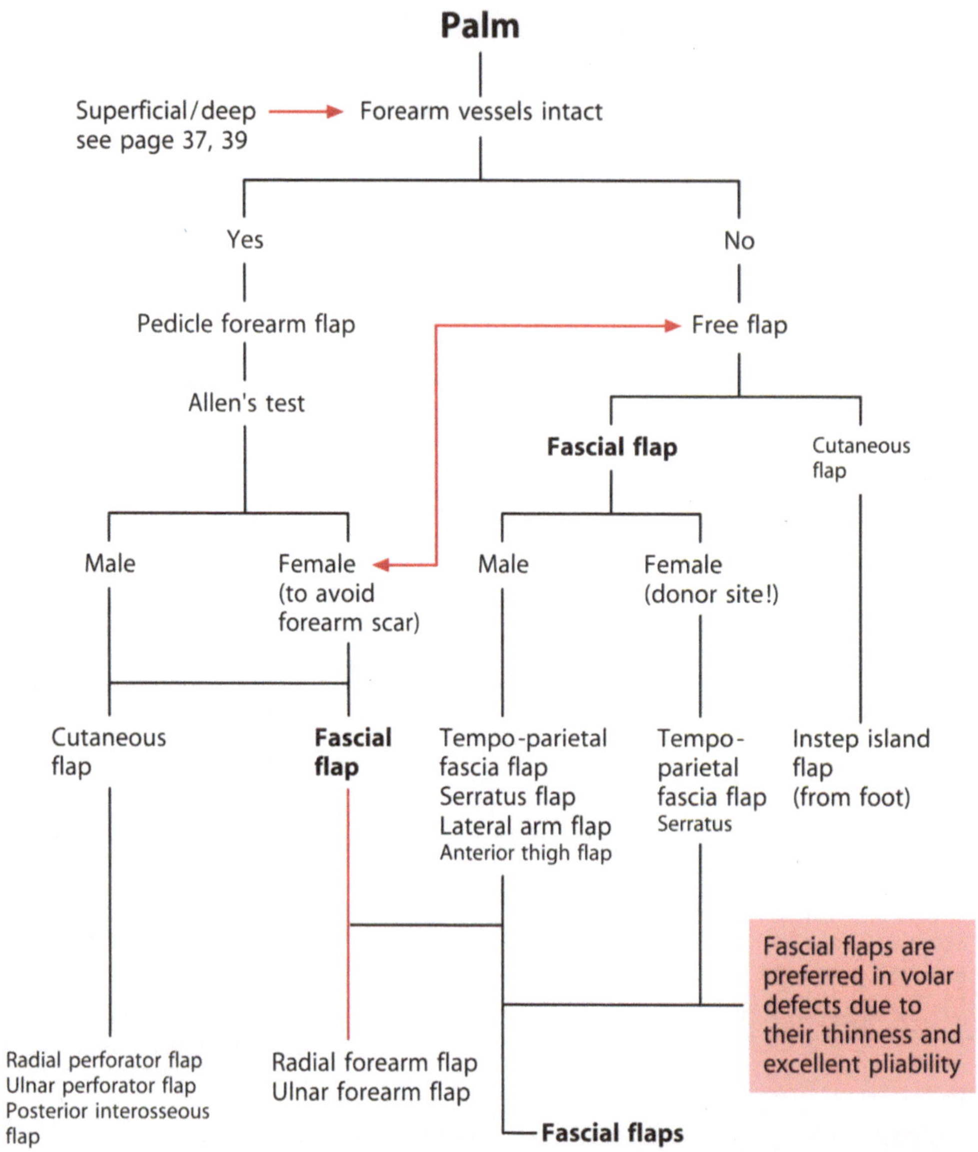

Palm

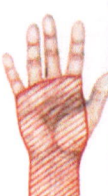

Superficial/deep ———▶ Forearm vessels intact
see page 37, 39

Yes   No

Pedicle forearm flap ————————————————▶ Free flap

Allen's test   **Fascial flap**   Cutaneous
                                                                  flap

Male   Female   Male   Female   Instep island
              (to avoid   (donor site!) flap
              forearm scar)   (from foot)

Cutaneous   **Fascial**   Tempo-parietal   Tempo-
flap   **flap**   fascia flap   parietal
                              Serratus flap   fascia flap
                              Lateral arm flap Serratus
                              Anterior thigh flap

Radial perforator flap   Radial forearm flap
Ulnar perforator flap   Ulnar forearm flap
Posterior interosseous
flap   **Fascial flaps**

Fascial flaps are
preferred in volar
defects due to
their thinness and
excellent pliability

Partial flap necrosis has been reported in all types of pedicle fascial
flaps so that delayed skin grafting should be considered if there are
signs of questionable flap viability!
Increased capillary bleeding may also been seen in fascial flaps. In
these cases secondary grafting is also recommended!

Tip: Harvest skin graft at primary operation
Storage in refrigerator
Leave catheter in brachial plexus for analgesia
Skin grafting after 2-3 days as "dressing room" procedure

Dorsal Hand Defects

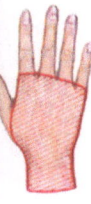

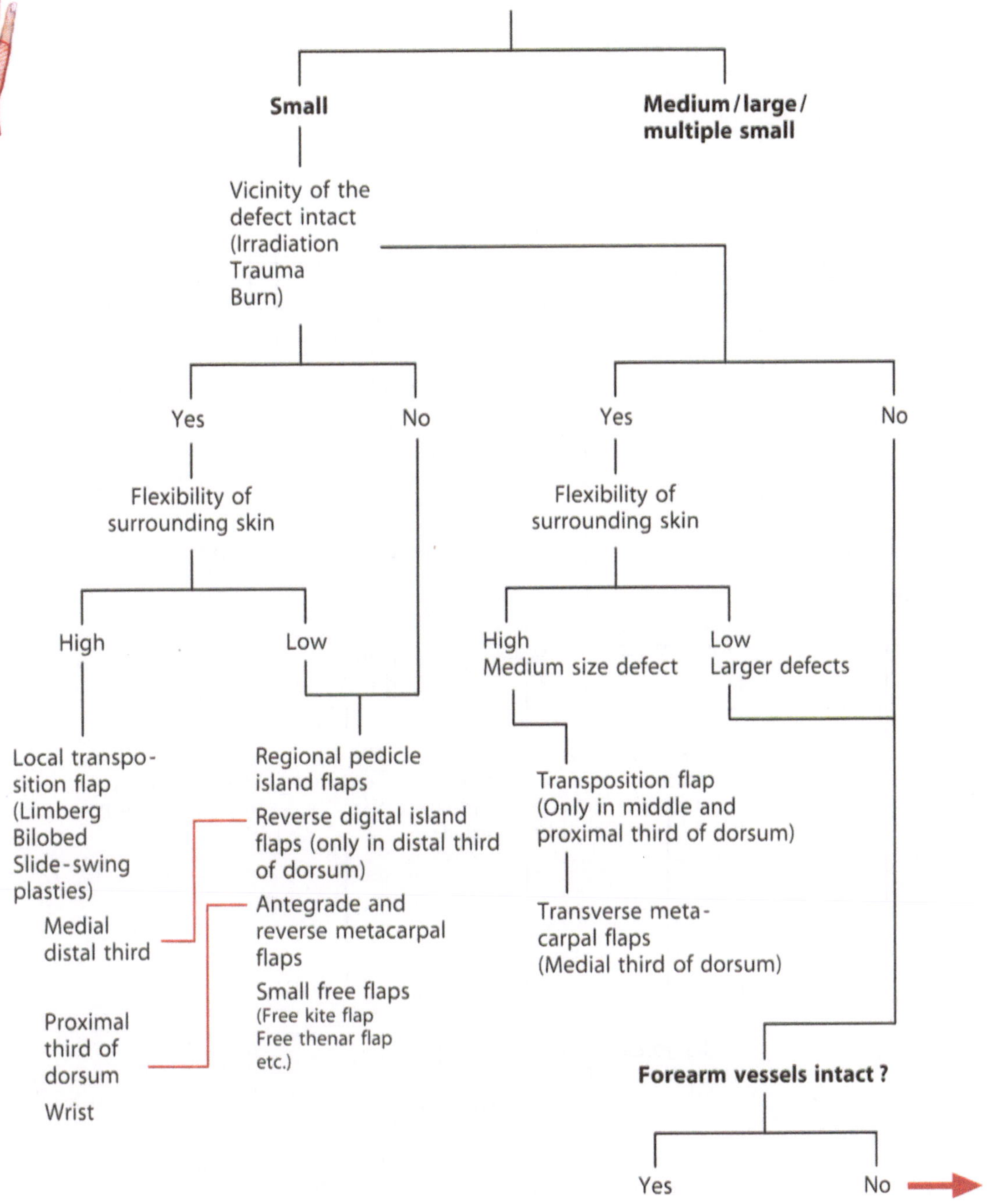

Small   **Medium/large/ multiple small**

Vicinity of the defect intact (Irradiation Trauma Burn)

Yes   **No**   **Yes**   **No**

Flexibility of surrounding skin   Flexibility of surrounding skin

High   **Low**   **High**   **Low**
                                            Medium size defect   Larger defects

Local transposition flap (Limberg Bilobed Slide-swing plasties)

Medial distal third

Proximal third of dorsum

Wrist

Regional pedicle island flaps

Reverse digital island flaps (only in distal third of dorsum)

Antegrade and reverse metacarpal flaps

Small free flaps (Free kite flap Free thenar flap etc.)

Transposition flap (Only in middle and proximal third of dorsum)

Transverse metacarpal flaps (Medial third of dorsum)

Forearm vessels intact?

Yes   **No** →

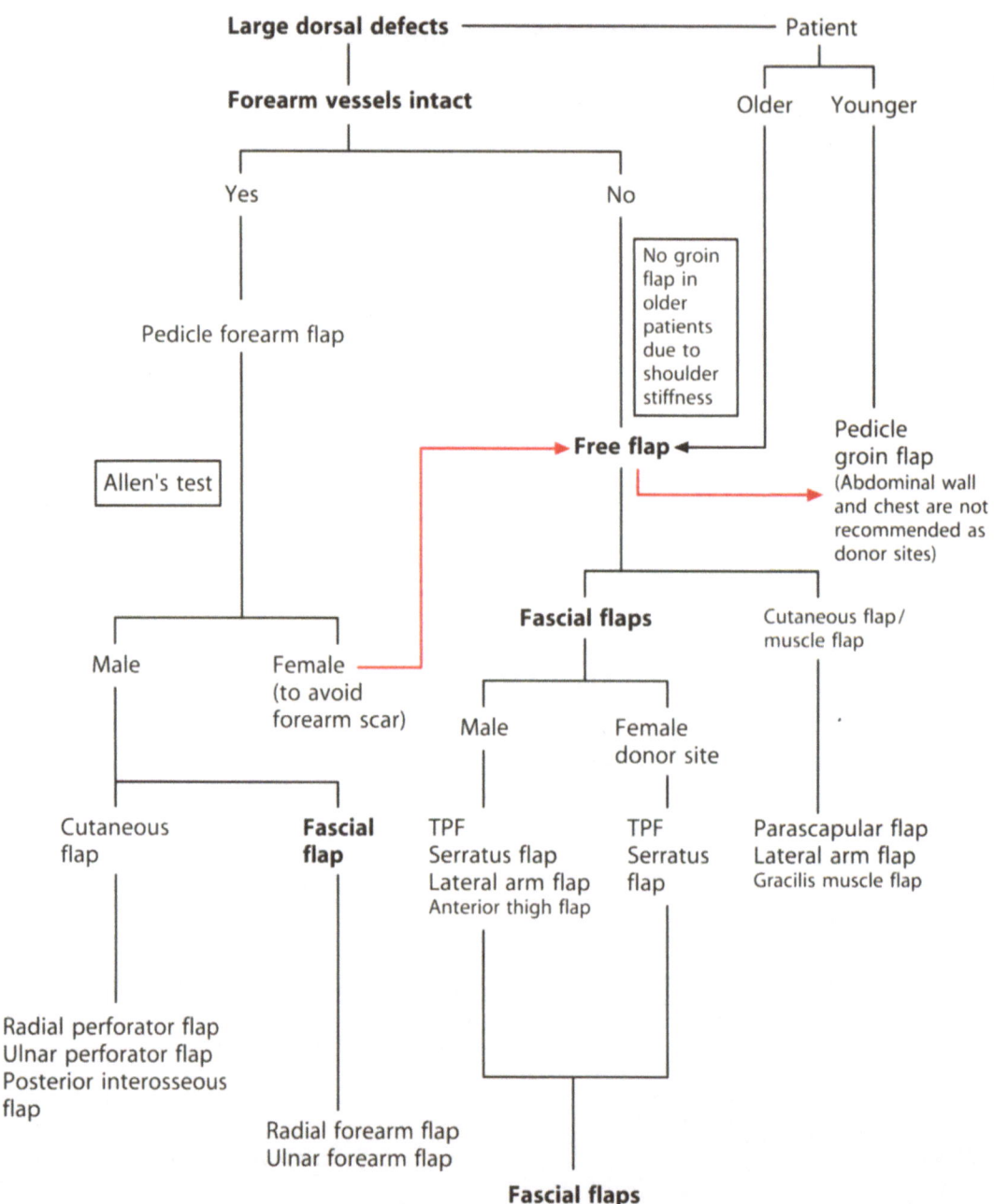

Large dorsal defects ———————————— Patient

Forearm vessels intact   Older   Younger

Yes   No

Pedicle forearm flap

┌─────────────────────────────┐
│ No groin flap in older patients due to shoulder stiffness │
└─────────────────────────────┘

Pedicle groin flap
(Abdominal wall and chest are not recommended as donor sites)

Free flap

┌─────────────┐
│ Allen's test │
└─────────────┘

Male   Female (to avoid forearm scar)

Fascial flaps   Cutaneous flap/ muscle flap

Male   Female donor site

Cutaneous flap   **Fascial flap**

TPF
Serratus flap
Lateral arm flap
Anterior thigh flap

TPF
Serratus flap

Parascapular flap
Lateral arm flap
Gracilis muscle flap

Radial perforator flap
Ulnar perforator flap
Posterior interosseous flap

Radial forearm flap
Ulnar forearm flap

Fascial flaps

Partial flap necrosis has been reported in all types of pedicle fascial flaps so that delayed skin grafting should be considered if there are signs of questionable flap viability!
Increased capillary bleeding may also been seen in fascial flaps. In these cases secondary grafting is also recommended!

Tip: Harvest skin graft at primary operation
Storage in refrigerator
Leave catheter in brachial plexus
Skin grafting after 2-3 days as "dressing room" procedure

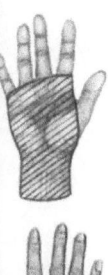

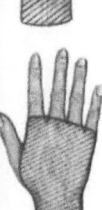

Complex Volar and Dorsal Defects

|

Reconstruction

|

Nerves   Tendons   Vessels

Single structure repair
and simultaneous
flap coverage

or

Multicomponent
"chimeric" flaps

|

Vascularized neuro-   Tendocutaneous flaps   Flow-through flap
cutaneous flap   Musculotendinous flaps

Choice of flaps depends on
vascular condition of the
forearm and the profile
of the patient

|

Forearm vessels intact?

(see page 145, 147)

Forearm – Distal Third and Wrist

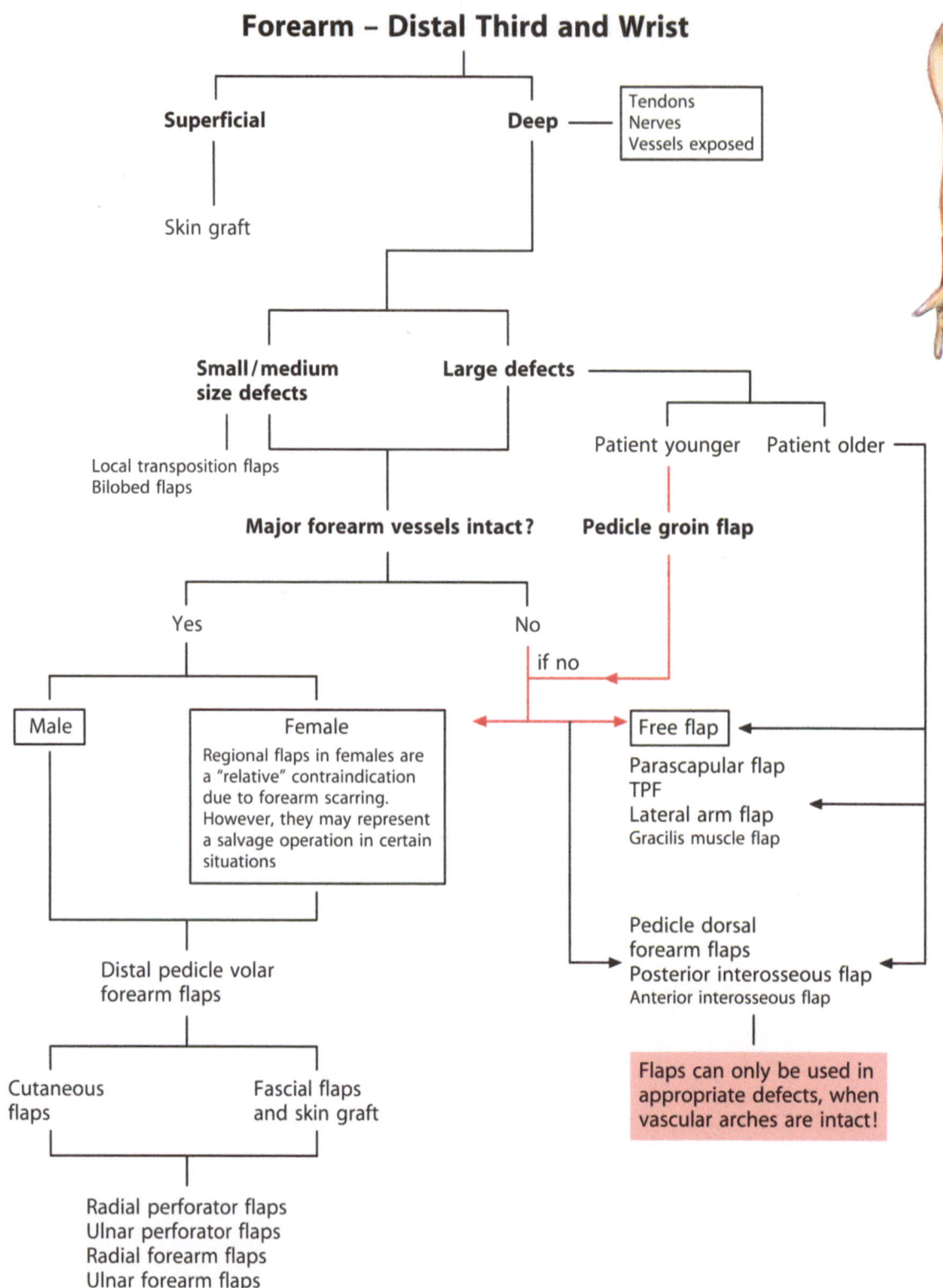

Superficial   **Deep** ——— | Tendons |
                                              | Nerves |
                                              | Vessels exposed |

Skin graft

Small/medium size defects   **Large defects** ———

                                                          Patient younger   Patient older ———

Local transposition flaps
Bilobed flaps

Major forearm vessels intact?   **Pedicle groin flap**

Yes   No

                                     if no

| Male | Female

                Regional flaps in females are
                a "relative" contraindication
                due to forearm scarring.
                However, they may represent
                a salvage operation in certain
                situations

                                     | Free flap |

                                     Parascapular flap
                                     TPF
                                     Lateral arm flap
                                     Gracilis muscle flap

Distal pedicle volar
forearm flaps

                                     Pedicle dorsal
                                     forearm flaps
                                     Posterior interosseous flap
                                     Anterior interosseous flap

Cutaneous   Fascial flaps
flaps   and skin graft

                                     Flaps can only be used in
                                     appropriate defects, when
                                     vascular arches are intact!

Radial perforator flaps
Ulnar perforator flaps
Radial forearm flaps
Ulnar forearm flaps

Forearm – Middle Third

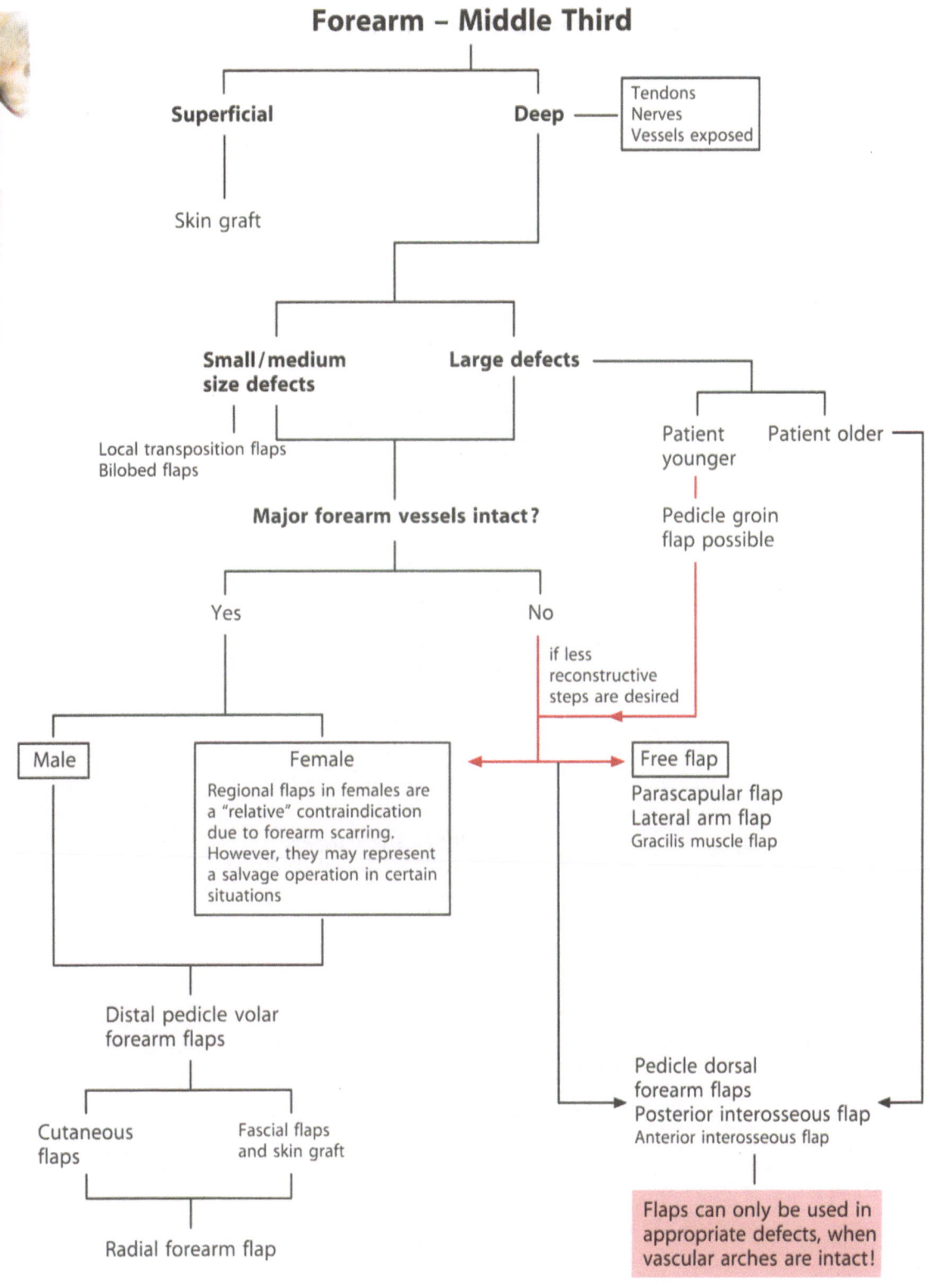

Superficial

Deep —— Tendons
Nerves
Vessels exposed

Skin graft

Small/medium size defects

Large defects

Local transposition flaps
Bilobed flaps

Patient younger   Patient older

Pedicle groin
flap possible

Major forearm vessels intact?

Yes

No

if less
reconstructive
steps are desired

Male

Female

Regional flaps in females are
a "relative" contraindication
due to forearm scarring.
However, they may represent
a salvage operation in certain
situations

Free flap

Parascapular flap
Lateral arm flap
Gracilis muscle flap

Distal pedicle volar
forearm flaps

Cutaneous
flaps

Fascial flaps
and skin graft

Pedicle dorsal
forearm flaps
Posterior interosseous flap
Anterior interosseous flap

Radial forearm flap

Flaps can only be used in
appropriate defects, when
vascular arches are intact!

Complex Forearm Defects

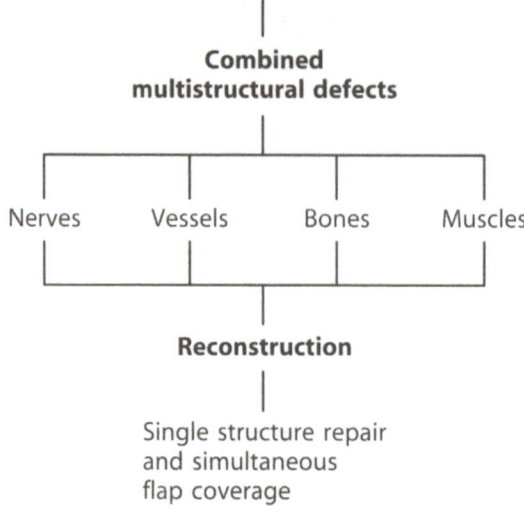

Combined multistructural defects

| Nerves | Vessels | Bones | Muscles |

Reconstruction

Single structure repair
and simultaneous
flap coverage

or

Multicomponent
"chimeric" flaps

Free flap

Vascularized neuro-
cutaneous flap

Flow-through flap

Osteocutaneous flaps

Fibula flap
Parascapula flap
Iliac crest flap

Vascularized tendon transfer

Free muscle transfer
(m. gracilis
m. latissimus dorsi)

Pedicle flap

Osteocutaneous posterior
interosseous flap

Osteocutaneous radial
forearm flap

Use of these
flaps depends
on volar versus
dorsal injury zones

Distal pedicle osteo-
cutaneous lateral arm flap

Tendocutaneous lateral
arm flap

Decision criteria
(see pp. 143-148)

Ventral Elbow and Proximal Forearm

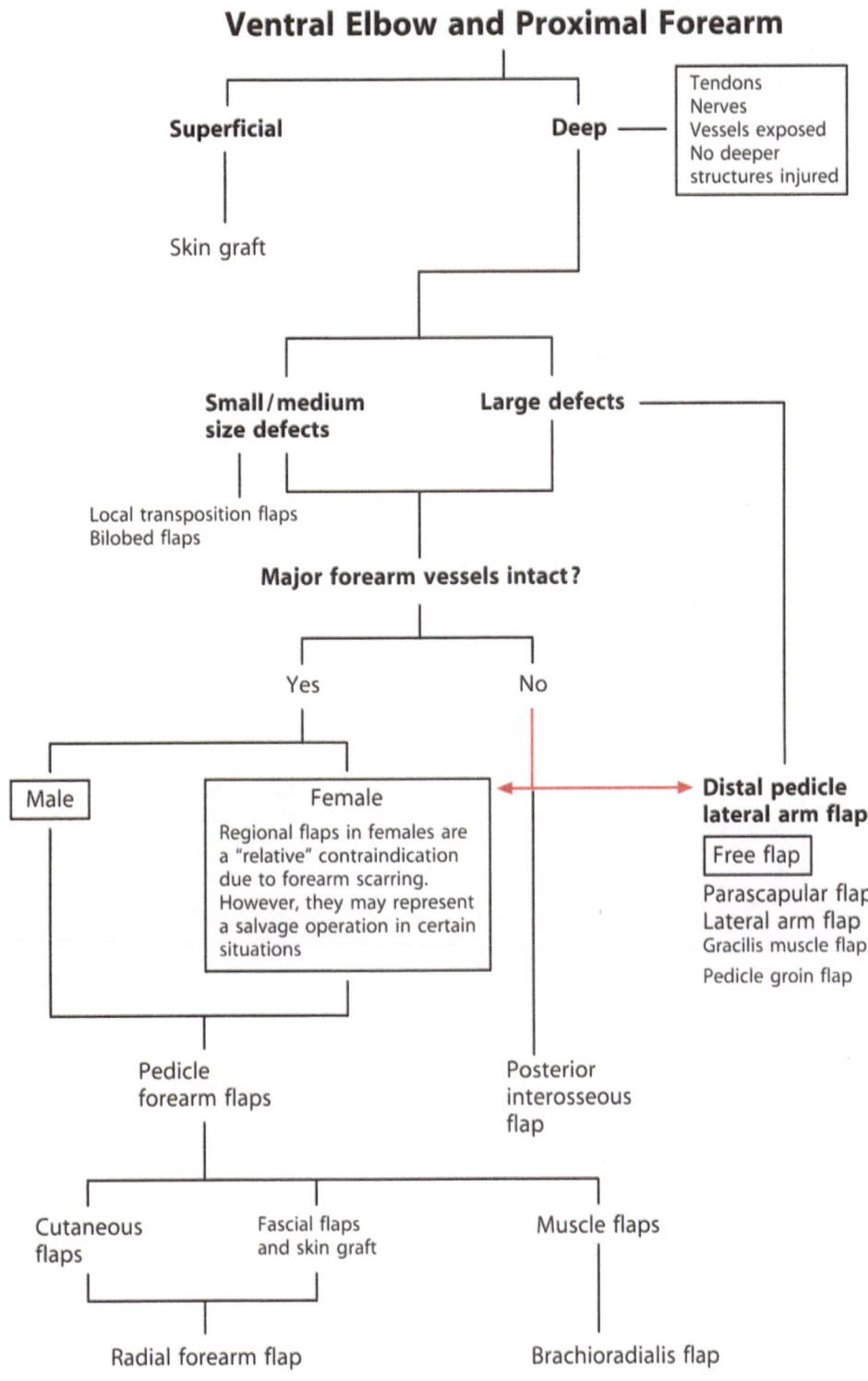

```
                                    ┌──────────────────┐
                                    │ Tendons          │
                                    │ Nerves           │
        Superficial        Deep ────│ Vessels exposed  │
                                    │ No deeper        │
                                    │ structures injured│
                                    └──────────────────┘
            │
        Skin graft
```

Superficial — Skin graft

Deep

Tendons
Nerves
Vessels exposed
No deeper
structures injured

Small/medium size defects

Local transposition flaps
Bilobed flaps

Large defects

Major forearm vessels intact?

Yes   No

Male

Female

Regional flaps in females are
a "relative" contraindication
due to forearm scarring.
However, they may represent
a salvage operation in certain
situations

Distal pedicle lateral arm flap

Free flap

Parascapular flap
Lateral arm flap
Gracilis muscle flap

Pedicle groin flap

Pedicle forearm flaps

Posterior interosseous flap

Cutaneous flaps

Fascial flaps and skin graft

Muscle flaps

Radial forearm flap

Brachioradialis flap

Elbow and Proximal Forearm

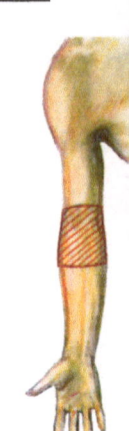

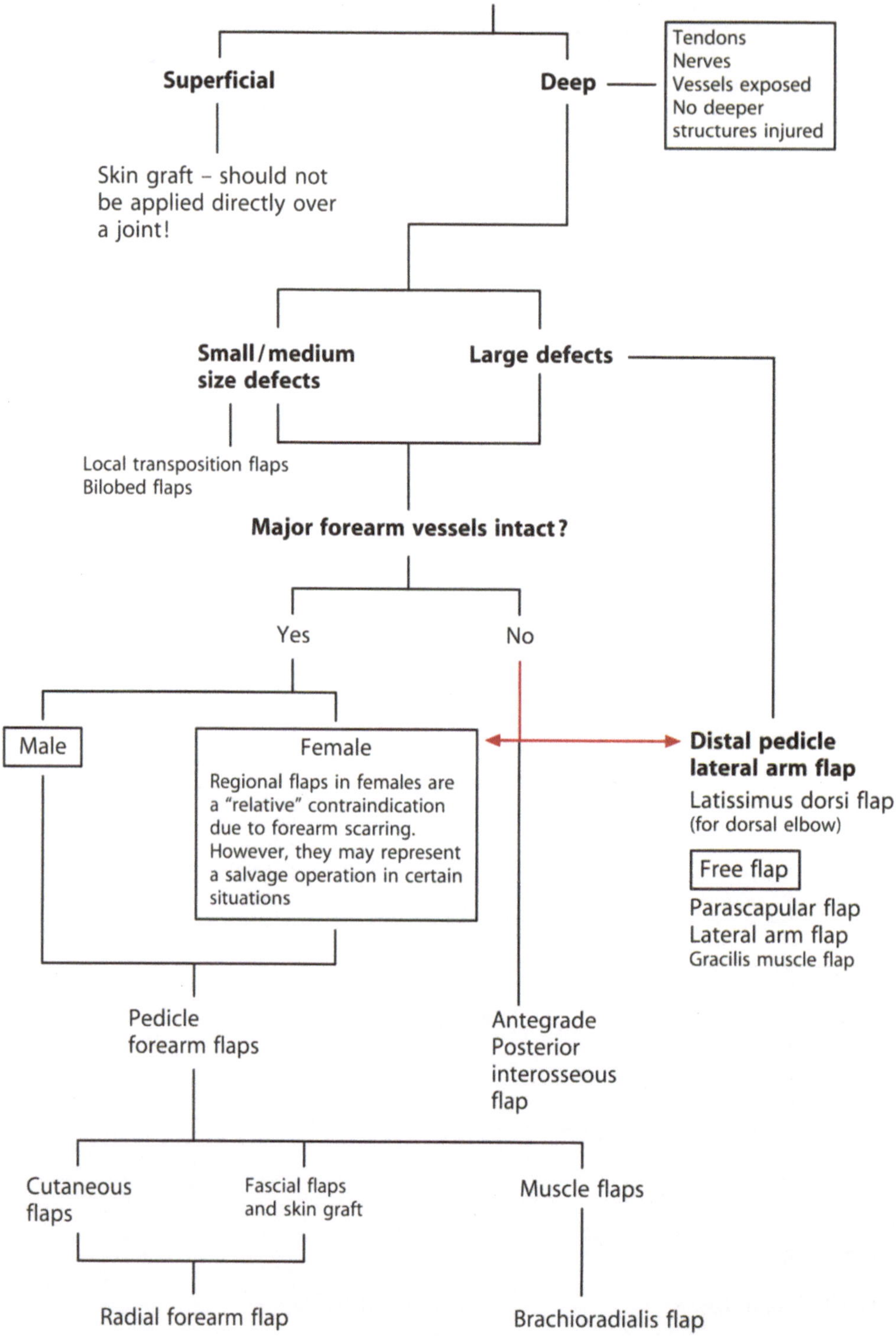

Superficial

Deep ——

> Tendons
> Nerves
> Vessels exposed
> No deeper
> structures injured

Skin graft – should not
be applied directly over
a joint!

**Small/medium
size defects**

Large defects ——

Local transposition flaps
Bilobed flaps

Major forearm vessels intact?

Yes

No

Male

Female

Regional flaps in females are
a "relative" contraindication
due to forearm scarring.
However, they may represent
a salvage operation in certain
situations

**Distal pedicle
lateral arm flap**

Latissimus dorsi flap
(for dorsal elbow)

Free flap

Parascapular flap
Lateral arm flap
Gracilis muscle flap

Pedicle
forearm flaps

Antegrade
Posterior
interosseous
flap

Cutaneous
flaps

Fascial flaps
and skin graft

Muscle flaps

Radial forearm flap

Brachioradialis flap

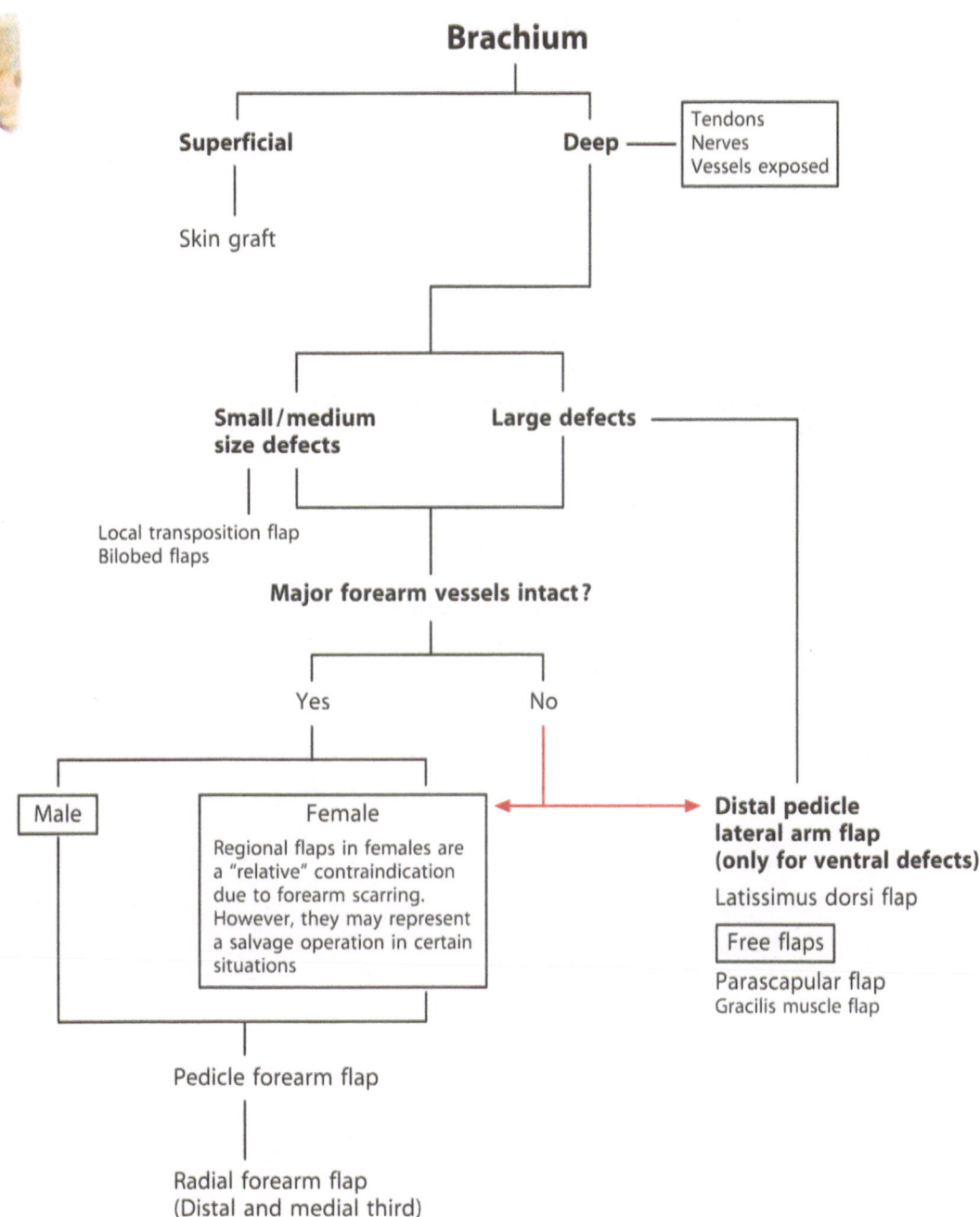

Brachium

Superficial

Skin graft

Deep —— Tendons
Nerves
Vessels exposed

**Small/medium
size defects**

Local transposition flap
Bilobed flaps

Large defects

Major forearm vessels intact?

Yes   No

Male

Female

Regional flaps in females are
a "relative" contraindication
due to forearm scarring.
However, they may represent
a salvage operation in certain
situations

Pedicle forearm flap

Radial forearm flap
(Distal and medial third)

**Distal pedicle
lateral arm flap
(only for ventral defects)**

Latissimus dorsi flap

Free flaps

Parascapular flap
Gracilis muscle flap

Shoulder and Proximal Brachium

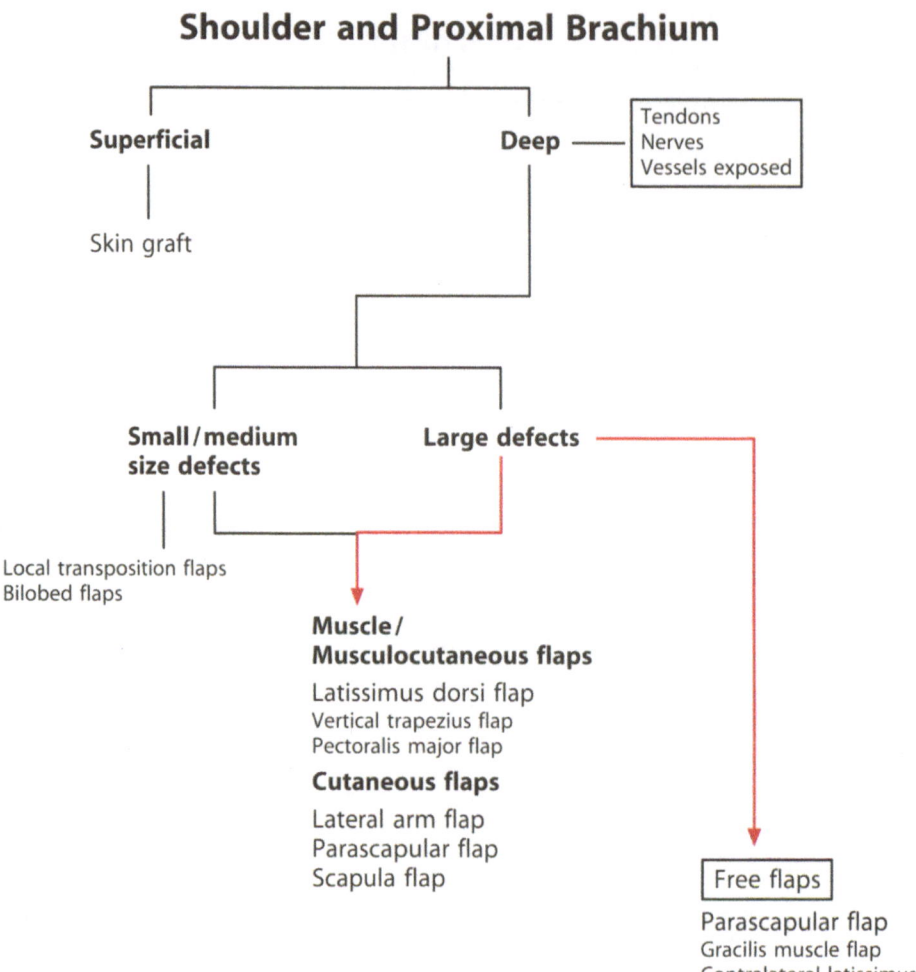
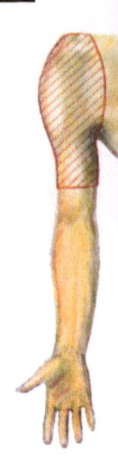

Superficial

Deep ——— Tendons
Nerves
Vessels exposed

Skin graft

**Small/medium
size defects**

Large defects

Local transposition flaps
Bilobed flaps

**Muscle/
Musculocutaneous flaps**

Latissimus dorsi flap
Vertical trapezius flap
Pectoralis major flap

Cutaneous flaps

Lateral arm flap
Parascapular flap
Scapula flap

Free flaps

Parascapular flap
Gracilis muscle flap
Contralateral latissimus
dorsi flap

Complex Defects of the Upper Arm

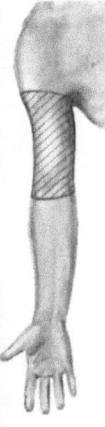

**Combined
multistructural defects**

| Nerves | Vessels | Bones | Muscles |

Reconstruction

Single structure repair
and simultaneous
flap coverage

or

Multicomponent
"chimeric" flaps

Free flap

Vascularized neuro-
cutaneous flap

Flow-through flap

Osteocutaneous flaps

Fibula flap
Parascapula flap
Iliac crest flap

Free muscle transfer
(m. gracilis
m. latissimus dorsi)

Tendon transfer

Pedicle flap

Multicomponent subscapular flaps:
  Latissimus dorsi
  Serratus
  Scapula bone
  Parascapular skin flaps
  etc.

Distal pedicle osteo-
cutaneous lateral arm flap
Tendocutaneous lateral
arm flap
Osteocutaneous radial
forearm flap
Vertical trapezius flap

CHAPTER IV
Clinical Examples
The Use of the Algorithms

Gunshot Wound

Case history:
23-year-old male: gunshot wound to hand

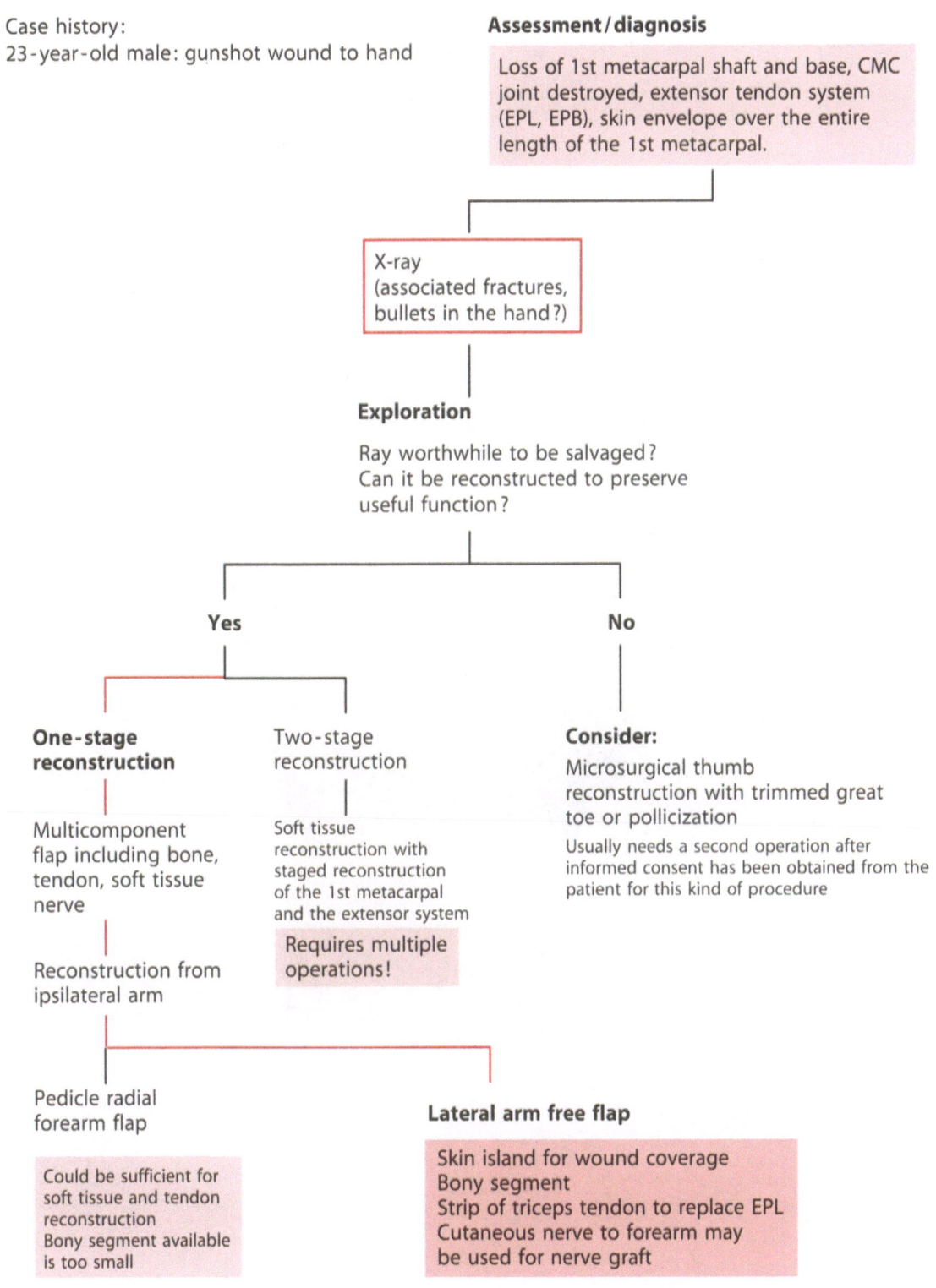

Assessment/diagnosis

Loss of 1st metacarpal shaft and base, CMC joint destroyed, extensor tendon system (EPL, EPB), skin envelope over the entire length of the 1st metacarpal.

X-ray
(associated fractures, bullets in the hand?)

Exploration

Ray worthwhile to be salvaged?
Can it be reconstructed to preserve useful function?

Yes   **No**

One-stage reconstruction   Two-stage reconstruction   **Consider:**

Multicomponent flap including bone, tendon, soft tissue nerve

Soft tissue reconstruction with staged reconstruction of the 1st metacarpal and the extensor system

Microsurgical thumb reconstruction with trimmed great toe or pollicization

Usually needs a second operation after informed consent has been obtained from the patient for this kind of procedure

Requires multiple operations!

Reconstruction from ipsilateral arm

Pedicle radial forearm flap

Lateral arm free flap

Could be sufficient for soft tissue and tendon reconstruction
Bony segment available is too small

Skin island for wound coverage
Bony segment
Strip of triceps tendon to replace EPL
Cutaneous nerve to forearm may be used for nerve graft

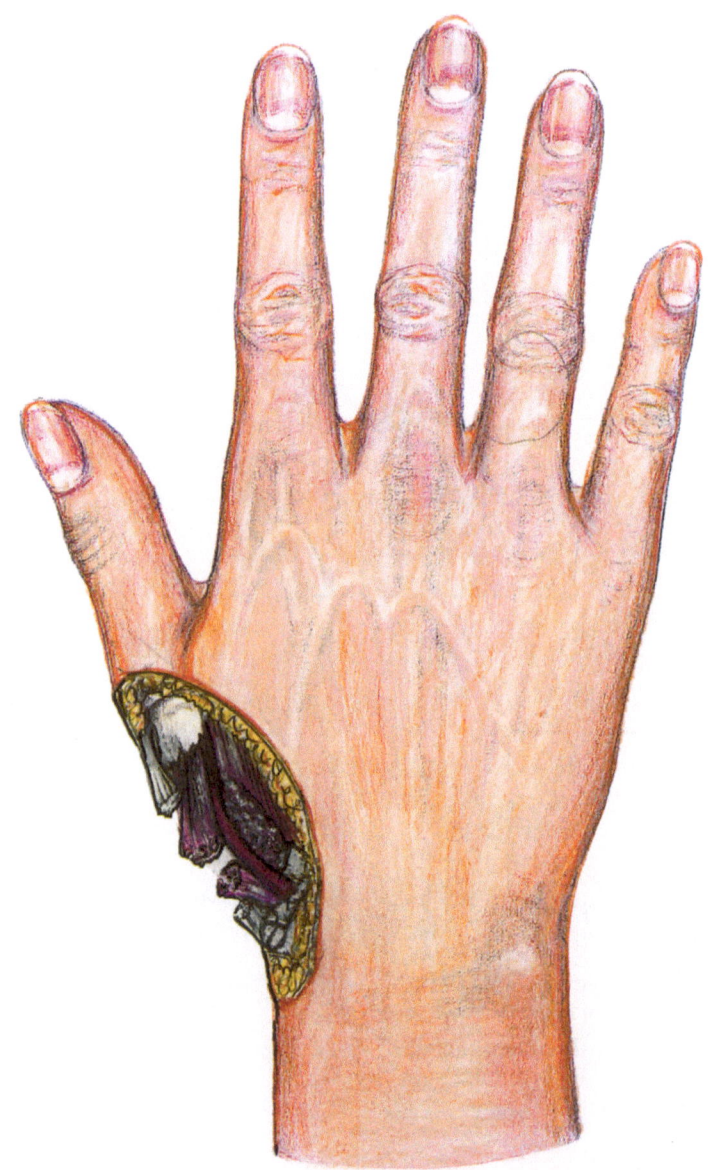

Friction Burn

Case history: 22-year-old female. 3° friction burn to dorsum of hand
              5% TBSA
              Left leg and thigh with 2° burns; spontaneous healing

Assessment/diagnosis

2° burn on left thigh and lower leg (will spontaneously heal)
3° burn to the hand
Index finger: MP, PIP joints exposed; paratenon preserved.
Ring finger: extensor hood exposed at MP joint, articular capsule
exposed at PIP joint
Long finger: extensor hood exposed at MP joint; PIP joint exposed
with paratenon preserved

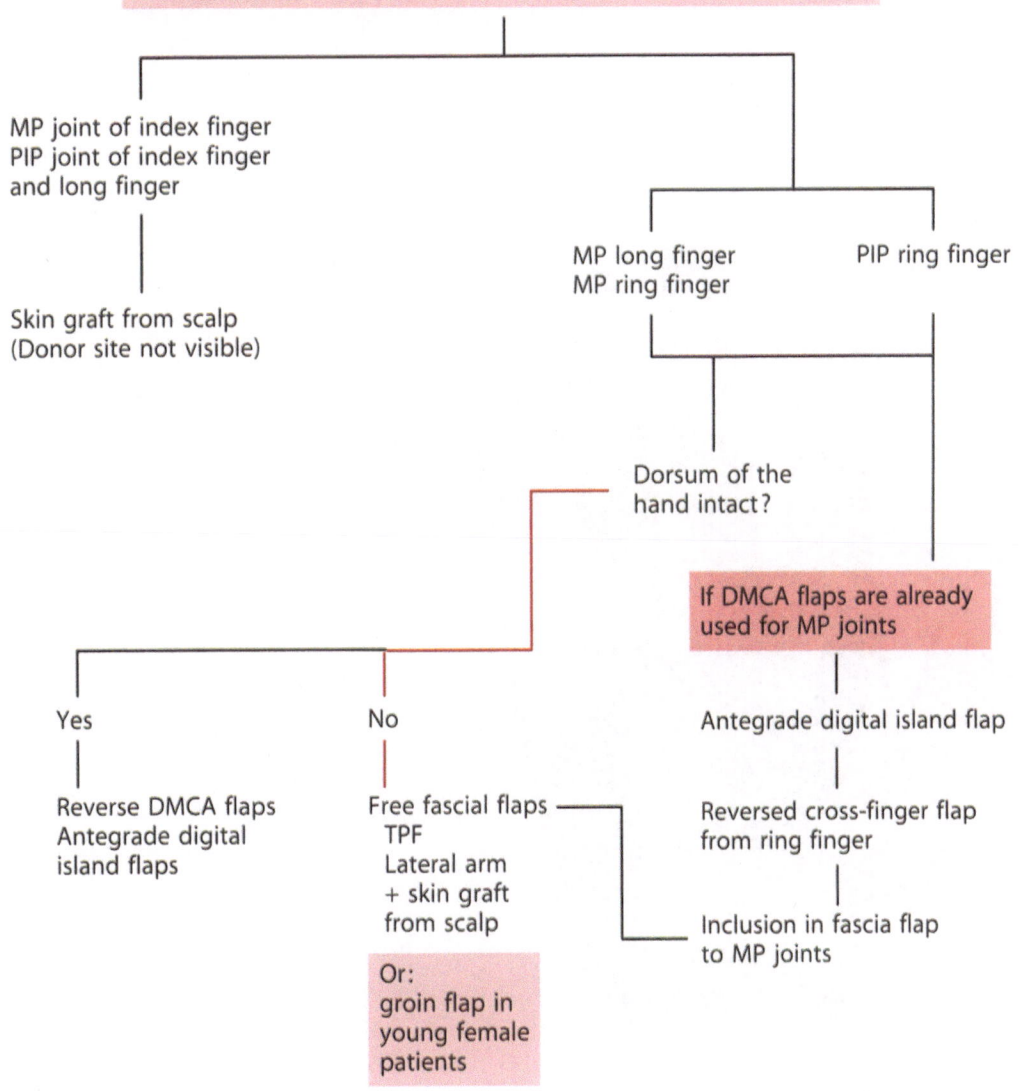

MP joint of index finger
PIP joint of index finger
and long finger

Skin graft from scalp
(Donor site not visible)

MP long finger
MP ring finger

PIP ring finger

Dorsum of the
hand intact?

If DMCA flaps are already
used for MP joints

Yes

No

Antegrade digital island flap

Reverse DMCA flaps
Antegrade digital
island flaps

Free fascial flaps
TPF
Lateral arm
+ skin graft
from scalp

Reversed cross-finger flap
from ring finger

Inclusion in fascia flap
to MP joints

Or:
groin flap in
young female
patients

At admission

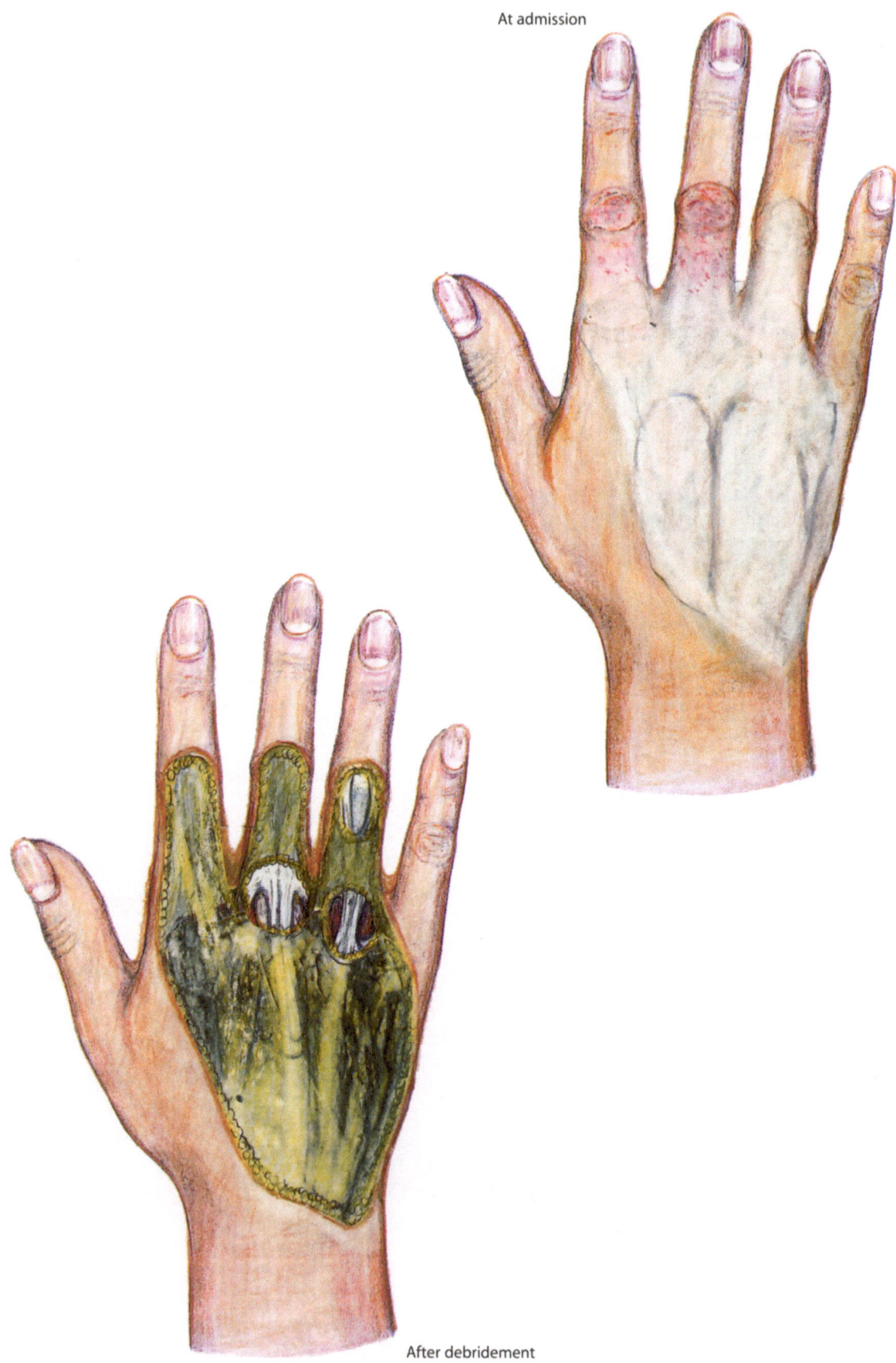

After debridement

Open Carpal Injury

Case history: 42-year-old male patient with open carpal injury sustained
in a MVA (convertible) with overlying soft tissue loss.

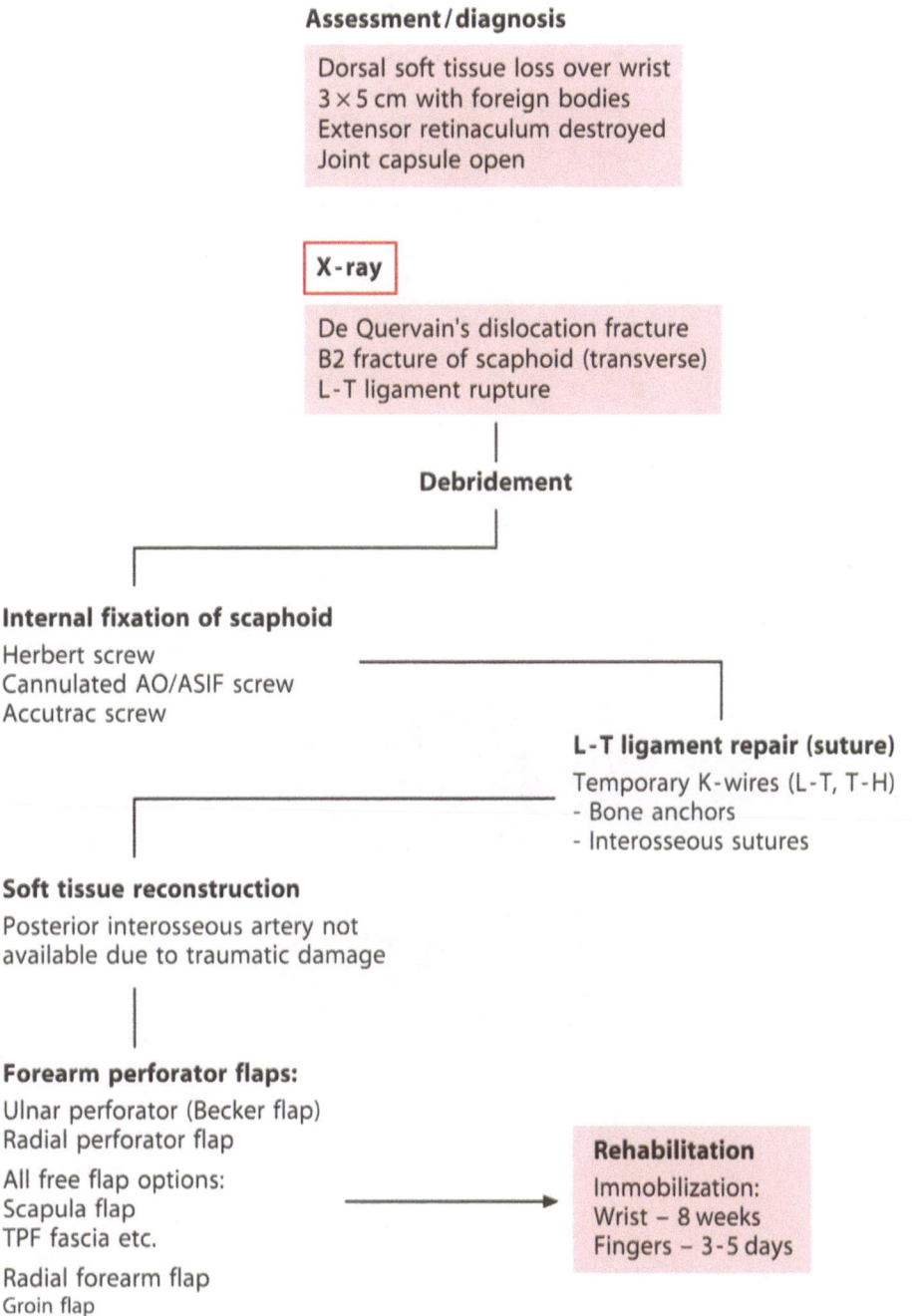

Assessment/diagnosis

Dorsal soft tissue loss over wrist
3 × 5 cm with foreign bodies
Extensor retinaculum destroyed
Joint capsule open

X-ray

De Quervain's dislocation fracture
B2 fracture of scaphoid (transverse)
L-T ligament rupture

Debridement

Internal fixation of scaphoid

Herbert screw
Cannulated AO/ASIF screw
Accutrac screw

L-T ligament repair (suture)

Temporary K-wires (L-T, T-H)
- Bone anchors
- Interosseous sutures

Soft tissue reconstruction

Posterior interosseous artery not
available due to traumatic damage

Forearm perforator flaps:

Ulnar perforator (Becker flap)
Radial perforator flap

All free flap options:
Scapula flap
TPF fascia etc.

Radial forearm flap
Groin flap

Rehabilitation

Immobilization:
Wrist – 8 weeks
Fingers – 3-5 days

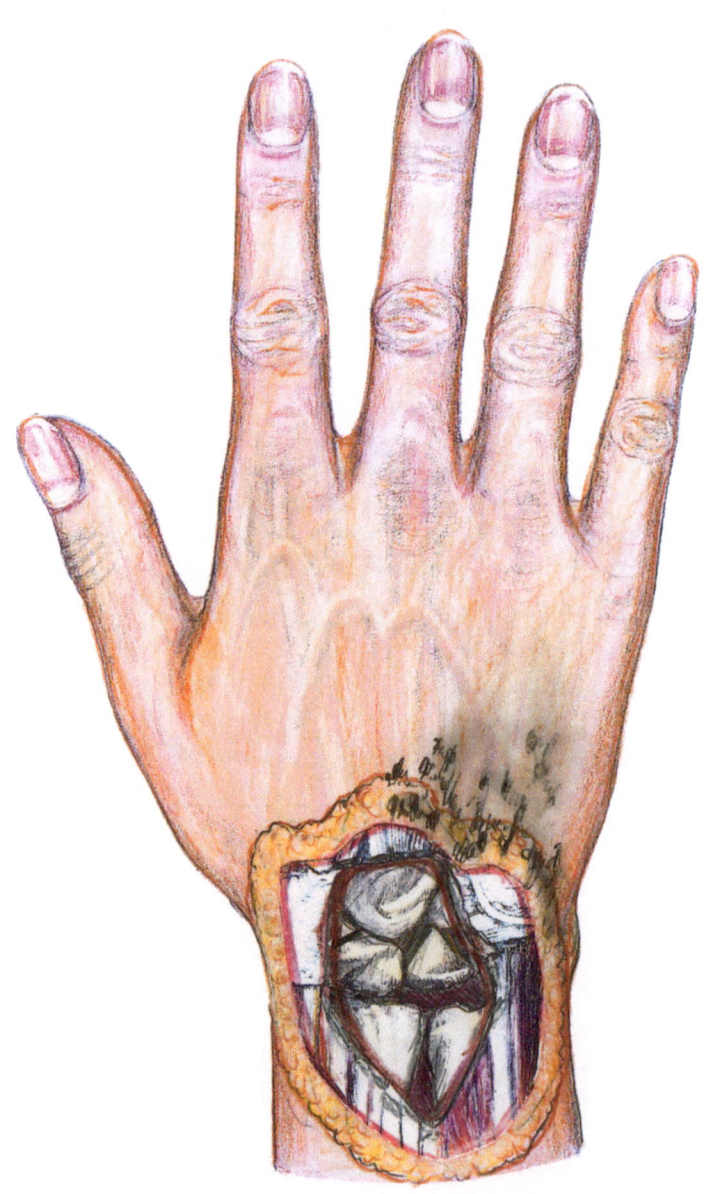

Crush Injury to Long Finger

Case history: 34-year-old male sustained an occupational
crush injury to distal phalanx of long finger

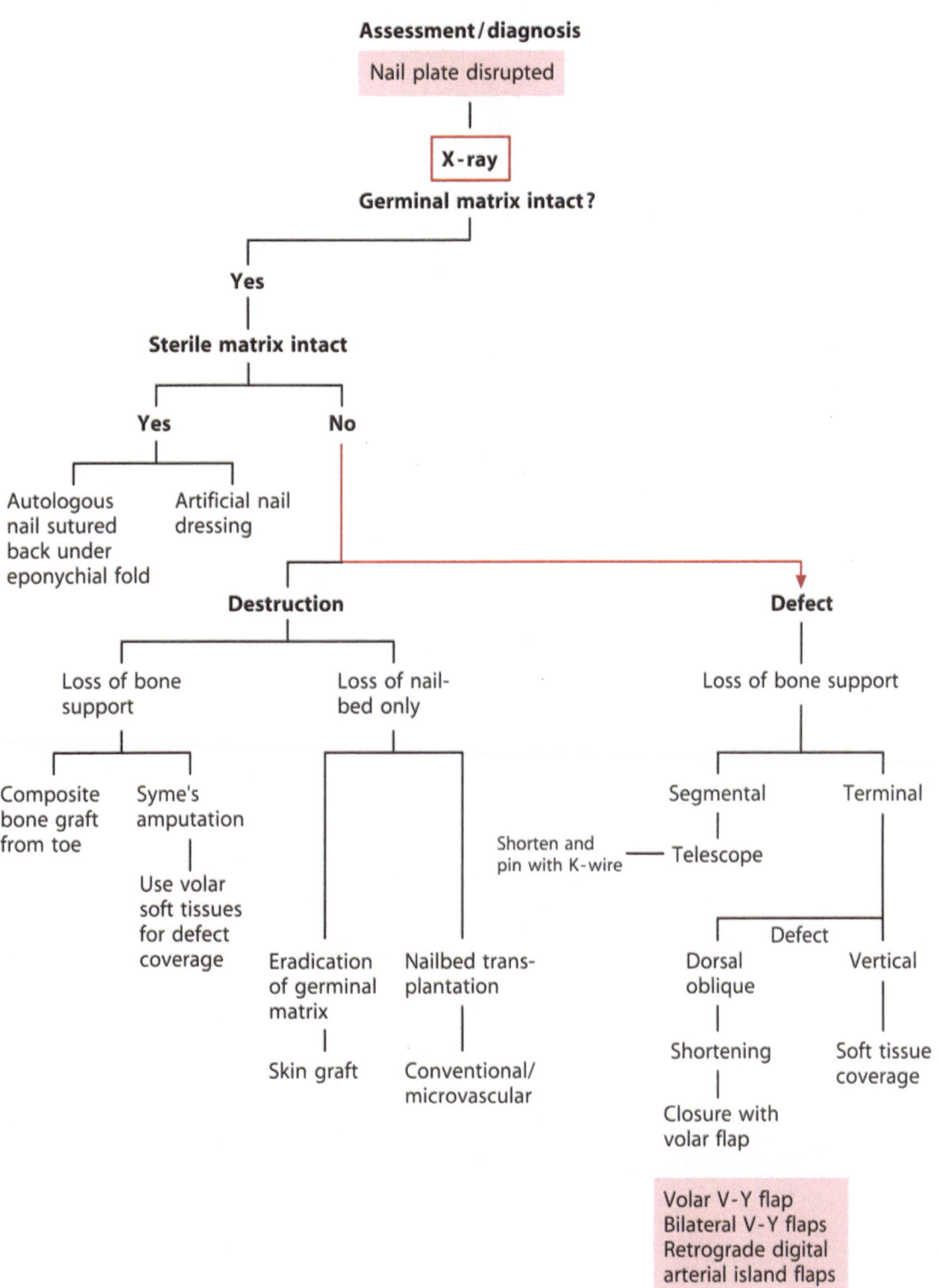

Assessment/diagnosis

Nail plate disrupted

X-ray

Germinal matrix intact?

Yes

Sterile matrix intact

Yes   No

Autologous   Artificial nail
nail sutured   dressing
back under
eponychial fold

Destruction   **Defect**

Loss of bone   Loss of nail-   Loss of bone support
support   bed only

Composite   Syme's   Segmental   Terminal
bone graft   amputation
from toe   Shorten and ── Telescope
             Use volar   pin with K-wire
             soft tissues   Defect
             for defect   Dorsal   Vertical
             coverage   Eradication   Nailbed trans- oblique
                              of germinal   plantation
                              matrix   Shortening   Soft tissue
                                                                                coverage
                              Skin graft   Conventional/   Closure with
                                            microvascular   volar flap

                                                           Volar V-Y flap
                                                           Bilateral V-Y flaps
                                                           Retrograde digital
                                                           arterial island flaps

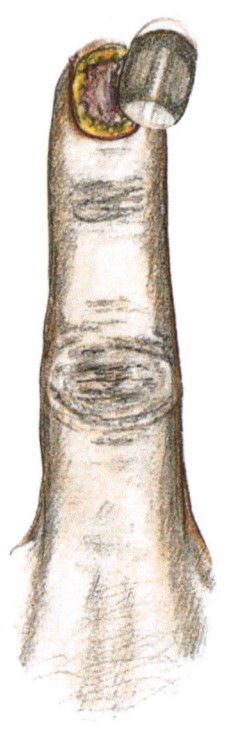

Tangential Cut

Case history: Occupational accident in a meat packing plant.
Tangential cut at dorsal aspect of ring finger

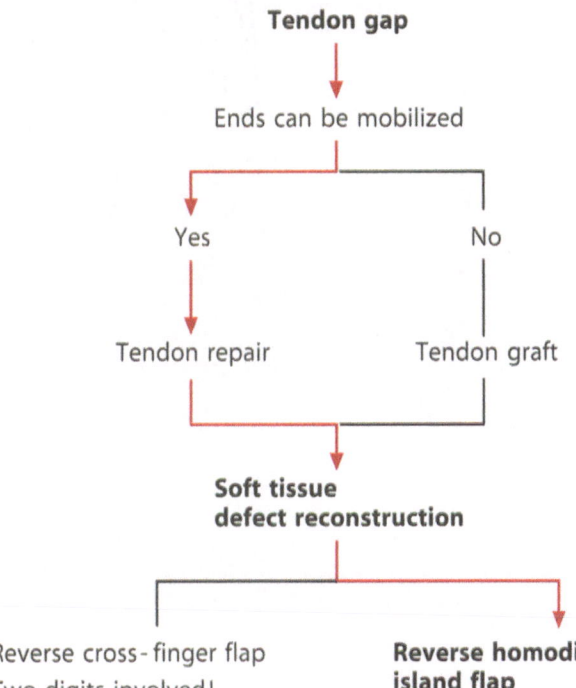

Assessment/diagnosis

Oval defect, tidy wound,
laceration of central slip with
tendon loss of 1.5 cm,
but distal stump that
is suitable for suture

Tendon gap

Ends can be mobilized

Yes   No

Tendon repair   Tendon graft

**Soft tissue
defect reconstruction**

Reverse cross-finger flap   **Reverse homodigital
                                     island flap**
Two digits involved!
This will delay early   Only one digit involved,
motion protocol   early motion protocol is possible

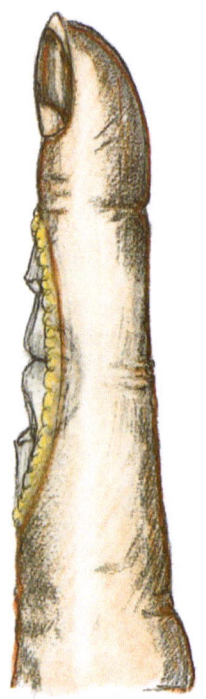
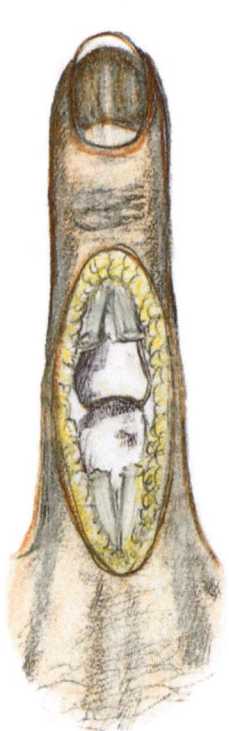

Crush Injury

Case history:
36-year-old female factory worker with
crush injury to thumb

Assessment/diagnosis

Open fracture of the IP joint of the thumb
Medium size soft tissue defect at dorsal
aspect (approx. 2 × 4 cm)

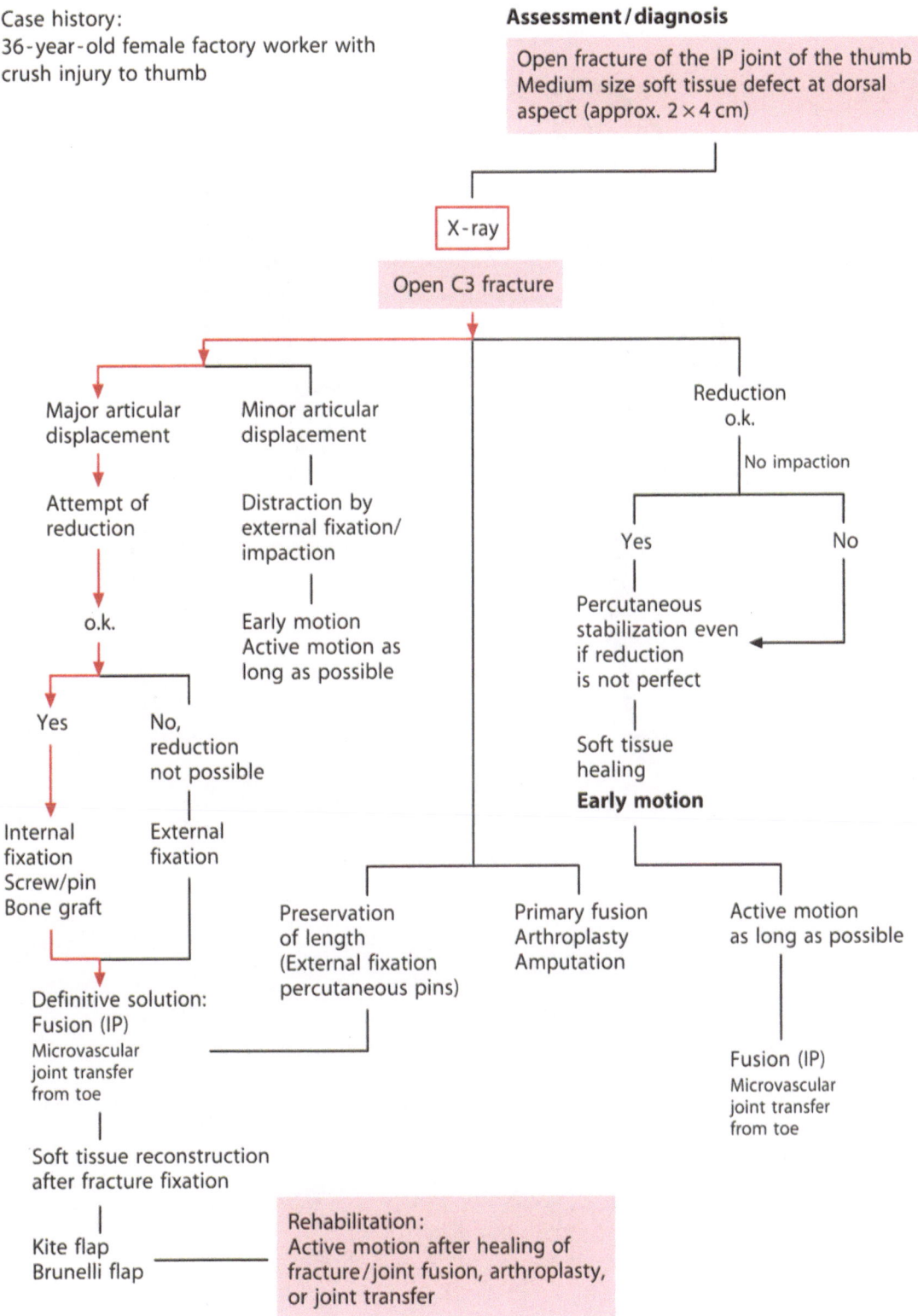

X-ray

Open C3 fracture

Major articular
displacement

Attempt of
reduction

o.k.

Yes   No,
           reduction
           not possible

Internal   External
fixation   fixation
Screw/pin
Bone graft

Definitive solution:
Fusion (IP)
Microvascular
joint transfer
from toe

Soft tissue reconstruction
after fracture fixation

Kite flap
Brunelli flap

Minor articular
displacement

Distraction by
external fixation/
impaction

Early motion
Active motion as
long as possible

Preservation
of length
(External fixation
percutaneous pins)

Primary fusion
Arthroplasty
Amputation

Reduction
o.k.

No impaction

Yes   No

Percutaneous
stabilization even
if reduction
is not perfect

Soft tissue
healing
Early motion

Active motion
as long as possible

Fusion (IP)
Microvascular
joint transfer
from toe

Rehabilitation:
Active motion after healing of
fracture/joint fusion, arthroplasty,
or joint transfer

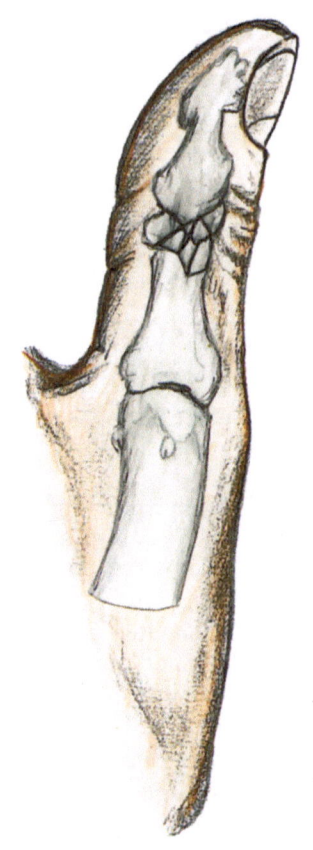
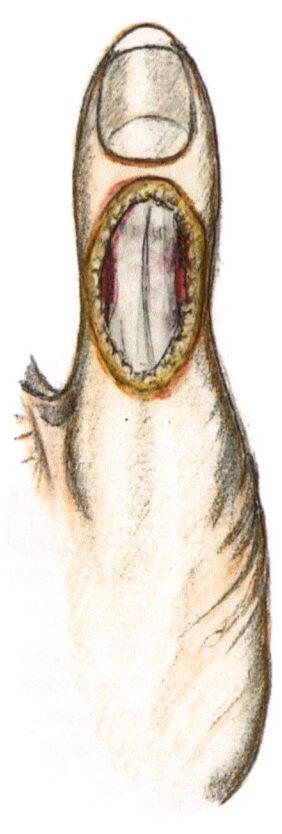

Abrasion Injury

Case history: 18-year-old female with abrasion injury of
dorsum of right hand after fall from motorcycle

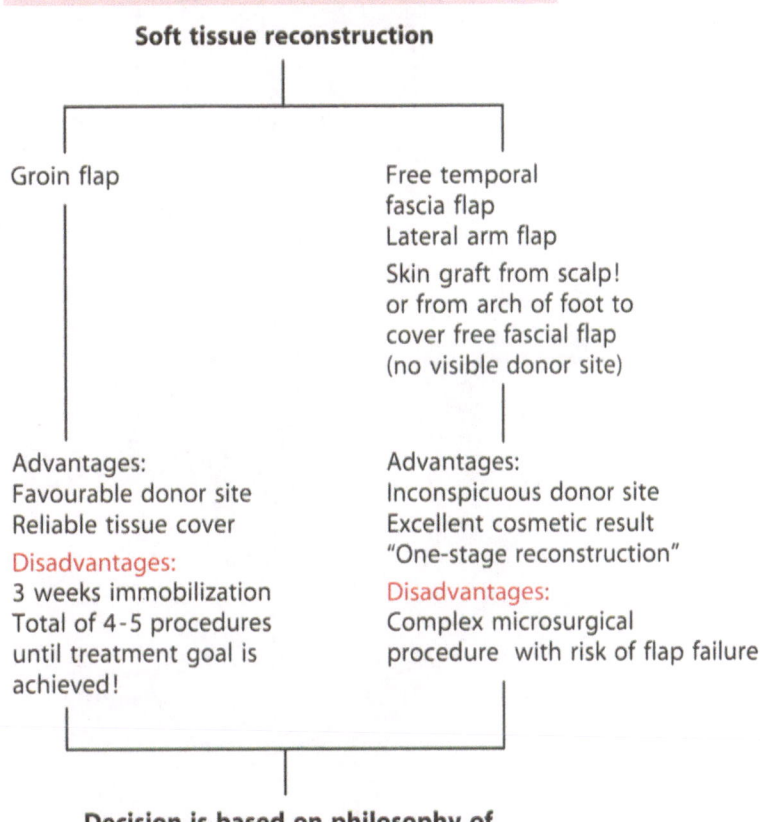

Assessment/diagnosis

Loss of skin and and subcutaneous tissue
Paratenon preserved – thick subcutaneous layer

Soft tissue reconstruction

Groin flap

Free temporal
fascia flap
Lateral arm flap

Skin graft from scalp!
or from arch of foot to
cover free fascial flap
(no visible donor site)

Advantages:
Favourable donor site
Reliable tissue cover
Disadvantages:
3 weeks immobilization
Total of 4-5 procedures
until treatment goal is
achieved!

Advantages:
Inconspicuous donor site
Excellent cosmetic result
"One-stage reconstruction"
Disadvantages:
Complex microsurgical
procedure with risk of flap failure

**Decision is based on philosophy of
the surgeon and the patient's request!**

A one-stage reconstruction should be attempted.
Primary skin graft is not recommended in this
case, since it leaves a contour and color deformity.
It also prolongs rehabilitation time and increases
treatment cost

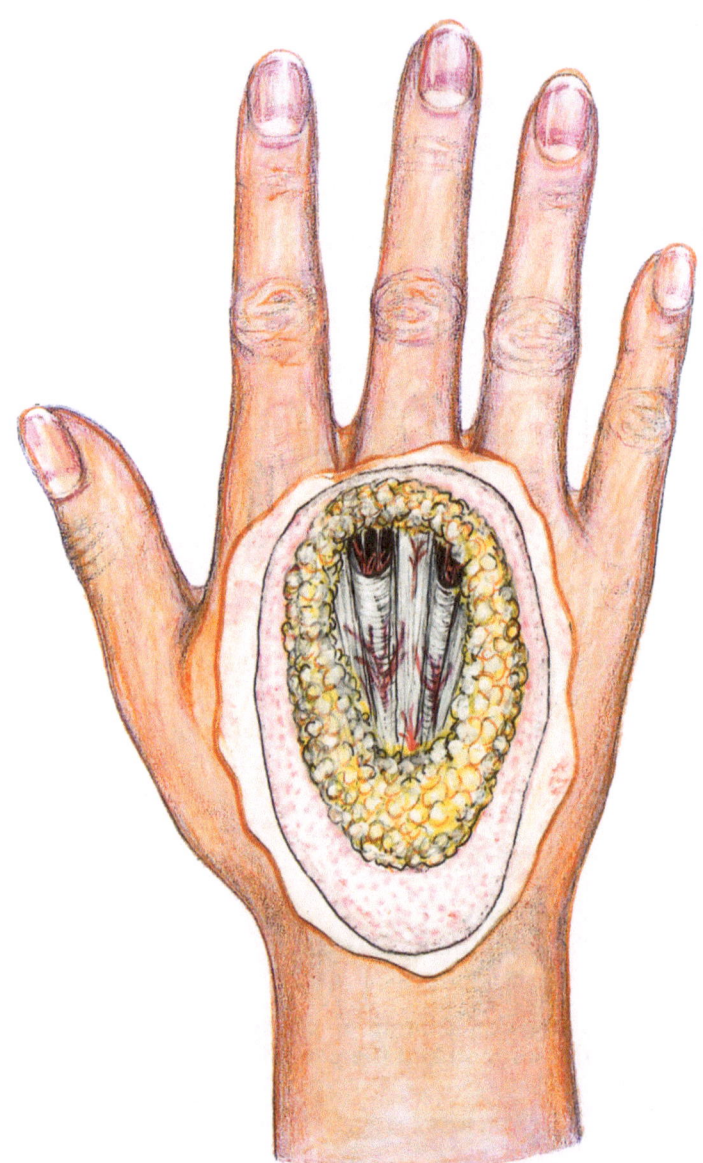

Palm Injury

Case history: Industrial grinder – 34-year-old female.
Injury to the palm with loss of functional structures

Assessment/diagnosis

Loss of entire volar skin,
Defects of FDP 2-4, FDS 2-4
Rupture of superficial volar arch with
destruction of common digital arteries 2-4
Loss (gap = 1 cm) of common digital nerves 2-4
Digits 2-4 avascular

Flexor tendon reconstruction

Avascular tendon grafts from
dorsum of the foot
(long extensor system)
or palmaris longus

Resection of FDS

Release of A1 pulleys

Simultaneous two
team approach

**Reconstruction of
superficial volar arch**

4 vein grafts
Volar or dorsum/
including depending
on vascular caliber

Alternatively:

Scapular fascial flap
Subscapular arterial
tree with branches
(very experienced
microsurgeon required)

Reconstruction of nerve gap

(Nerves were sharply lacerated)

Sural nerve grafts
Adjust diameters to
digital nerves!

Rehabilitation:

Wait until flap survival is
confirmed (3-5 days)
Then active motion protocol
for flexor tendons

Alternatively:

Primary soft tissue
coverage with
secondary structure
repair

Soft tissue reconstruction

Free temporal fascia flap +
Skin graft from scalp

Groin flap
Lateral arm flap

Consider delayed skin grafting
due to tendency of capillary
bleeding and swelling

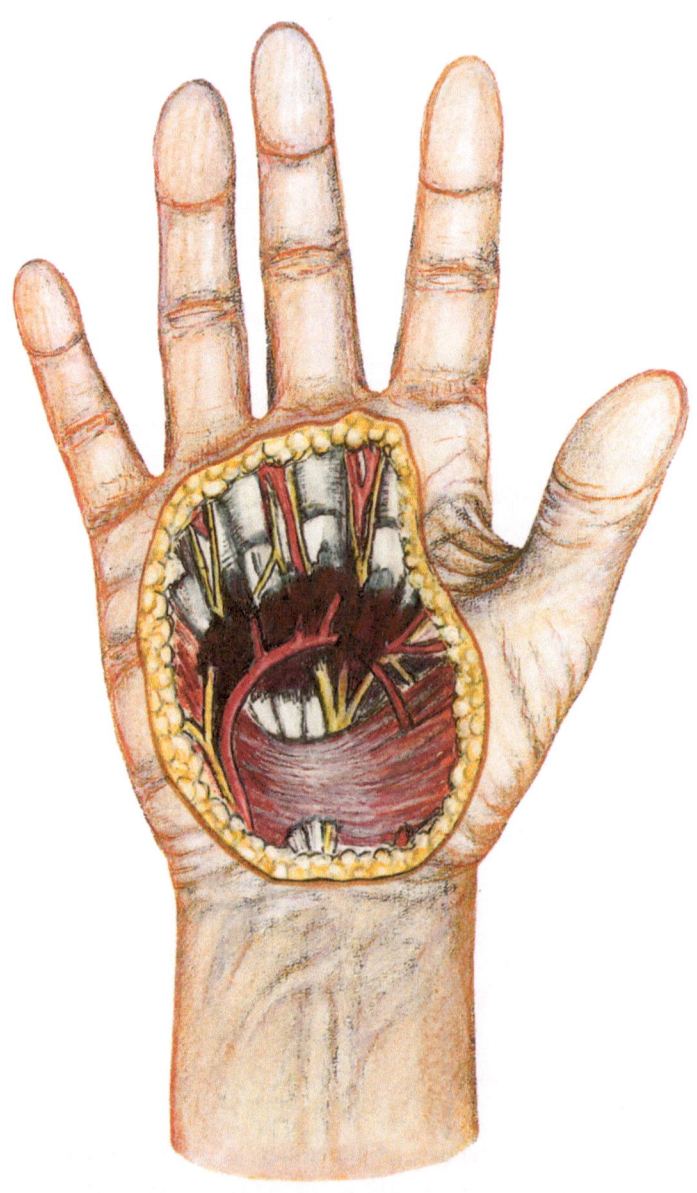

Circular Saw Injury

Case history: 23-year-old male worker with circular saw injury
               to dominant right long finger

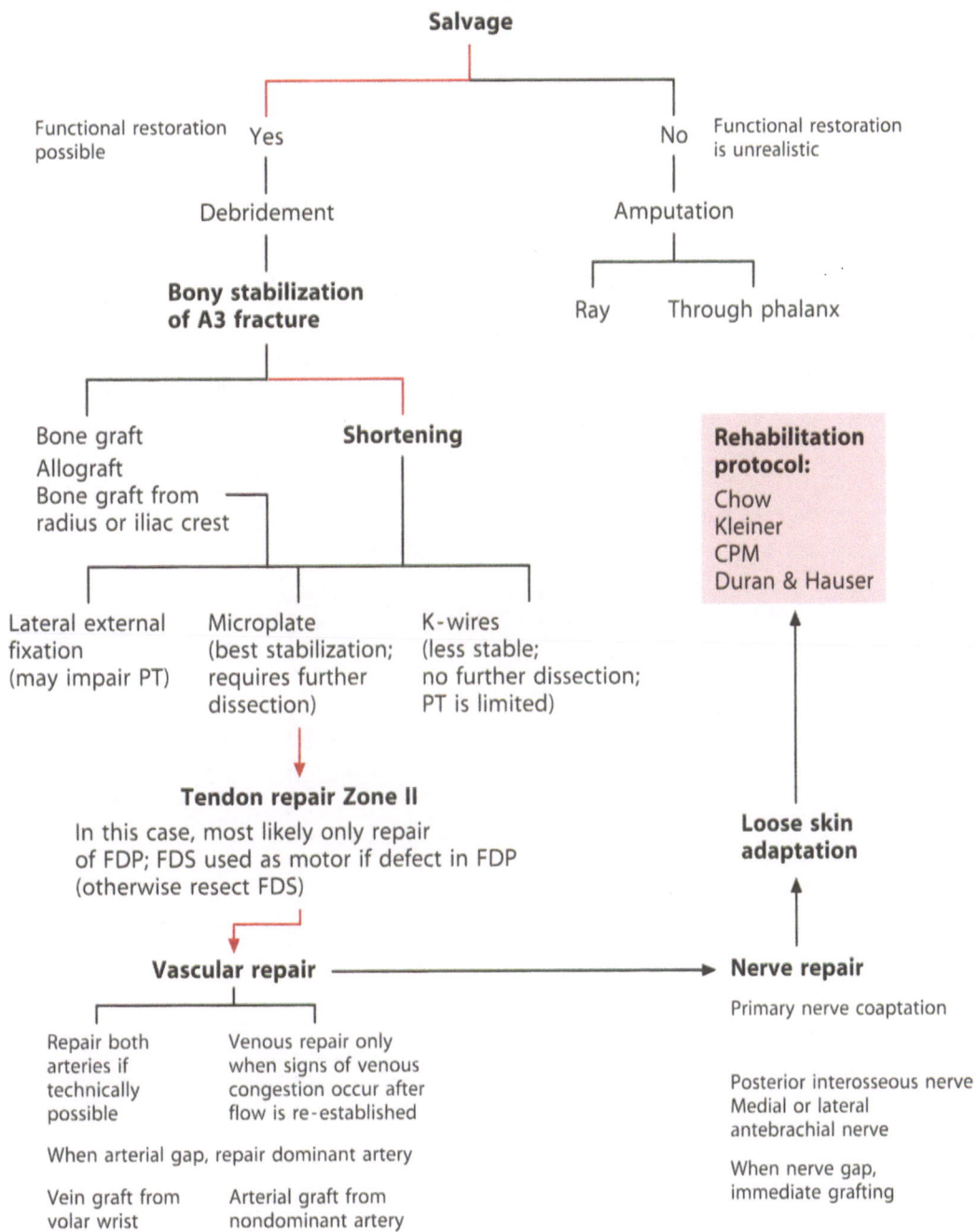

Assessment/diagnosis

Incomplete amputation of long finger through
middle of proximal phalanx
Comminuted A3 fracture with bone loss
Finger is avascular and insensitive

Salvage

Functional restoration   Yes   No   Functional restoration
possible   is unrealistic

Debridement   Amputation

**Bony stabilization
of A3 fracture**   Ray   Through phalanx

Bone graft   **Shortening**
Allograft
Bone graft from
radius or iliac crest

Lateral external   Microplate   K-wires
fixation   (best stabilization; (less stable;
(may impair PT)   requires further   no further dissection;
                     dissection)   PT is limited)

**Rehabilitation
protocol:**
Chow
Kleiner
CPM
Duran & Hauser

Tendon repair Zone II

In this case, most likely only repair
of FDP; FDS used as motor if defect in FDP
(otherwise resect FDS)

**Loose skin
adaptation**

Vascular repair ———————————→ **Nerve repair**

Repair both   Venous repair only   Primary nerve coaptation
arteries if   when signs of venous
technically   congestion occur after
possible   flow is re-established   Posterior interosseous nerve
                                                   Medial or lateral
When arterial gap, repair dominant artery   antebrachial nerve

Vein graft from   Arterial graft from   When nerve gap,
volar wrist   nondominant artery   immediate grafting

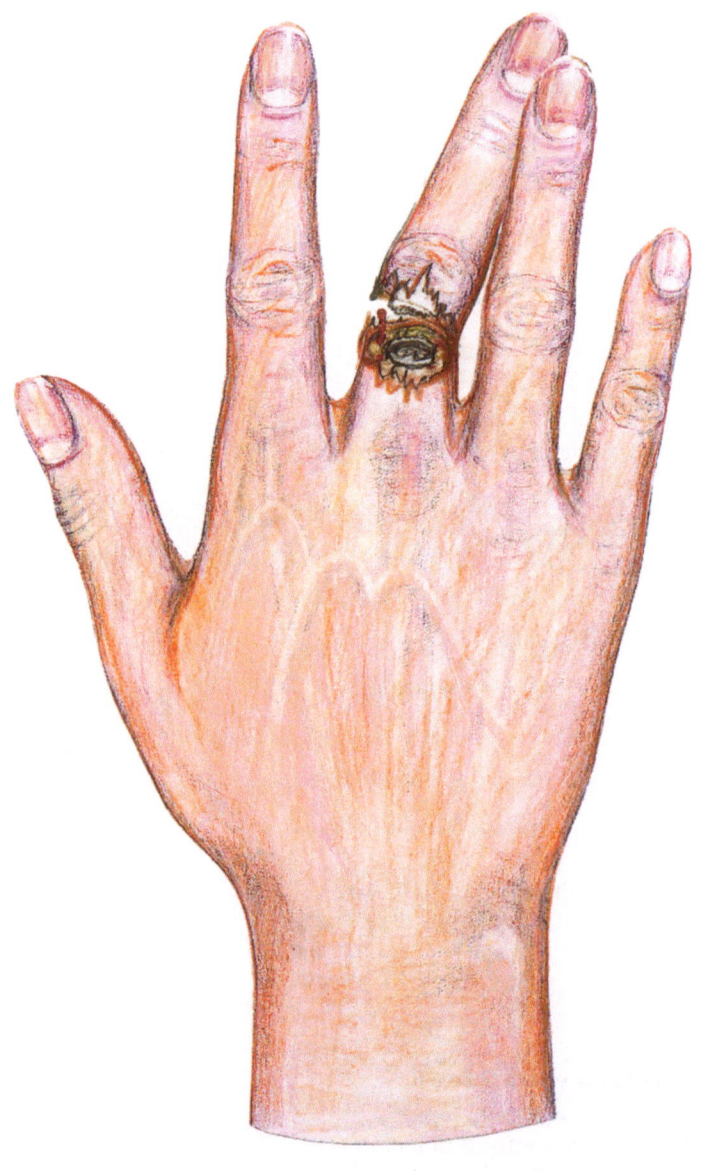

Chronic Volkmann's Contracture

Diagnosis: Chronic Volkmann's contracture secondary to compartment
syndrome in a 10-year-old girl after posterior dislocation of elbow

Treatment goal: restoration of active flexion

Clinical assessment

Joints			**Digital sensation**	

Mobile   Fixed   Present   Absent

                    Joint release
                    Capsulotomy
                                                          Anatomic   Physiologic
                                                          disruption   injury

                                                          Nerve   Nerve
                                                          grafting   decompression

          Return of mobility

                                              Return of sensation

          Reconstruction

Mild injury	Moderate injury	Severe injury

Direct excision   Tendon transfer   Functional free muscle transfer
of isolated necrotic   to restore flexion,
muscle segments   for example: Microvascular myocutaneous
                         ECRL, FDP   gracilis/latissimus flap

                                                  Coaptation of motor nerve
                                                  to FDP or FDS nerves

                                                  Anterior interosseous nerve to
                                                  obturator nerve

                                                  Skin island for replacement
                                                  of skin grafted areas

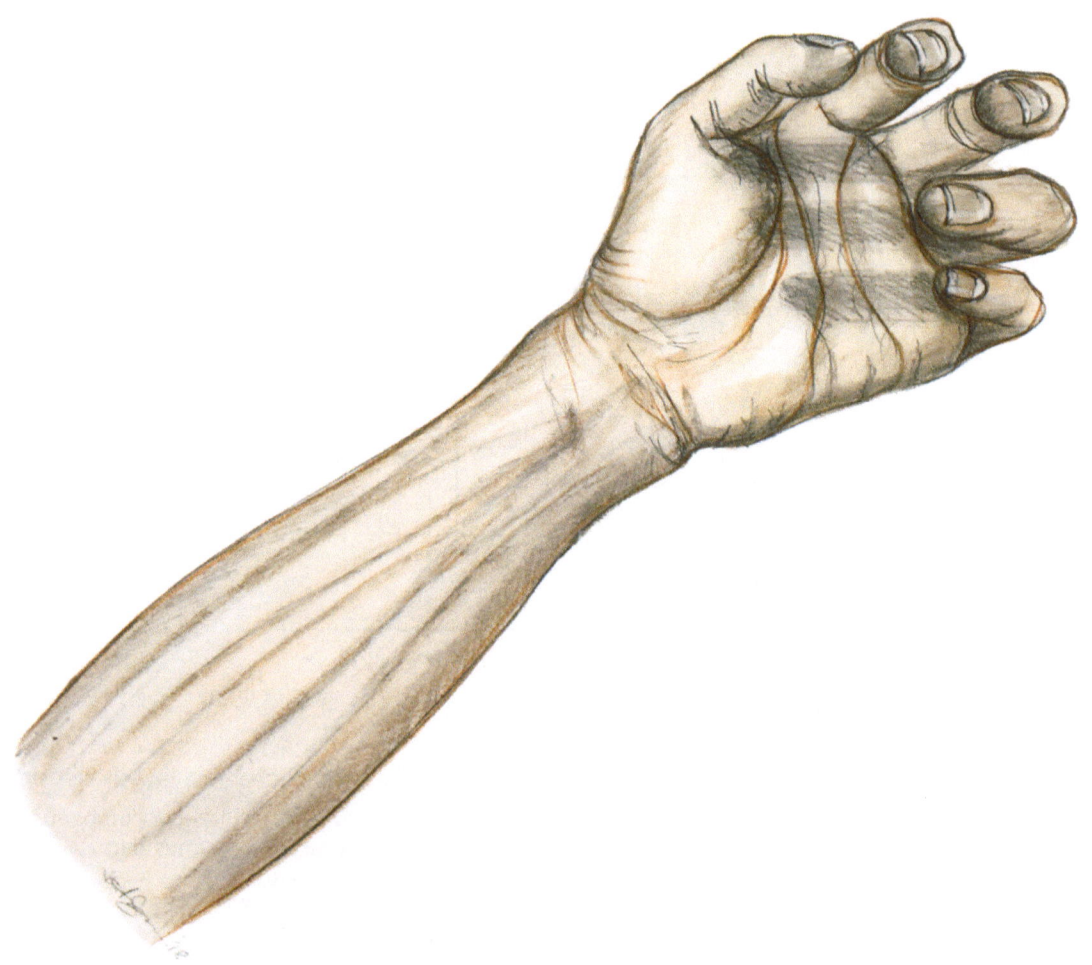

Tumor

Case history: 55-year-old male with mass in triceps muscle

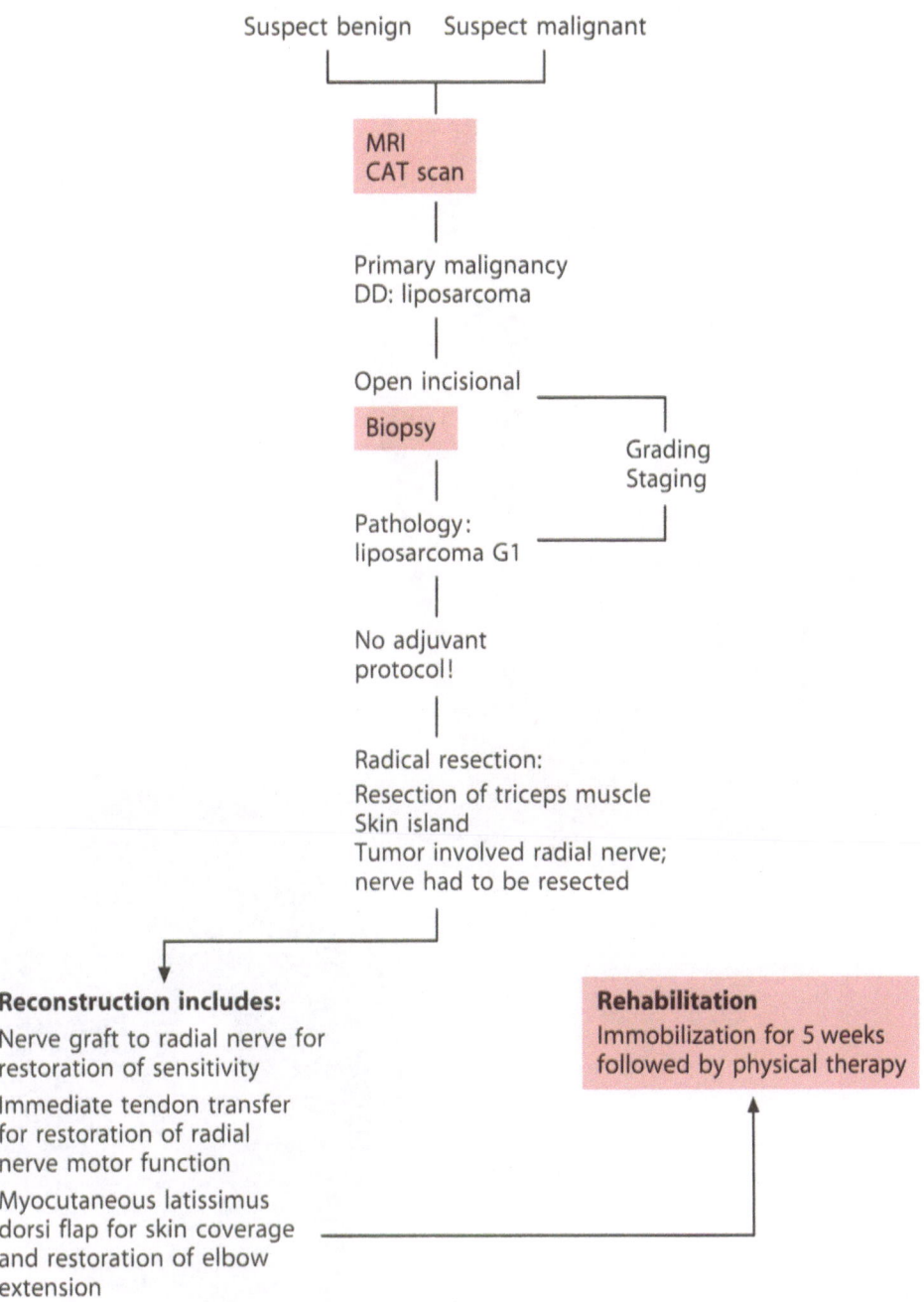

Clinical diagnosis

Suspect benign   Suspect malignant

MRI
CAT scan

Primary malignancy
DD: liposarcoma

Open incisional

Biopsy   Grading
                              Staging

Pathology:
liposarcoma G1

No adjuvant
protocol!

Radical resection:
Resection of triceps muscle
Skin island
Tumor involved radial nerve;
nerve had to be resected

Reconstruction includes: **Rehabilitation**
Nerve graft to radial nerve for   Immobilization for 5 weeks
restoration of sensitivity   followed by physical therapy

Immediate tendon transfer
for restoration of radial
nerve motor function

Myocutaneous latissimus
dorsi flap for skin coverage
and restoration of elbow
extension

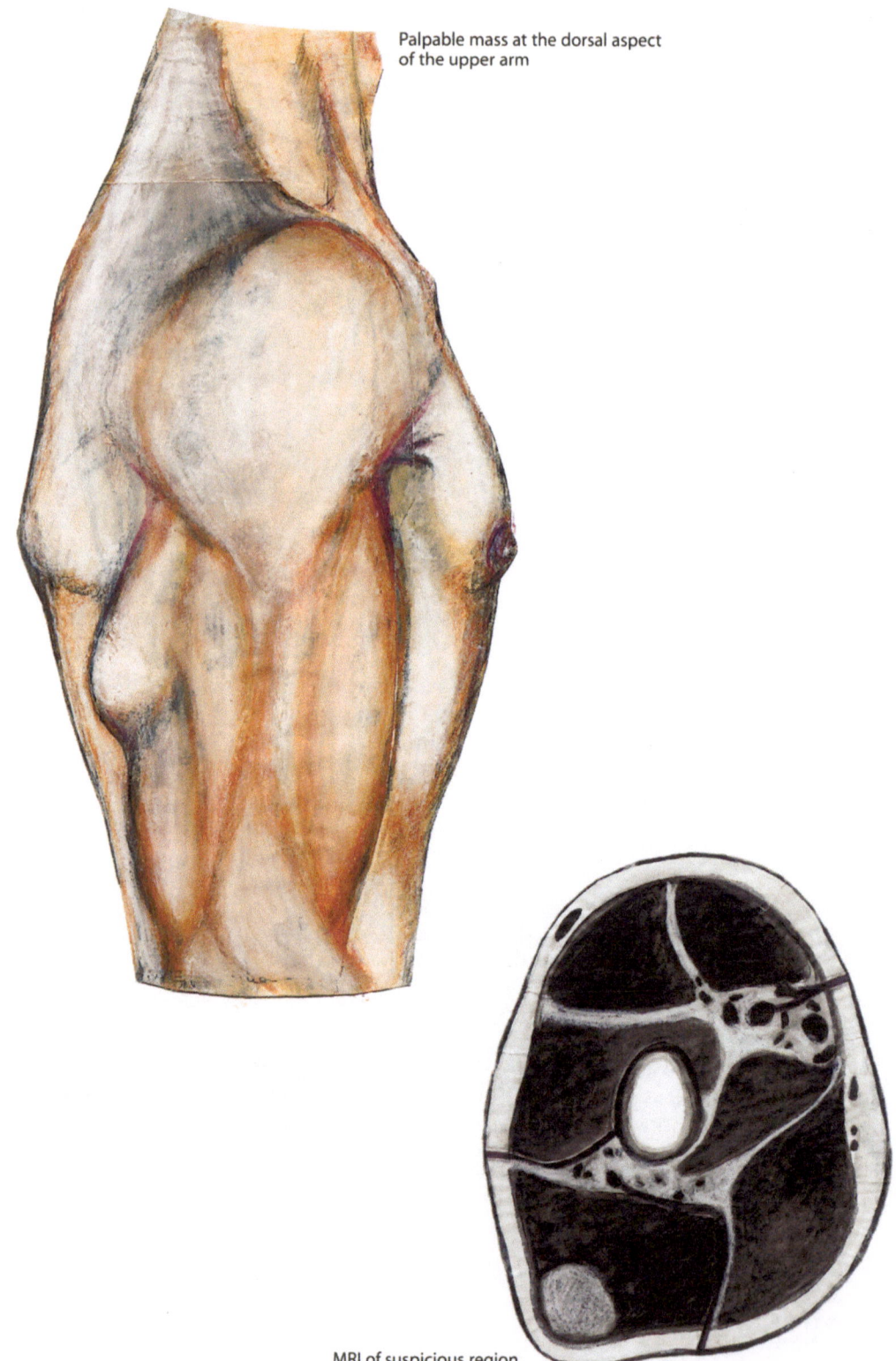

Palpable mass at the dorsal aspect
of the upper arm

MRI of suspicious region

Chronic Osteomyelitis

Case history: 17-year-old male with chronic osteomyelitis of radius.
Already 14 operations following internal fixation of a 2° open radius fracture

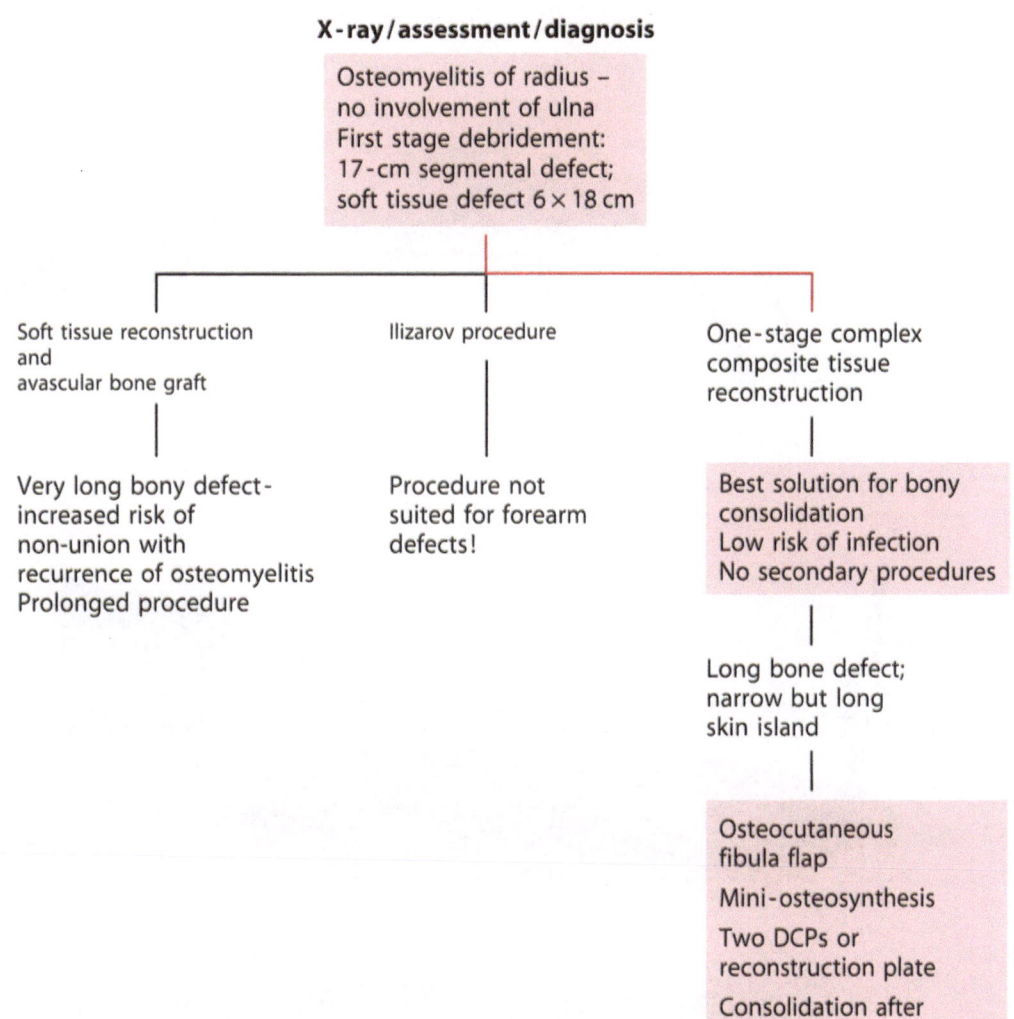

X-ray/assessment/diagnosis

Osteomyelitis of radius –
no involvement of ulna
First stage debridement:
17-cm segmental defect;
soft tissue defect 6 × 18 cm

Soft tissue reconstruction
and
avascular bone graft

Ilizarov procedure

One-stage complex
composite tissue
reconstruction

Very long bony defect-
increased risk of
non-union with
recurrence of osteomyelitis
Prolonged procedure

Procedure not
suited for forearm
defects!

Best solution for bony
consolidation
Low risk of infection
No secondary procedures

Long bone defect;
narrow but long
skin island

Osteocutaneous
fibula flap

Mini-osteosynthesis

Two DCPs or
reconstruction plate

Consolidation after
6-7 weeks

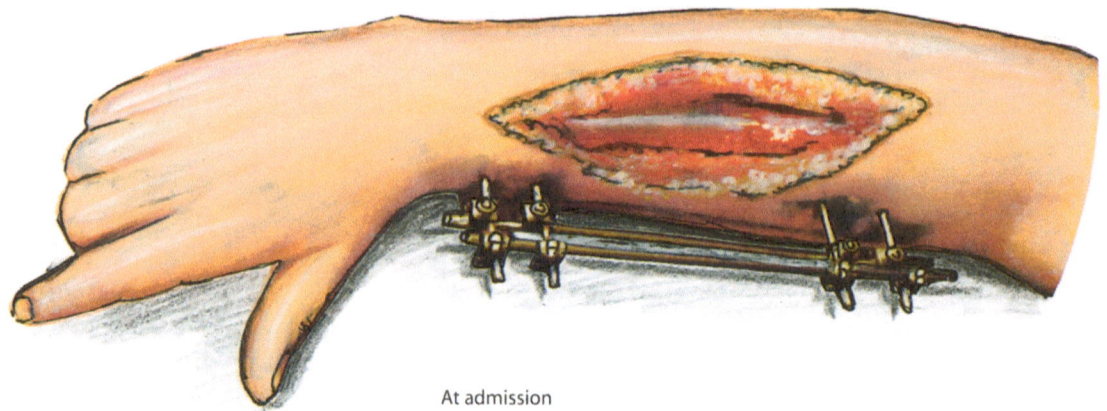

At admission

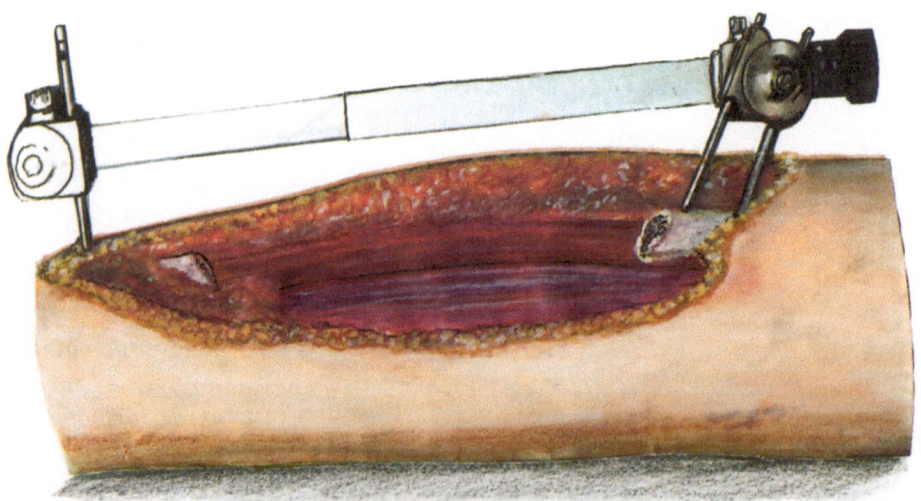

After radical debridement and before placement
and internal fixation of intercalary free
osteocutaneous fibula

CHAPTER V
Atlas of Flaps
Pearls and Pitfalls

Flap	**Cross-Finger Flap**
Tissue	Skin (conventional flap) or adipofascial tissue (reversed flap)
Course of the vessels	Axially in the subcutaneous tissue – no identifiable named vessel
Dimensions	2.5 × 2 cm in both versions
Extensions/combinations	
Anatomy: **Neurovascular pedicle** Artery Veins Length Diameter Nerve	**No defined pedicle**
Surgical technique **Preoperative examinations, markings**	Preferred donor site: Middle phalanx
Patient position	Arm on arm table – tourniquet ischemia
Dissection	Conventional flap: Incise at dorsolateral border of the digit, raise of flap in the plane above the tendon with preservation of paratenon; free laterovolar as far as possible without violating the neurovascular bundle, suturing the flap into the defect; skin graft to donor site Reversed flap: Incise flap; raise thin skin flap with preservation of subdermal plexus; raise flap of adipo-fascial tissue with preservation of paratenon; flip subcutaneous flap into defect; cover donor site with previously dissected skin flap
Advantages Dissection Flap size/shape Combinations	Simple, reliable Flap size sufficient for most typical defects over flexor or extensor tendons Refinement in design with axial vessel included (C-ring flap)
Disadvantages Flap size Donor site morbidity	Not optimally suited for longitudinal oval defect over several joints Skin graft for conventional flap may be conspicuous in the postoperative period, but improves with time
Tricks/pitfalls Dissection Contouring/corrections Clinical applications	Preservation of paratenon is of utmost importance for skin graft take; preservation of subdermal plexus guarantees excellent reconstruction of donor site in reversed flap Rarely required Conventional flap: volar digital defects Reversed flap: dorsal digital defects

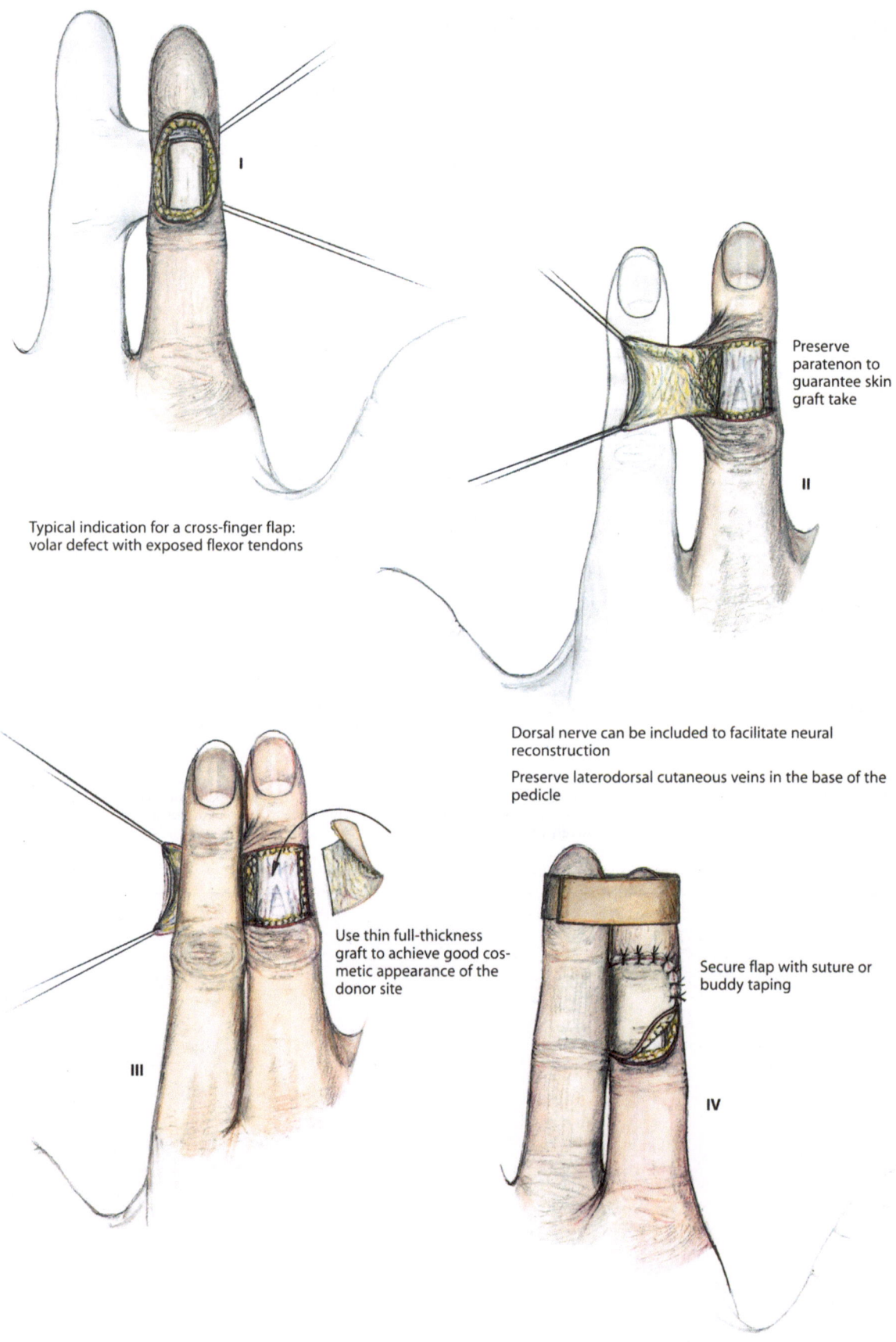

I

Typical indication for a cross-finger flap:
volar defect with exposed flexor tendons

II

Preserve
paratenon to
guarantee skin
graft take

Dorsal nerve can be included to facilitate neural
reconstruction

Preserve laterodorsal cutaneous veins in the base of the
pedicle

III

Use thin full-thickness
graft to achieve good cosmetic appearance of the
donor site

IV

Secure flap with suture or
buddy taping

Flap

V-Y Flap for Fingertips
Volar V-Y (Tanquilli – Leali, Atasoy)
Lateral V-Y (Geissendörfer, Kutler)

Tissue	Skin
Course of the vessels	In the subcutaneous tissue of the pulp
Dimensions	1 × 1.5 cm
Extensions/combinations	
Anatomy **Neurovascular pedicle** Artery Veins Length/arc of rotation Diameter Nerve	**No defined pedicle**
Surgical technique **Preoperative examinations, markings**	Slightly laterally curved triangular incision
Patient position	Arm on arm table, digital block or plexus anesthesia, tourniquet
Dissection	**Volar flap** Skin incision without violating subcutaneous tissue; release the fibrous septa from the pulp to the periosteum; trim bone; pull flap distally with Gillies hook; divide remaining septa; fixate flap in defect with needle; no distal suture **Lateral flap** Defect coverage with bilateral flaps; triangular flaps; limbs of the incision should meet at distal flexor crease; incise skin; do not injure subcutaneous tissue; release fibrous septa from periosteum; trim bone; pull flap medially with Gillies; release remaining septa; fixate flap to contralateral flap with sutures or use two needles
Advantages Dissection Flap size/shape Donor site	 Dissection is easy Flap is reliable, small defects of the fingertip can be covered with sensate skin Primary closure in V-Y technique or loose approximation of the skin
Disadvantages Flap size	 Flap is sometimes too small
Tricks/pitfalls Dissection Contouring/corrections Clinical applications	 Do not injure the subcutaneous tissue; do not suture the flap distally – this will impair blood supply; flap is frequently pale after release of the tourniquet; wait and rinse with warm saline Very rarely required Small defects of the fingertips

Use Gillies' hooks to pull flap
gently distally

Divide all septa to facilitate advancement
of the flap

Design flap large enough!!

Use needle for distal fixation to reduce
tension on the suture line –
Do not close too tightly

Flap	Volar Advancement Flap (Moberg); O'Brien Modification; Lateral Advancement Flap (Venkataswami)
Tissue	Skin
Course of the vessels	Underneath the flap
Dimensions	Can reach the dimension of the entire volar surface of a digit or the thumb
Anatomy **Neurovascular pedicle** Artery Veins Length/arc of rotation Nerve	 Proper digital artery Concomitant veins of digital artery Maximal defect size – longitudinal mobilization: 1.5 – 2 cm Proper digital nerves
Surgical technique **Preoperative examinations, markings**	 Midlateral skin markings, digital Allen-test recommended
Patient position	Hand on arm table, tourniquet ischemia
Dissection	**Moberg** Mid-lateral incision; identification of neuro-vascular bundles; unilateral preservation of dorsal branches; volar advancement; distal flap fixation with needle!; frequently flexion of the digit is necessary to allow closure of the defect **O'Brien modification** Bilateral dissection of neuro-vascular bundles; volar flap advancement; skin graft to donor site (dissection site of vessels) **Venkataswami** Mid-lateral triangle based on proper digital vessels; leave septum to neuro-vascular bundle intact; V-Y closure of donor site
Advantages Flap Dissection Vascular pedicle Flap size/shape	 Sensate flap to restore sensibility of the pulp Strightforward – easy Reliable Pulp defects of 1.5 – 2 cm
Disadvantages Flap Donor site morbidity	 Only small-midsize defects Flexion contracture, especially in the thumb!!
Tricks/pitfalls Dissection Contouring/corrections Clinical applications	 Preserve dorsal collaterals on one side; fixate flap distally only with needle to avoid further tension and impairment of distal flap supply; rather relaxing incision at the base of the thumb or convert in into O'Brien modification to reduce risk of flexion contracture especially in older patients; Insert Z-plasty in regular Moberg's to avoid tension at flap base Extremely rare Defects of the pulp of the thumb, but also appropriate for digital defects; oblique defects (lateral advancement flap)

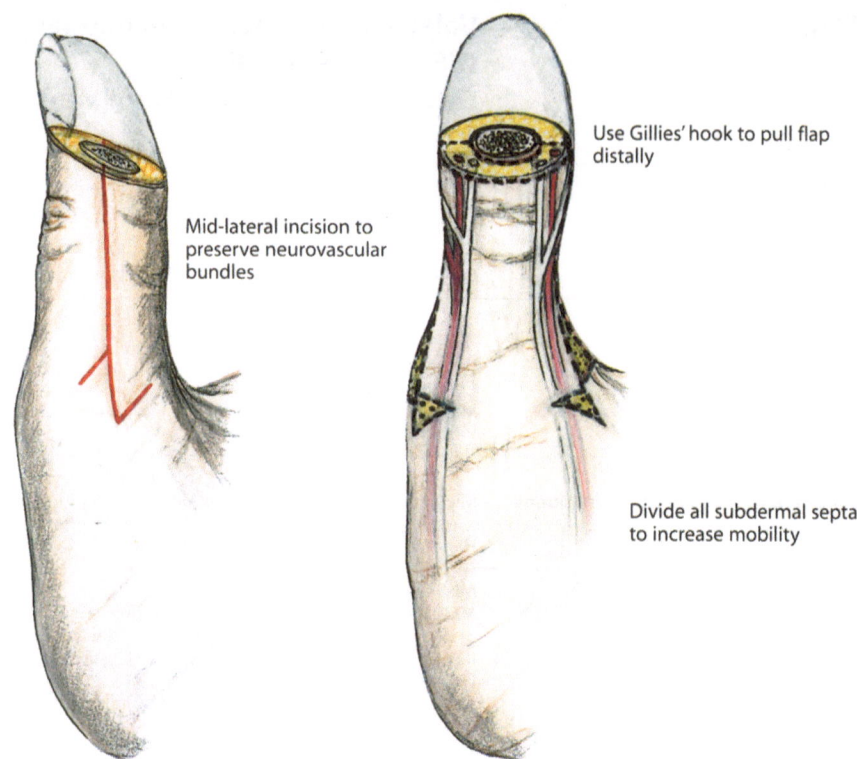
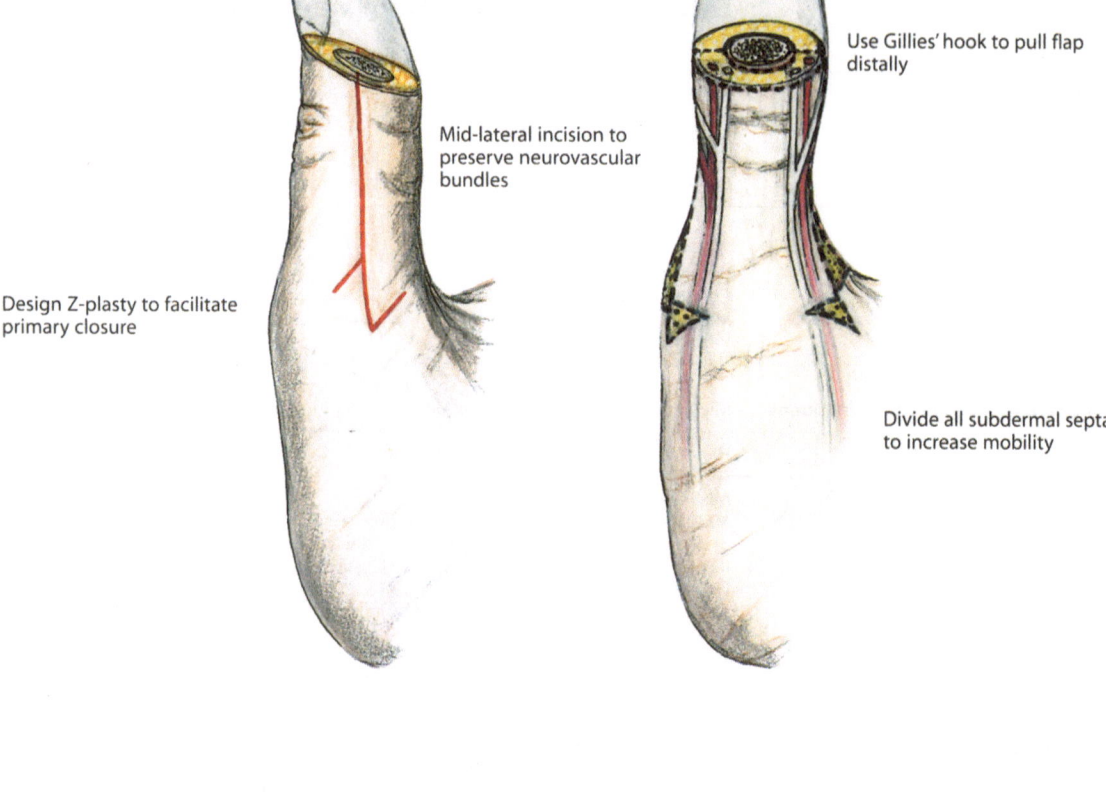

Design Z-plasty to facilitate primary closure

Mid-lateral incision to preserve neurovascular bundles

Use Gillies' hook to pull flap distally

Divide all subdermal septa to increase mobility

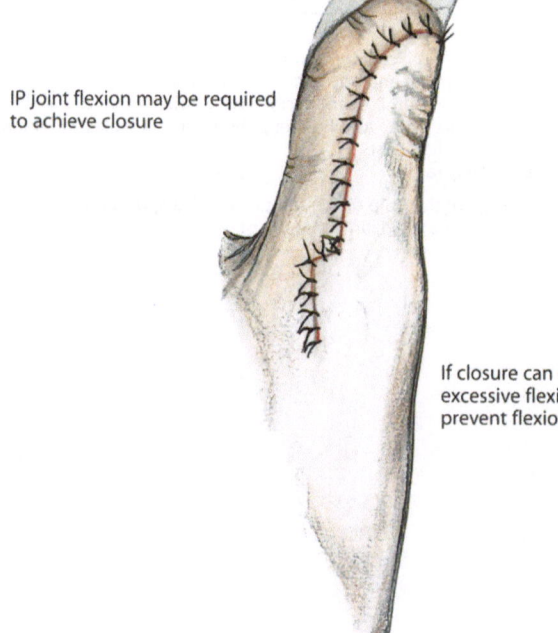

IP joint flexion may be required to achieve closure

If closure can only be achieved with excessive flexion, use other option to prevent flexion contracture

Flap	Axial Digital Island Flap
Tissue	Skin
Course of the vessels	Axial in the center of the flap
Dimensions	1.5 × 2.5 cm
Extensions/combinations	Inclusion of the nerve to restore sensibility at the defect site
Anatomy **Neurovascular pedicle** Artery Veins Length Diameter Nerve	 Proper digital artery Accompanying veins of digital artery 3–4 cm Proper digital nerve can be included
Surgical technique **Preoperative examinations, markings**	 Digital Allen's test is mandatory
Patient position	Arm on arm table; tourniquet ischemia
Dissection	Incise skin; identify neurovascular bundle proximal to flap; dissect flap down to artery and accompanying veins; spare nerve; preserve delicate septum between skin island and neurovascular bundle; apply micro-clamp proximally and distally to flap; open tourniquet; remove proximal clamp; check perfusion of digit and flap; when intact transpose flap
Advantages Vascular pedicle Flap zise/shape	 Reliable pedicle; sufficient arc of rotation Sufficient for typical homodigital dorsal defects, especially over exposed joints (MP and PIP joints)
Further options	Heterodigital flap in special situations when injured finger does not allow homo-digital flap
Disadvantages Dissection Donor site morbidity	 Difficult dissection; delicate septum between flap and neurovascular bundle Acceptable – early contour defect that improves with time
Tricks/pitfalls Dissection Contouring/corrections Clinical applications	 Use loops and microsurgical instruments when dissecting the nerve from the pedicle; do not forget digital Allen's test; check for venous congestion; apply leeches early when there are signs of congestions after transposition of flap into defect; do not inset too tightly; use FTSG for donor site Rarely required Proximal homodigital dorsal defects (PIP, MP joints, or tendons exposed)

Center flap over neurovascular bundle

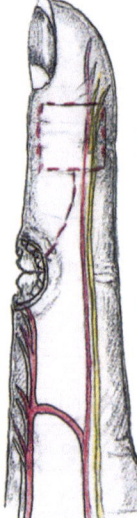

If sensate flap is required, include proper digital nerve

If only skin coverage is required, free the nerve carefully from the artery

If a "Littler flap" is designed, split common digital nerve intraneurally to increase pedicle length

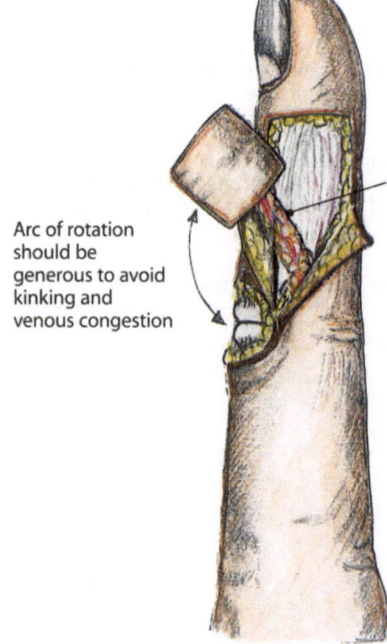

Arc of rotation should be generous to avoid kinking and venous congestion

Preserve areolar tissue around the artery to maintain venous outflow

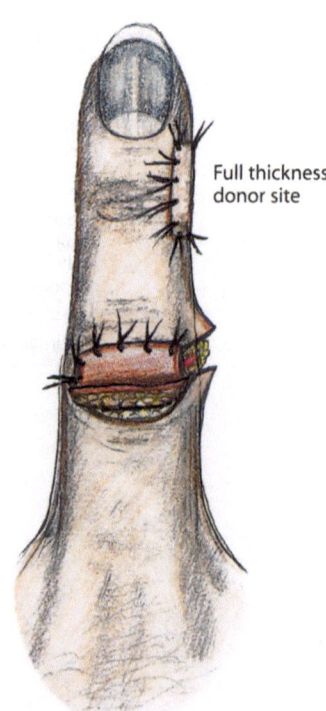

Full thickness skin graft for donor site

Flap   **Reverse Axial Digital Island Flap**

Tissue	Skin
Course of the vessels	Axial in the center of the flap
Dimensions	1.5 × 2.5 cm
Extensions/combinations	Very rarely inclusion of the nerve to restore sensation at the defect site by coapting the proximal stump to a lacerated contralateral digital nerve
Anatomy **Neurovascular pedicle** Artery Length Diameter Nerve	Proper digital artery Accompanying veins of digital artery 3–4 cm Proper digital nerve can be included
Surgical technique **Preoperative examinations, markings**	Digital Allen's test is mandatory; distal digital arterial arch in the pulp must be intact
Patient position	Arm on arm table; tourniquet ischemia
Dissection	Incise skin; identify neurovascular bundle proximal to flap; dissect flap down to artery and accompanying veins; spare nerve; preserve delicate septum between skin island and neurovascular bundle; apply micro-clamp proximally to pedicle; open tourniquet; remove proximal clamp; check perfusion of digit and flap; when intact transpose flap
Advantages Vascular pedicle Flap size/shape **Further options**	Reliable pedicle; sufficient arc of rotation (PIP and DIP joints) Sufficient for typical homodigital dorsal defects, especially over exposed joints Heterodigital flap in special situations when injured finger does not allow homo-digital solution
Disadvantages Flap/pedicle Dissection Donor site morbidity	Flap has a tendency for venous congestion; do not kink the pedicle; do not make the arc of rotation too narrow Difficult dissection; delicate septum between flap and neurovascular bundle Acceptable – early contour defect that improves with time
Tricks/pitfalls Dissection Contouring/corrections Clinical applications	Use loops and microsurgical instrument when dissecting the nerve from the pedicle; do not forget digital Allen's test; check for venous congestion; apply leeches early when there are signs of congestions after transposition of flap into defect; make arc of rotation wide enough to avoid venous kinking; do not inset the flap too tightly Rarely required Distal homodigital dorsal defects (PIP joints or tendons exposed)

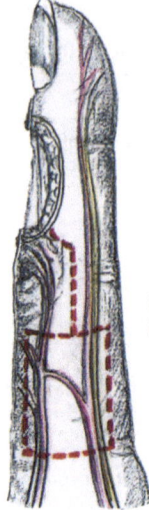

If sensate flap is required,
include proper digital nerve

Center flap over neurovascular bundle

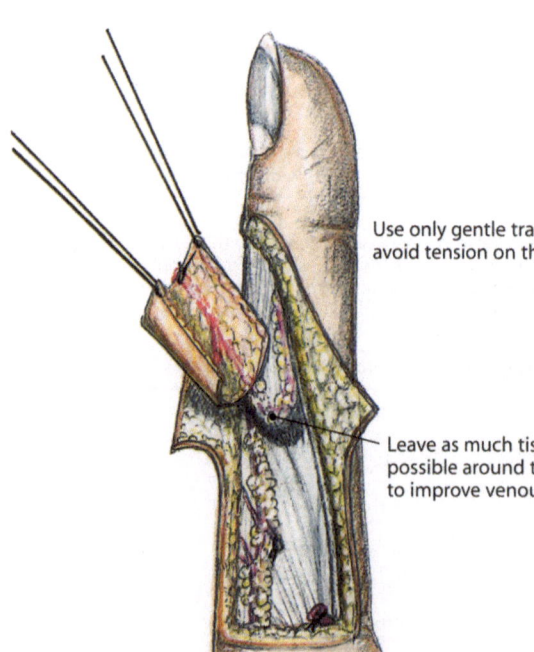

Use only gentle traction to
avoid tension on the pedicle

Leave as much tissue as
possible around the pedicle
to improve venous outflow

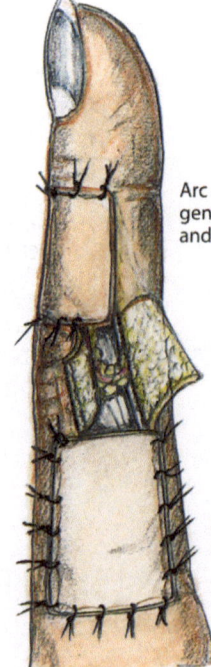

Arc of rotation should be
generous to avoid kinking
and venous congestion

Full thickness skin graft for
donor site

Flap	First Dorsal Metacarpal Artery Flap – Neuro-Fascioseptocutaneous Flap – "Kite" Flap
Tissue	Skin
Course of the vessels	In intermuscular septum
Dimensions	2 × 4–6 cm, pedicle or free flap located on proximal phalanx of the index finger
Extensions/combinations	Rarely tendon strips from proper extensor indicis; terminal branch from superficial radial nerve
Anatomy **Neurovascular pedicle** Artery Veins Length/Arc of rotation Diameter Nerve	 Dorsal metacarpal artery nourished from the princeps pollicis artery Small Vv. comitantes; larger subcutaneous vein 3–3.5 cm (artery) 3–6 cm (vein) 2–3 mm (artery at the level of princeps pollicis); vein: 3–5 mm Terminal branch of superficial radial nerve
Surgical technique **Preoperative examinations, markings**	 Preoperative Doppler examination for presence of vessels is mandatory; mark couse of vessels on skin; vessels are always more radially than presumed!!
Patient position	Supine with arm on arm table; tourniquet ischemia
Dissection	Incise skin along markings; incise interosseous muscle fascia; preserve intermuscular septum and raise fascio-cutaneous flap including the fascia; take care to include nerve; create deepithelialized pedicle; leave approx. 0.5 to 1 cm fatty tissue around artery; preserve paratenon above extensor hood; open tourniquet; check for perfusion; inset flap at recipient site; wait for normal perfusion; skin graft donor site (medium or full thickness skin graft); be careful with tunneling
Advantages Tissue Vascular pedicle Flap size/shape Combinations	 Sensate thin and pliable flap Reliable pedicle with wide arc of rotation, large caliber vessel when used as a free flap Can cover large defects without sacrifice of a proper digital artery Inclusion of a tendon strip of the extensor indicis muscle possible; bony segment of 2nd metacarpal may be future option
Disadvantages Pedicle Donor site morbidity	 Flap is often white during the first few minutes after opening the tourniquet; venous congestion may occur if flap is passed through a tunnel to the recipient site Donor site is conspicuous at first but improves significantly over time
Tricks/pitfalls Dissection Extensions/combinations Contouring/corrections Clinical applications	 Do not make arc of rotation too narrow – venous congestion may occur; preserve paratenon of extensor tendons for perfect skin graft take for donor site; when tunnel for the flap seems too narrow – skin graft pedicle; apply leeches early when venous congestion occurs; avoid any tension on pedicle; when flap does not show adequate reperfusion after opening of the tourniquet; rinse with warm saline; it may take 20 minutes to re-establish flow Bony segment from metacarpal may be possible Rarely required – flap shrinks with time **Pedicle flap** Small and medium size dorsal defects of the thumb; restoration of sensation of the pulp of the thumb **Free flap** Small and medium size defects wherever local flaps are not possible or appropriate

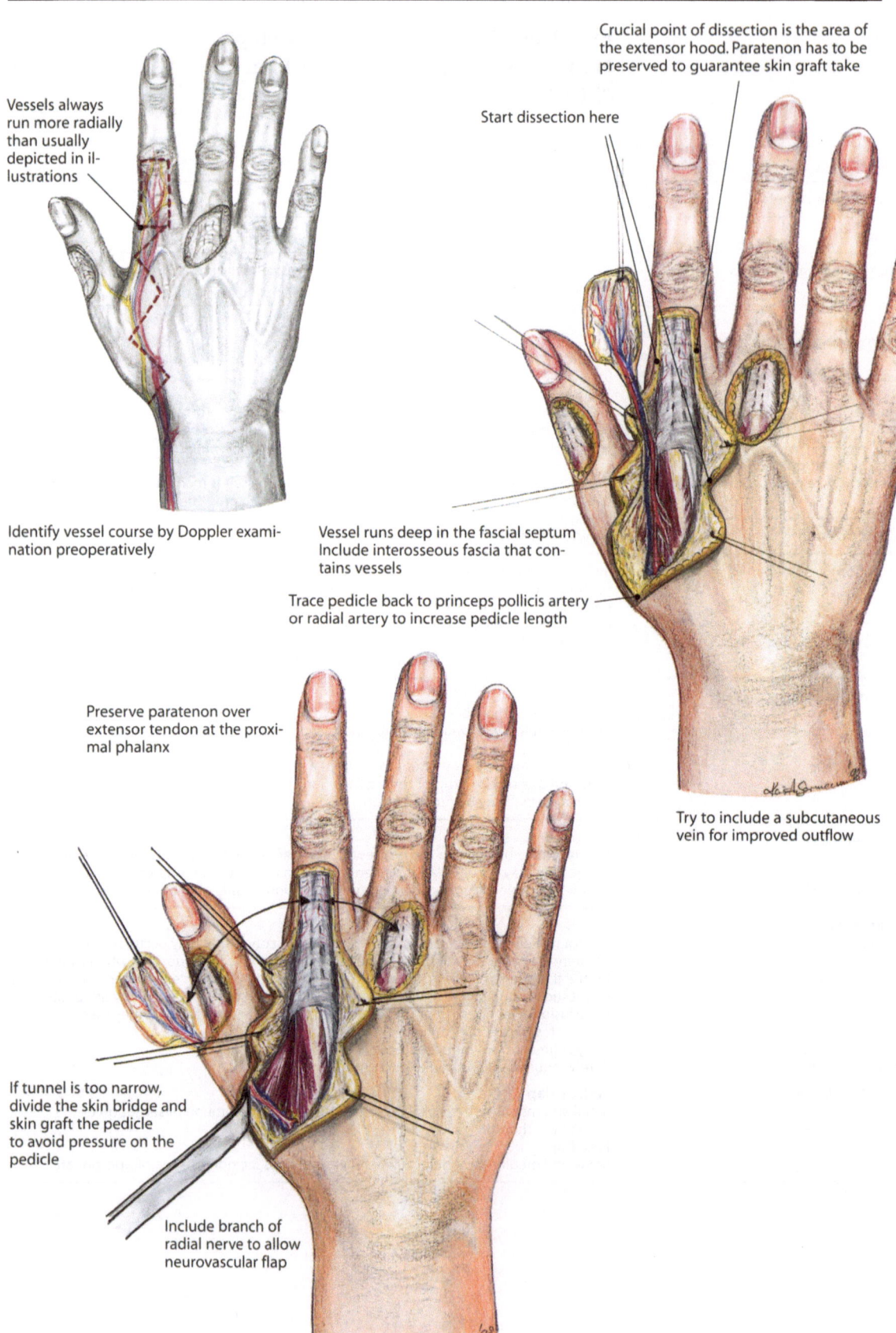

Vessels always run more radially than usually depicted in illustrations

Identify vessel course by Doppler examination preoperatively

Crucial point of dissection is the area of the extensor hood. Paratenon has to be preserved to guarantee skin graft take

Start dissection here

Vessel runs deep in the fascial septum Include interosseous fascia that contains vessels

Trace pedicle back to princeps pollicis artery or radial artery to increase pedicle length

Try to include a subcutaneous vein for improved outflow

Preserve paratenon over extensor tendon at the proximal phalanx

If tunnel is too narrow, divide the skin bridge and skin graft the pedicle to avoid pressure on the pedicle

Include branch of radial nerve to allow neurovascular flap

Flap	**Dorsal Metacarpal Artery Flap (2 – 4)**

Tissue	Skin
Course of the vessels	In intermuscular septum
Dimensions	2 × 4 cm; Reverse flap located over prosimal metacarpals; antegrade flap over proximal phalanx
Extensions/combinations	Rarely tendon strips from proper extensor indicis or proper extensor digitus minimus
Anatomy **Neurovascular pedicle** Artery Veins Length/Arc of rotation Diameter Nerve	 Dorsal metacarpal artery nourished from dorsal arterial arch or through volar-dorsal perforator from volar arch Small vv. comitantes Reverse pedicle flap reaches PIP joint; antegrade flap reaches proximal wrist extensor crease
Surgical technique **Preoperative examinations, markings**	 Preoperative Doppler examination for presence of vessels is mandatory; reliability declines from radial to ulnar aspect; DMCA 4 is only present in approx. 80 % of the cases
Patient position	Supine with arm on arm table; tourniquet ischemia
Dissection	**Reverse pedicle** Incise skin along markins; incise interosseous muscle fascia; preserve intermuscular septum and raise fasciocutaneous flap including the fascia; create de-epithelialized pedicle towards volar-dorsal preforator at the level of the metacarpal head; leave approx. 0.5 to 1 cm fatty tissue around artery; ligate proximal pedicle; open tourniquet; check for perfusion; rotate and inset flap into recipient site; wait for normal perfusion **Antegrade pedicle** Incise skin along markings; incise interosseous muscle fascia; preserve intermuscular septum and raise fasciocutaneous flap including the fascia; create de-epithelialized pedicle towards volar-dorsal perforator at the level of the metacarpal head; leave approx. 0.5 to 1 cm fatty tissue around artery; ligate distal pedicle; open tourniquet; check for perfusion; inset flap at recipient site; wait for normal perfusion

Continuation see p. 196

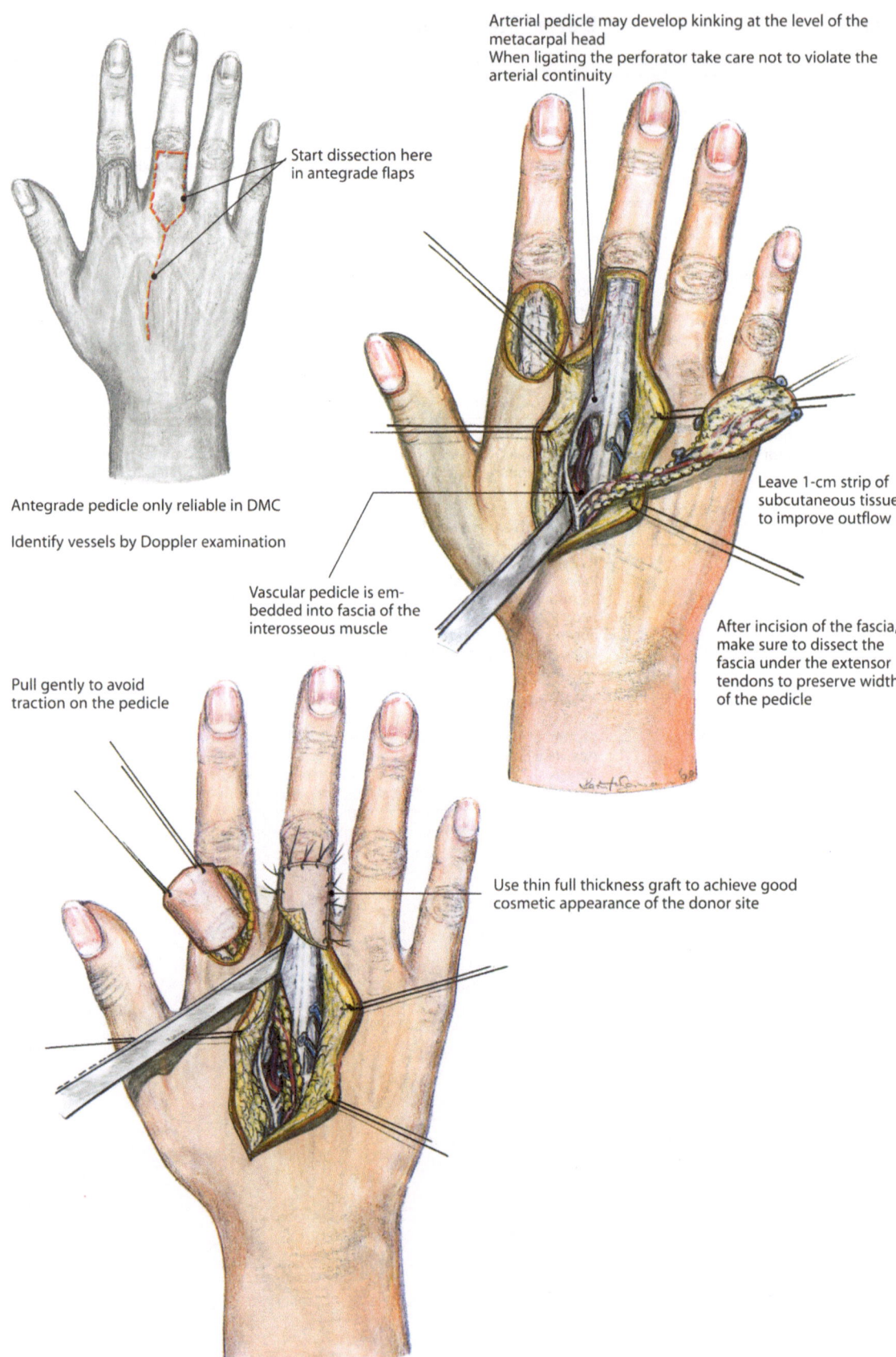

Start dissection here
in antegrade flaps

Arterial pedicle may develop kinking at the level of the
metacarpal head
When ligating the perforator take care not to violate the
arterial continuity

Antegrade pedicle only reliable in DMC

Identify vessels by Doppler examination

Vascular pedicle is em-
bedded into fascia of the
interosseous muscle

Leave 1-cm strip of
subcutaneous tissue
to improve outflow

After incision of the fascia,
make sure to dissect the
fascia under the extensor
tendons to preserve width
of the pedicle

Pull gently to avoid
traction on the pedicle

Use thin full thickness graft to achieve good
cosmetic appearance of the donor site

Flap

Dorsal Metacarpal Artery Flap (2 – 4)

Advantages

Tissue	Flap is thin and pliable
Vascular pedicle	Reliable pedicle with wide arc of rotation (for both pedicles)
Flap size/shape	Can cover even larger digital defect
Combinations	Can be combined with adjacent DMCA flaps for multidigital injuries

Disadvantages

Pedicle	Veins cannot be identified in most cases; flap often appears ischemic during the first few minutes after deflating the tourniquet; venous congestion may occur
Donor site morbidity	Only donor site of smaller flaps can be closed primarily, skin graft on dorsum of the hand can be conspicuous, contour defect improves with time

Tricks/pitfalls

Dissection	Don't make arc of rotation too narrow; venous congestion may occur; preserve paratenon of extensor tendons for perfect skin graft take for donor site; when tunnel for the flap seems too narrow – skin graft pedicle; apply leeches early when venous congestion occurs; avoid any tension on pedicle; when flap does not show adequate reperfusion after opening of the tourniquet, rinse with warm saline; it may take 20 min to re-establish flow
Extensions/combinations	Bony segment from metacarpal may be possible
Contouring/corrections	Rarely required – flap shrinks with time
Clinical applications	**Reserve pedicle flap**
	Small and medium size dorsal digital defects as far as the PIP joint

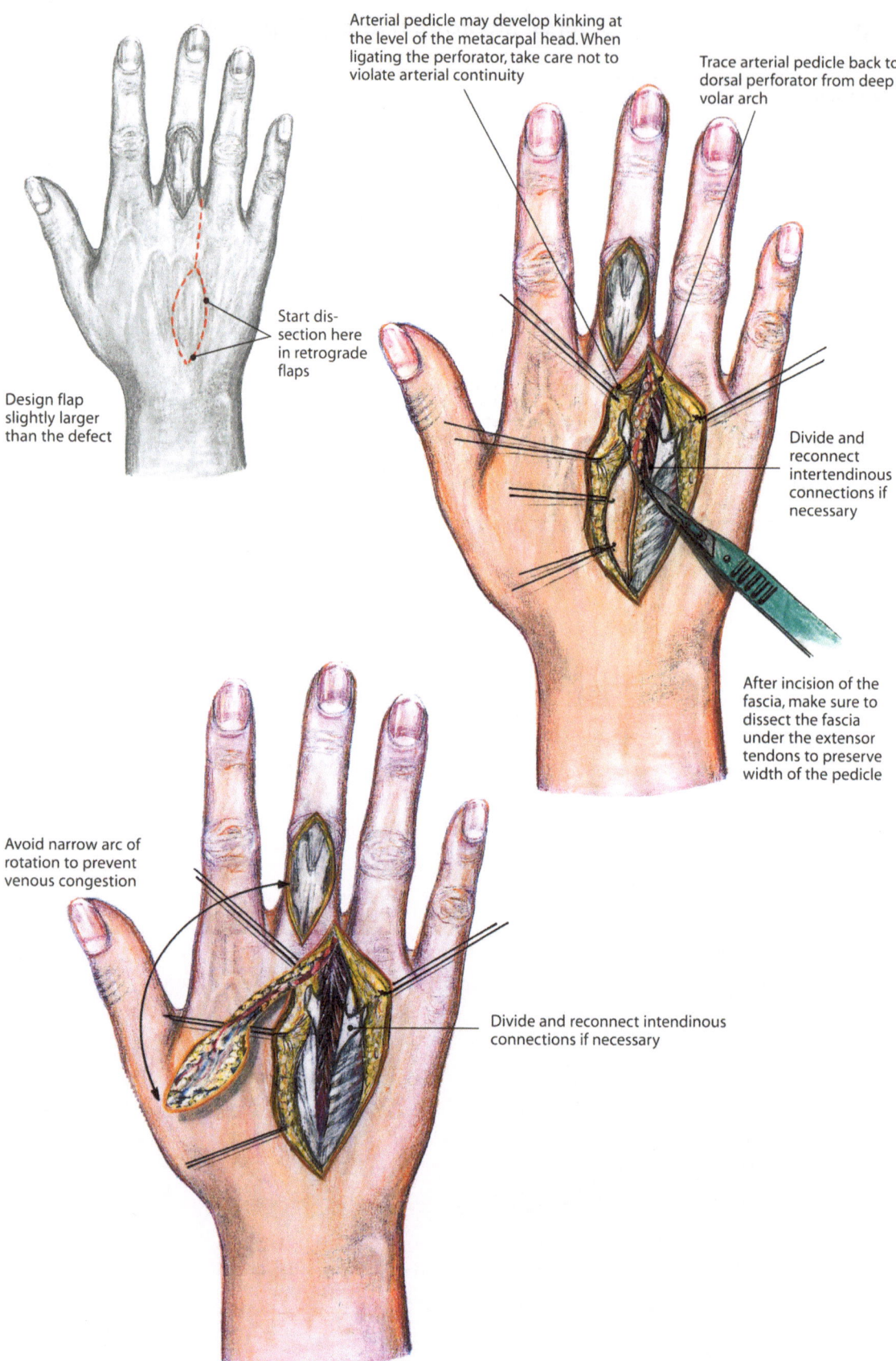

Design flap slightly larger than the defect

Start dis-section here in retrograde flaps

Arterial pedicle may develop kinking at the level of the metacarpal head. When ligating the perforator, take care not to violate arterial continuity

Trace arterial pedicle back to dorsal perforator from deep volar arch

Divide and reconnect intertendinous connections if necessary

After incision of the fascia, make sure to dissect the fascia under the extensor tendons to preserve width of the pedicle

Avoid narrow arc of rotation to prevent venous congestion

Divide and reconnect intendinous connections if necessary

Flap	**Radial Forearm Flap**
Tissue	Pedicle or free flap – distal or proximal pedicle Potentially innervated fasciocutaneous flap with little hair; also possible as fascial flap
Course of the vessels	At the bottom of a fascial septum along the brachioradialis muscle as the leading structure
Dimensions	Maximum 8 × 20 cm
Extensions/combinations	Can be combined with strip of brachioradialis or palmaris longus tendon, a bony segment of the radius, or a second proximal skin island based on a perforator vessel
Anatomy **Neurovascular pedicle** Artery Veins Length Diameter Nerve	 Radial artery Two concomitant veins or cephalic system Depends on flap location on the forearm; up to 15 cm Artery 3–4 mm, veins 3–5 mm (in the case of a free flap) Lateral antebrachial cutaneous nerve
Surgical technique **Preoperative examinations, markings**	 Identify course of radial artery by Doppler examination; Allen's test!
Patient position	Supine position with arm on arm board
Dissection	Mark the flap centered over the course of the vessel; Skin incision and subfascial dissection towards the vessel; stay under the vessels and isolate the pedicle distally; include a cuf of subcutaneous fat and a subcutaneous vein if the flap is raised as a distal pedicle flap; for experienced surgeons – suprafascial dissection possible Distal pedicle flap: Raise flap from distal to proximal; isolate vessels proximally; put vessel clamp on proximal pedicle; check for perfusion or signs of venous congestion; wait for 15 min; leave a subcutaneous vein long; ligate proximal vessels and rotate flap to distal site; check again for perfusion and venous congestion; if congested, connect vein to forearm vein (turbocharging) Proximal pedicle: Put vessel clamp on distal pedicle after isolating the flap; check perfusion; ligate distal vessels
Advantages Dissection Vascular pedicle Flap size/shape Combinations	 Donor and recipient site can be dissected simultaneously Long, reliable pedicle with large caliber vessels; atheroscleosis is rare; can be used as „flow-through" flap when used as a free flap Large flap; can be raised as a multi-island flap with strips of de-epithelialized subcutaneous tissue and fascia between the skin islands; many shapes possible; usually thin and pliable even in obese patients Can be combined with extensions or second skin islands based on perforators, strips of tendons and bony segments of the radius
Disadvantages Pedicle Donor site morbidity	 Sacrifice of a major forearm artery Very conspicuous donor site with potential impairment of tendon function; indication has to be carefully weighed especially in women; graft take can be impaired distally
Tricks/pitfalls Dissection Extensions/combinations Contouring/corrections Clinical applications	 Avoid separating the fascial septum from the vessels! Maintain connections to bone and tendons when combined flaps are raised Flap has only little tendency to sag – corrections are rarely required Defects where flat, thin, and supple flaps are indicated – forearm, dorsum of the hand, donor site appearance can be improved with suprafascial dissection

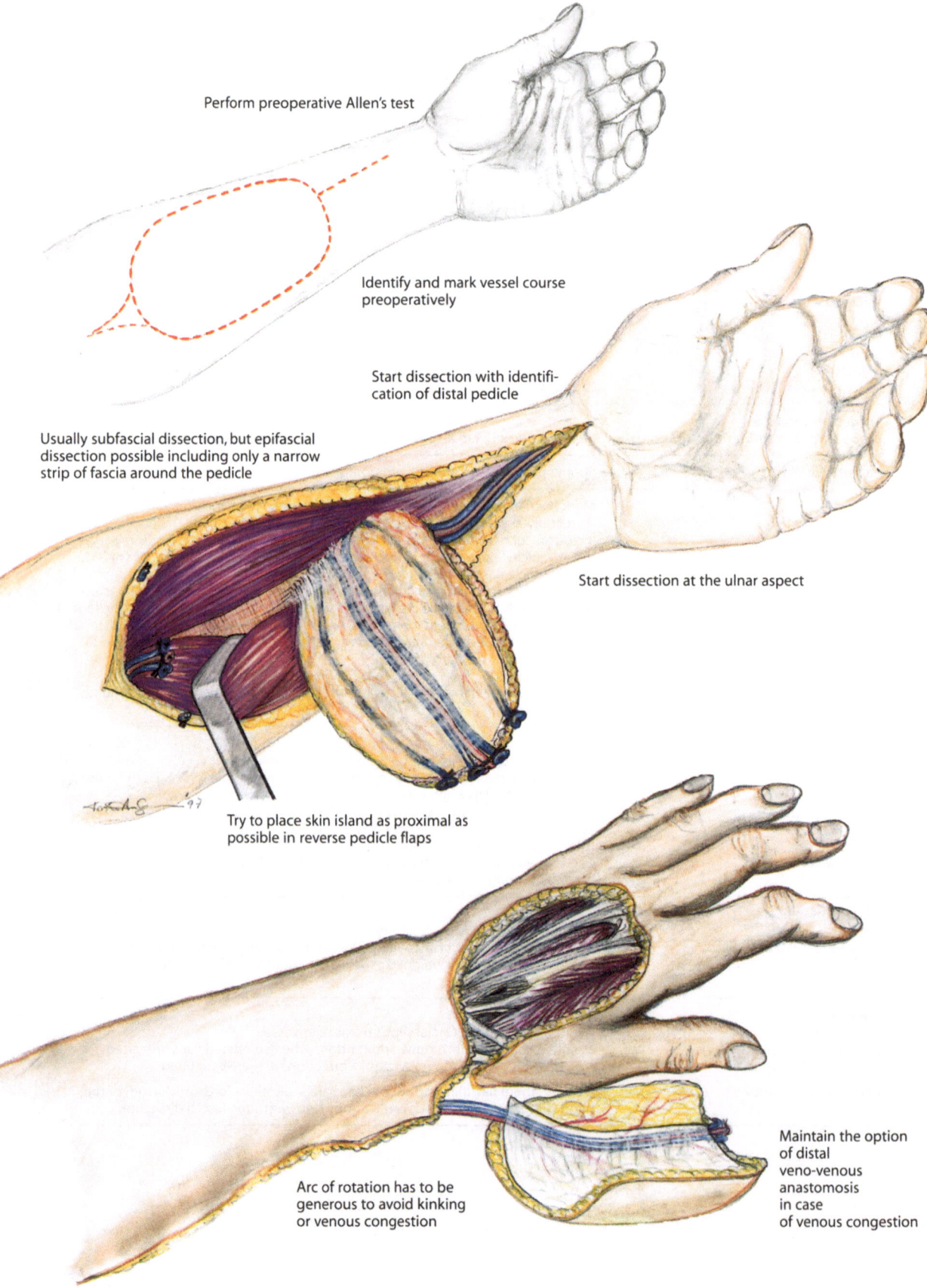

Perform preoperative Allen's test

Identify and mark vessel course
preoperatively

Start dissection with identification of distal pedicle

Usually subfascial dissection, but epifascial
dissection possible including only a narrow
strip of fascia around the pedicle

Start dissection at the ulnar aspect

Try to place skin island as proximal as
possible in reverse pedicle flaps

Arc of rotation has to be
generous to avoid kinking
or venous congestion

Maintain the option
of distal
veno-venous
anastomosis
in case
of venous congestion

Flap	**Posterior Interosseous Flap (Reverse Pedicle Flap)**
Tissue	Skin, fascia
Course of the vessels	Deep to flap surface in a fascial septum. Antegrade vessels in the free flap, recurrent vessels in pedicle flap
Dimensions	8 × 15 cm, flaps of less than 4 cm width should be closed primarily
Extensions/combinations	Tendon strip from ECU, bony segments from radius
Anatomy **Neurovascular pedicle**	
Artery	Posterior interosseous artery; recurrent vessels via anastomosis with anterior interosseous artery through interosseous membrane
Veins	Vv. comitantes
Length	
Diameter	Artery 1–1.5 mm, vein 1 mm
Nerve	Ulnar cutaneous antebrachial branch
Surgical technique **Preoperative examinations, markings**	Draw line from lateral epicondyle to dorsal center of the wrist; identify the two main perforators at the proximal third of the forearm; outline flap centered over the line
Patient position	Supine with arm on arm table; tourniquet ischemia
Dissection	Lateral incision along the marking; incision of muscle fascia; subfascial dissection until fascial septum between EDQ and ECU can be identified; medial incision; subfascial dissection until septum is identified from the other side; free septum from periosteum from distally → cephalad; raise flap and pedicle can be traced to radial artery; apply micro-clamp to proximal pedicle; watch out for nerve branches supplying wrist extensors; open tourniquet; check for adequate perfusion; rotate flap after ligation of pedicle and inset flap in recipient site
Advantages	
Flap size/shape	Donor site of flap of less than 4 cm in width can be closed primarily; subcutaneous fat can provide excellent gliding tissue for tendon reconstructions
Combinations	Inclusion of tendon strip and bone segments enhance versatility
Disadvantages	
Pedicle	Pedicle can contain very small concomitant veins; a tendency for venous congestion has been reported; nerve transection may be required if motor branches cross between main perforators
Bulkiness	Can be bulky in strong patients with fleshy forearms
Donor site morbidity	Donor site can be very conspicuous – not first choice in younger patients and females
Tricks/pitfalls	
Dissection	Try to spare motor nerve; avoid too narrow arc of rotation – flap has a tendency for venous congestion; include a proximal subcutaneous vein for emergency turbo-charging; include a wide segment of dorsal fascia with pedicle; identify arterial anastomosis to anterior interosseous artery first; 5% of all patients do not have this anastomosis
Extensions/combinations	Include tendon strip in subfascial dissection; stay very close to periosteum to avoid injury to the pedicle
Contouring/corrections	Secondary corrections may be required in many cases
Clinical applications	Dorsal defects of the hand; defects of the first web space; defects around the wrist

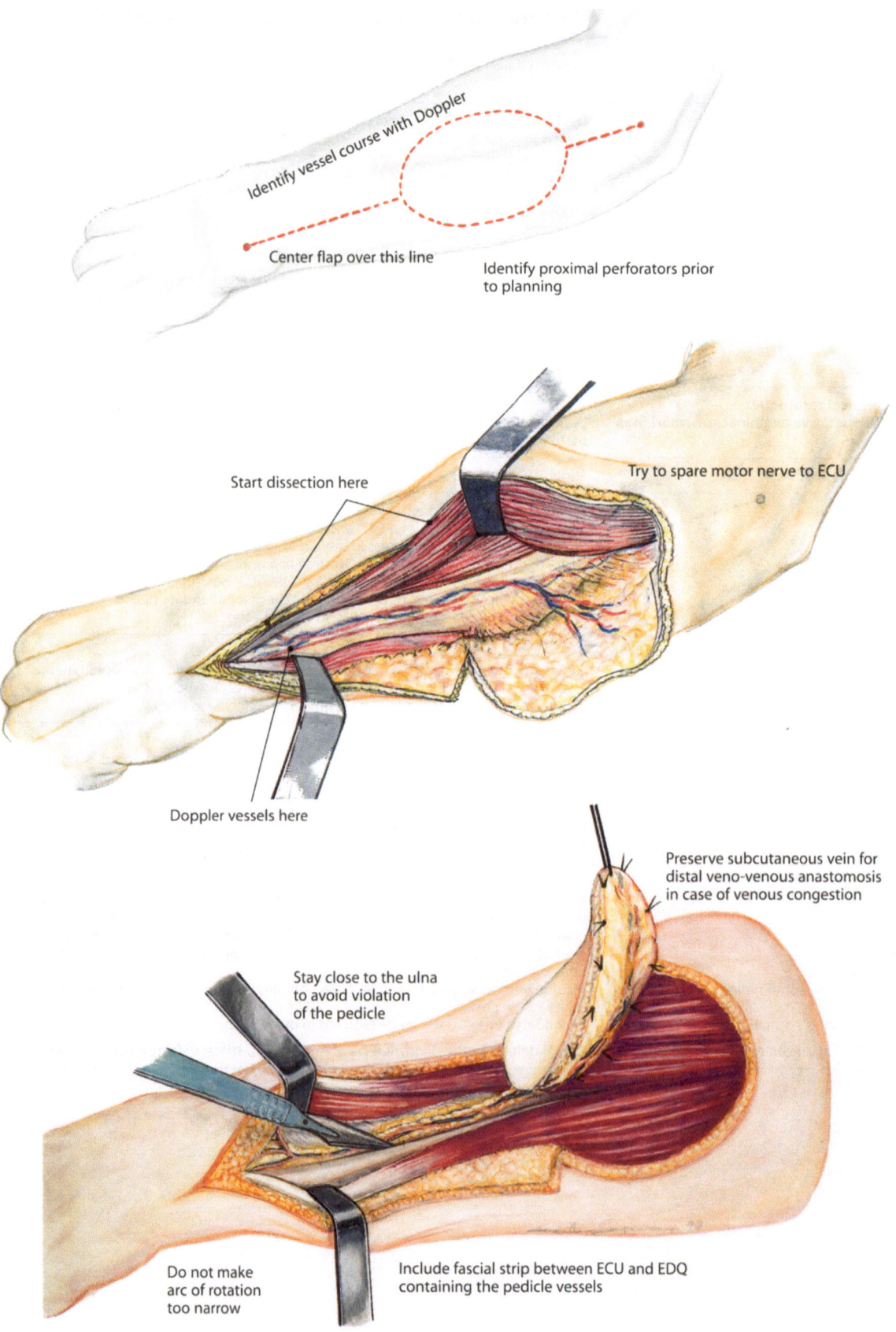

Identify vessel course with Doppler

Center flap over this line

Identify proximal perforators prior to planning

Start dissection here

Try to spare motor nerve to ECU

Doppler vessels here

Preserve subcutaneous vein for distal veno-venous anastomosis in case of venous congestion

Stay close to the ulna to avoid violation of the pedicle

Do not make arc of rotation too narrow

Include fascial strip between ECU and EDQ containing the pedicle vessels

Flap	**Posterior Interosseous Flap** **(Free Flap and Antegrade Pedicle Flap)**
Tissue	Skin, fascia
Course of the vessels	Deep to flap surface in a fascial septum; antegrade vessels in the free flap
Dimensions	8 × 15 cm, flaps of less than 4 cm width should be closed primarily
Extensions/combinations	Tendon strip from ECU; bony segments from radius
Neurovascular pedicle Artery Veins Length Diameter Nerve	Posterior interosseous artery; antegrade vessel from radial artery Vv. comitantes Pedicle length: 3–4 cm Artery 2–3 mm; vein 2.5–3.5 mm Ulnar cutaneous antebrachial branch
Surgical technique **Preoperative examinations, markings**	Draw line from lateral epicondyle to dorsal center of the wrist; identify the two main perforators at the proximal third of the forearm; outline flap centered over the line
Patient position	Supine with arm on arm table; tourniquet ischemia
Dissection	Lateral incision along the marking; incision of muscle fascia; subfascial dissection until fascial septum between EDQ and ECU can be identified; medial incision; subfascial dissection until septum is identified from the other side; free septum from periosteum from distally cephalad; ligate pedicle distally; raise flap until pedicle branches off in direction to radial artery; watch out for nerve branches supplying wrist extensors; open tourniquet; check for adequate perfusion; rotate flap or ligate pedicle and inset flap in recipient site

Advantages	
Vascular pedicle	Adequate caliber
Flap size/shape	Donor site of flap of less than 4 cm in width can be closed primarily; subcutaneous fat can provide excellent gliding tissue for tendon reconstructions
Combinations	Inclusion of tendon strip and bone segments enhance versatility
Disadvantages	
Pedicle	Pedicle is short; nerve transsection may be required if motor branches cross between main perforators
Bulkiness	Can be bulky in strong patients with fleshy forearms
Donor site morbidity	Donor site can be very conspicuous – not first choice in younger patients and females
Tricks/pitfalls	
Dissection	Try to spare motor nerve; avoid too narrow arc of rotation – flap has a tendency for venous congestion; include a proximal subcutaneous vein for emergency turo-charging; include a wide segment of dorsal fascia with pedicle; identify arterial anastomosis to anterior interosseous artery first; 5% of all patients do not have this anastomosis
Extensions/combinations	Include tendon strip in subfascial dissection; stay very close to periosteum to avoid injury to the pedicle
Contouring/corrections	Secondary corrections may be required in many cases
Clinical applications	Forearm defects; dorsal hand defects; complex reconstructions with free non-vascularized tendon grafts; defect around the elbow when used as a proximal pedicle flap

Flap	**Reverse Ulnar Perforator Flap**
Tissue	Skin or fascia
Course of the vessels	Underneath the flap in scarpa's fascia; passes laterally under FCU
Dimensions	4 × 15 cm at the ulnar aspect of the forearm
Extensions/combinations	
Anatomy **Neurovascular pedicle** Artery Veins Length/arc of rotation	Distal perforator (4 cm from wrist) of ulnar artery Vv. comitantes Flap reaches proximal palm of the wrist joint
Surgical technique **Preoperative examinations, markings**	Doppler identification of perforator vessel; flap centered over the lateral ulnar aspect of the forearm
Patient position	Supine with arm on arm table; tourniquet ischemia
Dissection	Skin incision along the markings; subfascial dissection with sparing of ulnar artery and nerve; preservation of extensor paratenon; identify distal perforator; distal skin incision when taken as an island flap; otherwise leave distal skin bridge intact; open tourniquet; check flap for perfusion; rotate into defect
Advantages Dissection Vascular pedicle Flap size/shape Combinations	Dissection is easy and straightforward Reliable and easy to identify Large flap possible Inclusion of tendon strip (FCU) possible
Disadvantages Flap Bulkiness Donor site morbidity	Flap leaves dog-ear at pivot point frequently requiring secondary corrections; donor site has to be skin grafted in the majority of cases Flap may be bulky Skin grafted area may be conspicuous, impairment of tendon gliding rarely encountered
Tricks/pitfalls Dissection Extensions/combinations Contouring/corrections Clinical applications	Do not violate paratenon; identify perforator prior to dissection; frequently check integrity of perforator when proceeding distally with the dissection Inclusion of tendon strip (FCU) Contouring after 6 months; frequently smaller dog-ears – smooth out Long, narrow defects around the wrist

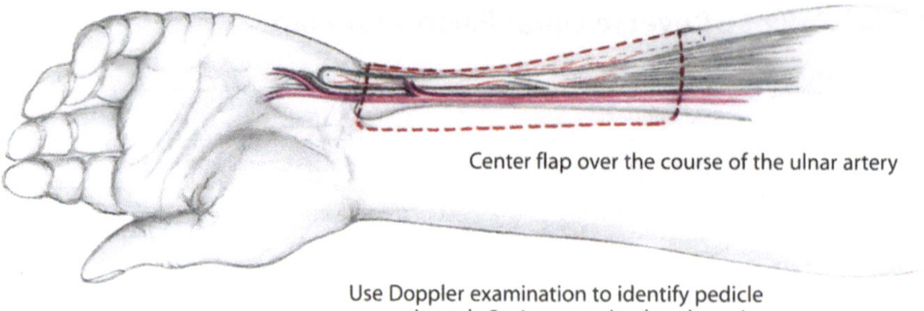

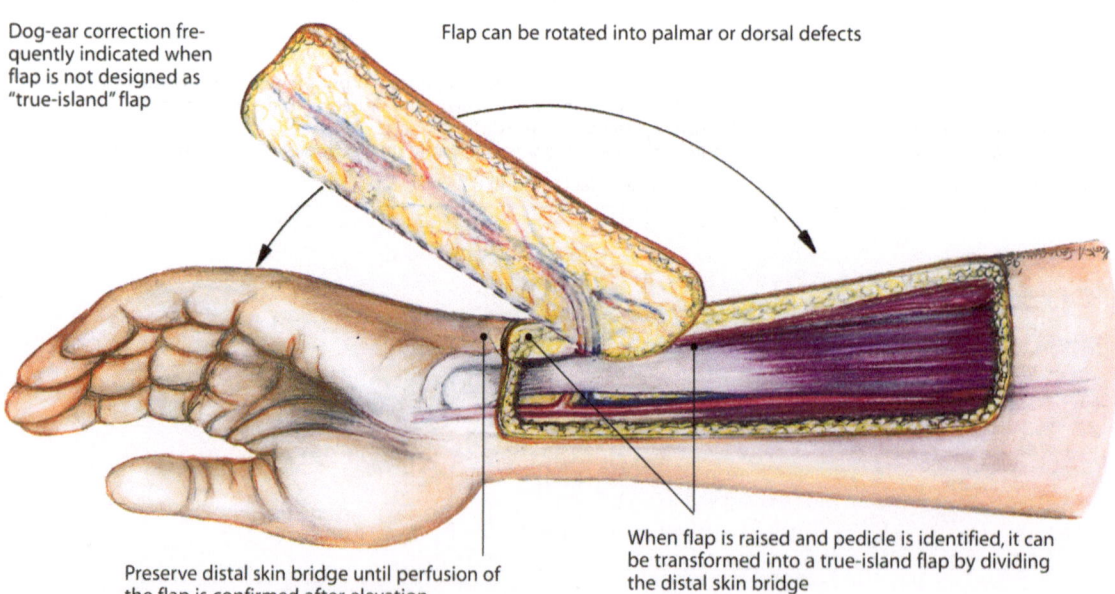

Center flap over the course of the ulnar artery

Use Doppler examination to identify pedicle approximately 3–4 cm proximal to the wrist crease

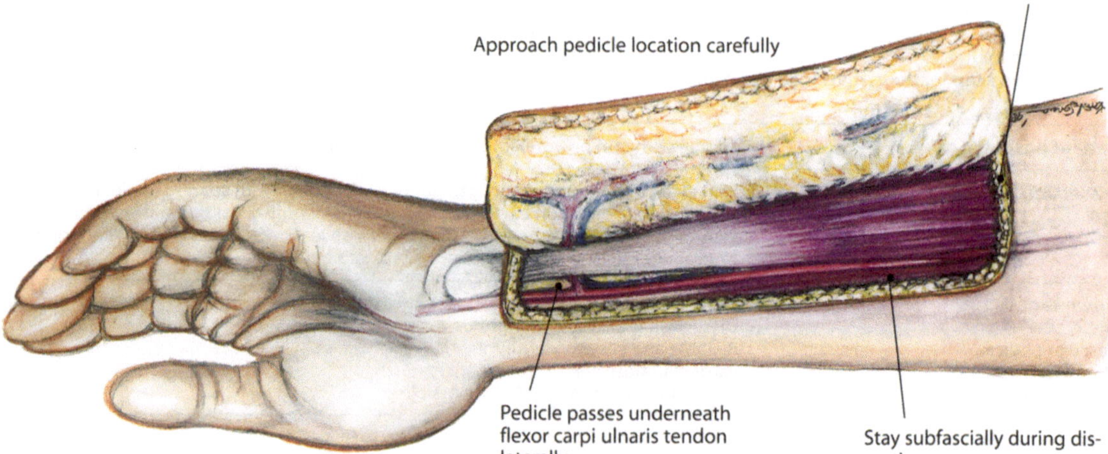

Approach pedicle location carefully

Start with dissection proximally, proceed distally

Pedicle passes underneath flexor carpi ulnaris tendon laterally

Stay subfascially during dissection

Dog-ear correction frequently indicated when flap is not designed as "true-island" flap

Flap can be rotated into palmar or dorsal defects

Preserve distal skin bridge until perfusion of the flap is confirmed after elevation

When flap is raised and pedicle is identified, it can be transformed into a true-island flap by dividing the distal skin bridge

Flap	Lateral Arm Flap
	Pedicle or free flap, antegrade or reverse pedicle
Tissue	Innervated cutaneous flap, frequently non-hair-bearing, also de-epithelialized as subcutaneous fascial flap
Course of the vessels	In a fascial plane deep along the humerus; perforators enter the flap via a delicate septum from the undersurface
Dimensions	Up to 15 × 8 cm (primary closure only possible up to 6 × 12 cm)
Extensions/combinations	Flap can be harvested as osteocutaneous flap with a segment from the humerus; can include a fasciocutaneous forearm extension
Anatomy **Neurovascular pedicle** Artery Veins Length Diameter Nerve	 Posterior radial collateral artery (branch of the profunda brachii artery – PRCA); distal flow from recurrent radial collateral artery from the articular network around the elbow Two concomitant veins and cephalic system Up to 8 cm Artery 1.5–2 mm, veins 2–2.5 mm Posterior cutaneous forearm nerve from the radial nerve
Surgical technique **Preoperative examinations, markings**	 Doppler identification of vessel course recommended; mark insertion of deltoid muscle and lateral condyle; outline flap dimensions centered over this line
Patient position	Supine; arm draped to allow free movement; lying on an arm table or fixed across the chest; tourniquet recommended, but sometimes hard to hold in place
Dissection	**Free flap and antergrade pedicle flap** Start with posterior incision down to muscle fascia; raise subfascially and tack fascia to skin to prevent sheering; continue to anterior border of triceps muscle; here fascia dives deep and inserts into humerus; perforators are seen in the septum; anterior incision down to fascia; subfascial dissection including the flexor muscles fascia; pursuit of fascia down to humerus; ligate distal continuation of PRCA; separate fascial septum as close as possible to the periosteium; follow the pedicle proximally under the triceps muscle into the spiral groove; separate lower cutaneous nerve from radial nerve **Reverse pedicle flap** Proceed with dissection as in the free flap dissection; ligate proximal inflow; pursue distal pedicle in direction to the elbow; Fasciocutaneous forearm extension: Flap can be extended 5 cm distal to the elbow; width is similar to lateral arm flap; raise extension also subfascially; include recurrent pedicle as long as possible
Advantages Dissection Vascular pedicle Flap size/shape Combinations	 Flap dissection is rapid for experienced surgeons; simultaneous two-team approach possible Reliable constant pedicle with moderate diameter Thin flap of various shapes, optimal shape is oval Very versatile due to optional combinations with bone, tendon strip from the triceps, or forearm fascia extension
Disadvantages Flap Donor site morbidity Pedicle	 Depending on the patient, the flap can be bulky due to the subcutaneous layer Scar is conspicuous; only donor sites up to 6 cm flap width can be closed primarily; otherwise skin graft is required; no functional loss except numbness on the lateral forearm Pedicle is short; vascular diameter can be small, especially in women
Tricks/pitfalls Dissection Extensions/combinations Contouring/corrections Clinical applications	 Do not confuse the nerve branches; stay extremely close to the periosteum of the humerus in order to preserve the delicate septum; tack fascia to the skin to prevent shear forces; repair tendon donor site in the triceps muscle Try to center a perforator over the strip of periosteum taken with the bony segment; Posterior cutaneous nerve can be harvested as a vascularized nerve graft Flap shows a tendency to sag – contour corrections are frequently needed Defects of the dorsum of the hand; the first web space; defects around the elbow and the shoulder region when used as a distal or proximal pedicle flap

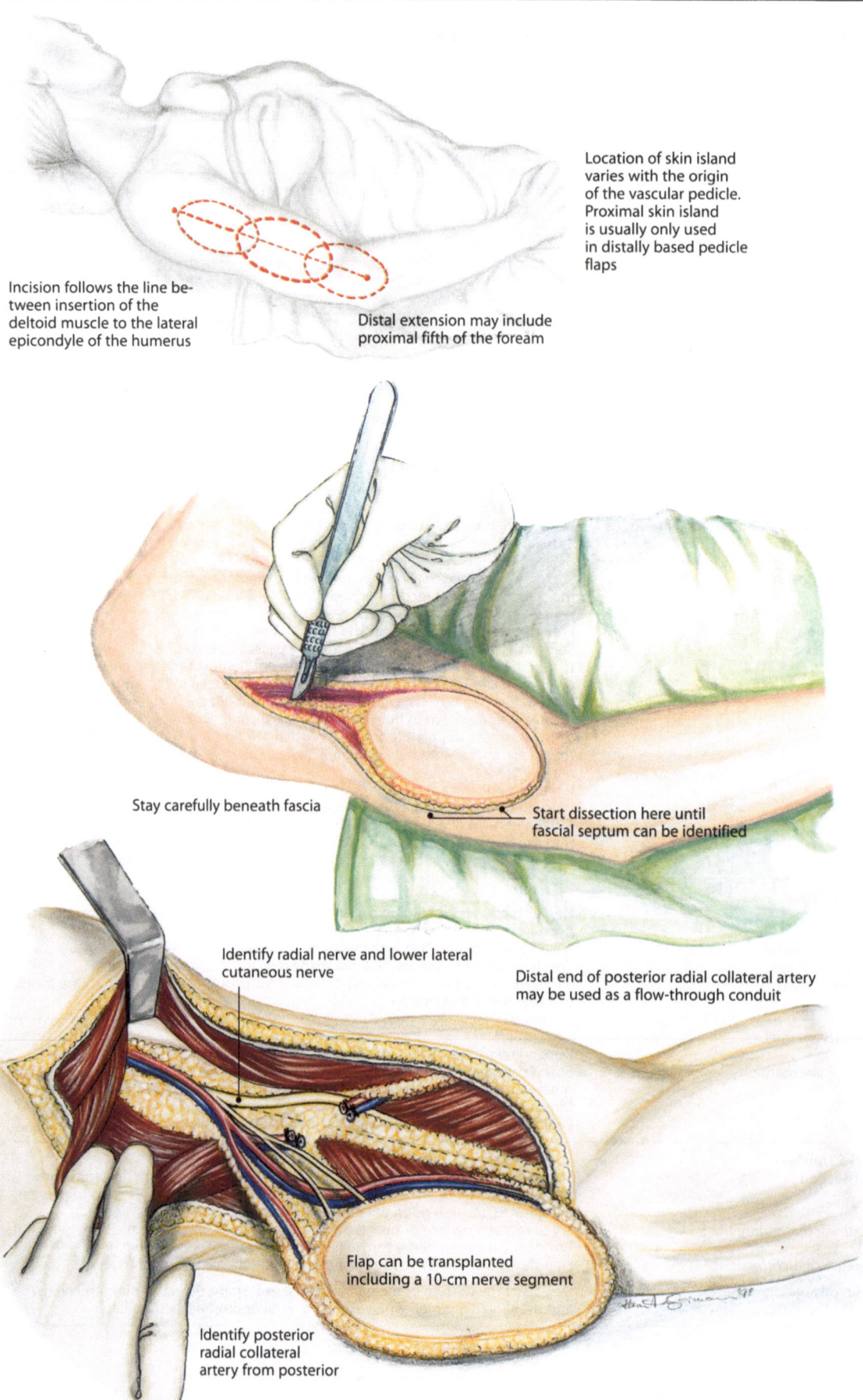

Location of skin island
varies with the origin
of the vascular pedicle.
Proximal skin island
is usually only used
in distally based pedicle
flaps

Incision follows the line between insertion of the
deltoid muscle to the lateral
epicondyle of the humerus

Distal extension may include
proximal fifth of the foream

Stay carefully beneath fascia

Start dissection here until
fascial septum can be identified

Identify radial nerve and lower lateral
cutaneous nerve

Distal end of posterior radial collateral artery
may be used as a flow-through conduit

Flap can be transplanted
including a 10-cm nerve segment

Identify posterior
radial collateral
artery from posterior

Flap	Parascapular/Scapular Flap
Tissue	Cutaneous flap, non-hair-bearing, can also be de-epithelialized as subcutaneous fascial flap – pedicle or free
Course of the vessels	Parallel to the skin above the deep fascia
Dimensions	8–10 × 20–25 cm (parascapular flap) 10–15 × 12–25 cm (scapula flap)
Extensions/combinations	Fascial extensions; any combination with other flaps from the subscapular system
Anatomy **Neurovascular pedicle** Artery Veins Length Diameter Nerve	 Constant branch of the circumflex scapular artery (CSA); vertical branch for parascapular flap; horizontal branch for scapular flap Two concomitant veins 6–10 cm Artery: 1.5–3 mm; veins: 2–4 mm No sensory nerve
Surgical technique **Preoperative examinations, markings**	 Doppler identification of vessels (horizontal and vertical branch), identification and marking of triangular space, tip of the scapula, scapula spine, spine, border of latissimus dorsi muscle
Patient position	Midlateral or oblique prone position
Dissection	**Parascapular flap** Start with low medial incision (retrograde evlevation); identification of epifascial plane; proceed cranially to the area of the triangular space; complete skin incision; identify fatty tissue around the pedicle; carefully retract flap medially; ligate or clip muscle and bone branches very carefully; follow pedicle into the triangular space; identify thoraco-dorsal or subscapular artery; check flap perfusion; pedicle transsection or flap transfer Some authors favor the identification of the vascular pedicle as the first step of the dissection! **Scapula flap** Same strategy of dissection as for the parascapular flap – Start dissection laterally and proceed towards triangular space. As in the parascapular flap, the vascular pedicle can also be identified first in the course of the dissection!
Advantages Vascular pedicle Flap size/shape Combinations	 Long; reliable; large caliber; arc of rotation as a pedicle flap reaches the axillary fold and the dorsal brachium Large flaps possible with medial and lateral extensions, scapular fascial extension; uniform thickness of flap; can also be used as a "burried flap" when de-epithelialized Possible with all flaps from the subscapular system; very valuable: combination with bone parts for segmental forearm defects; bone segments can be harvested medially and laterally
Further options	Leaves most of the other flaps from the subscapular system available
Disadvantages Bulkiness Donor site morbidity	 Thickness depends on patient's body habitus – sometimes too bulky No functional loss; conspicuous scarring when scar widens; only donor sites of 8–12 cm width can be closed primarily!!
Tricks/pitfalls Dissection Extensions/combinations Contouring/corrections Clinical applications	 Watch out for fatty tissue around the pedicle; put some stay sutures in for careful flap retraction; **Do not severe large muscular/bony branch** (comes very soon after the pedicle dives deep); have the patient deeply relaxed during pedicle dissection (facilitates dissection into the axilla); use long blade retractors to open triangular space When fascial extension is raised; take alveolar and subcutaneous tissue with the deep muscle fascia; otherwise fascia is avital!! most combined flaps can be raised without altering patient position, do not violate bony/muscular branch when taking a bone segment; include a muscle cuff!! axillary incision only required when flap is combined with other flaps from the subscapular system; in the case of combined flaps, do not transect the pedicle before anatomic variations have been excluded! May be necessary – Flap tends to sag – Debulking may be required (Liposuction can be difficult due to the structure of the dorsal fatty tissue) Resurfacing of forearm and dorsum of the hand; provision of skin coverage and gliding tissue for flexor and extensor tendons, when fascial extension is included; perfect for segmental defects of the forearm; defects of the shoulder area and the dorsal brachium when used as a pedicle flap

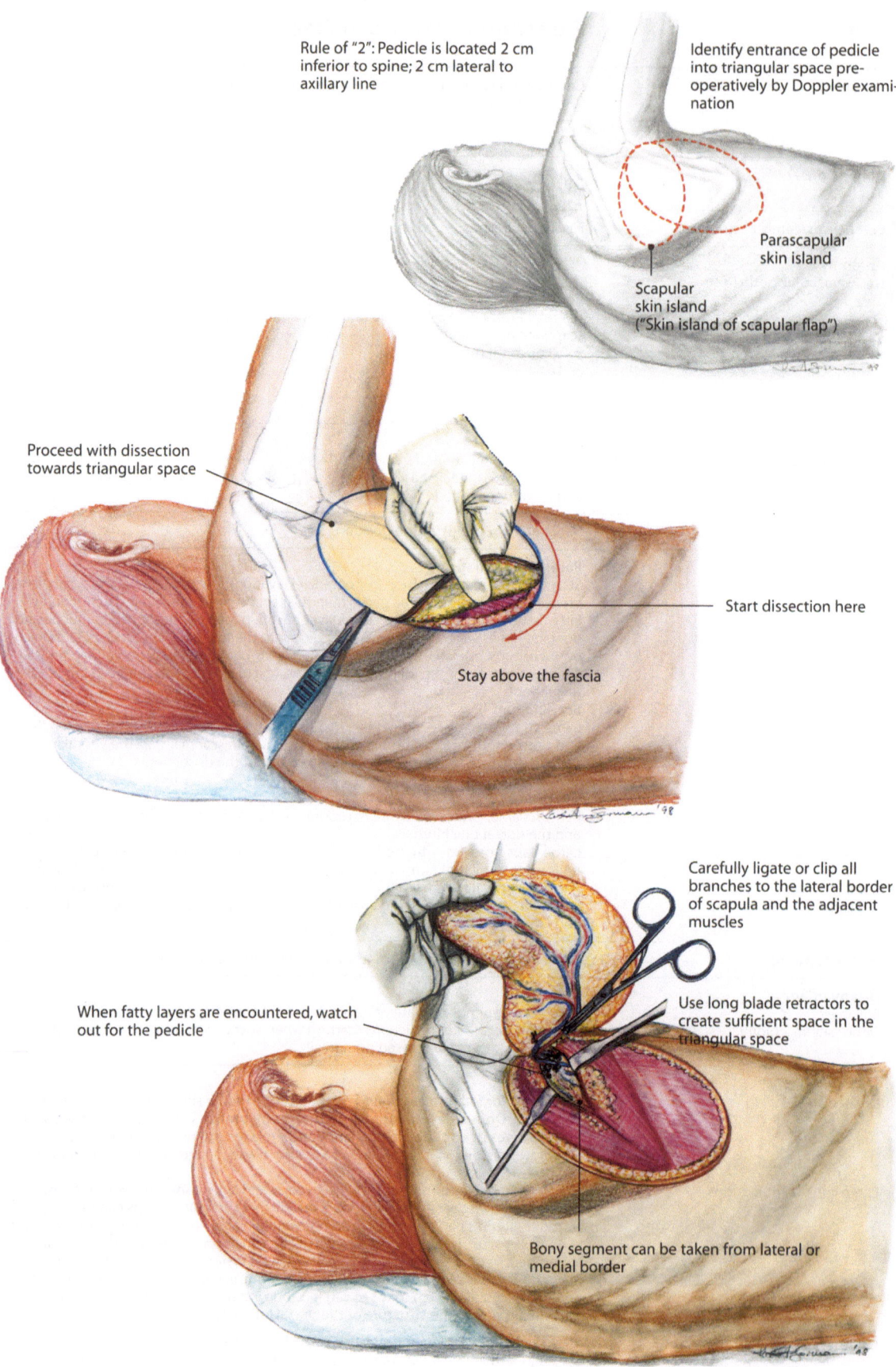

Rule of "2": Pedicle is located 2 cm inferior to spine; 2 cm lateral to axillary line

Identify entrance of pedicle into triangular space pre-operatively by Doppler examination

Parascapular skin island

Scapular skin island ("Skin island of scapular flap")

Proceed with dissection towards triangular space

Start dissection here

Stay above the fascia

Carefully ligate or clip all branches to the lateral border of scapula and the adjacent muscles

When fatty layers are encountered, watch out for the pedicle

Use long blade retractors to create sufficient space in the triangular space

Bony segment can be taken from lateral or medial border

Flap	**Latissimus Dorsi Flap**
Tissue	Muscle or musculocutaneous flap – pedicle or free
Course of the vessels	From the axilla along the anterior border of the muscle. Enters the muscle from underneath; spreads into three major branches at the undersurface of the muscle
Dimensions	Can be tailored to almost any size; maximum dimensions 20 × 35 cm
Extensions/combinations	Can be raised as muscle, musculocutaneous, and perforator flap. Combinations are possible with any component from the subscapular system (bone, skin, fascia, muscle)
Neurovascular pedicle Artery Veins Length Diameter Nerve	 Thoracodorsal artery One vein usually originating from the subscapular vein Up to 15 cm, branches of the subscapular system; anatomical variations in 3%–5% Artery: 2–4 mm; vein: 2–5 mm Motor nerve; some studies report deep sensation 18 months after coaptation to sensory recipient
Surgical technique **Preoperative examinations, markings**	 No vessel identification necessary. In cases of previous axilla dissection or radiation, check muscle function; if muscle function is intact vessels are usually not violated; mark anterior muscle border and tip of the scapula to outline flap borders
Patient position	Mid-lateral; arm elevated 90°
Dissection	Mark flap dimensions; start with incision along muscle border; identify muscle border and branch to serratus muscle; identify pedicle and follow pedicle to origin; free anterior border of the muscle and raise flap from ventral in dorsal direction to the spine; take care to coagulate or ligate the perforating vessels; divide muscle distally as required; divide muscle at the spine insertions; raise muscle in cranial direction; ligate serratus branches; check perfusion; divide pedicle
Advantages Vascular pedicle Flap size/shape Combinations	 Long; reliable; large-caliber vessels Any flap size possible; the latissimus dorsi is the largest muscle in the body Numerous combinations possible; multicomponent flaps with other flaps from the subscapular system; vascularized bone can be harvested as rib grafts with the latissimus or on a connected pedicle from the scapula; fascia can be added from the serratus muscle
Further options	Scapular flaps are still available if latissimus is harvested correctly; serratus muscle is available, but vessels are small
Disadvantages Bulkiness Donor site morbidity	 Muscle can be bulky; skin islands in musculocutaneous flaps are usually bulky and require secondary contour correction Donor scar rather conspicuous; functional loss of shoulder function of approximately 7%
Tricks/pitfalls Dissection Extensions/combinations Contouring/corrections Clinical applications	 Watch out for constant large perforator vessels at the tip of the scapula (ligate); finalize dissection of the pedicle by splitting the fascial leaf that separates the latissimus from the teres muscles from dorsal; ligate branch to the scapula; do not confuse it with second branch to the muscle; take skin island as a monitoring island even in pure muscle flaps; harvest additional skin; store in the refrigerator; take skin island off after 5 days and transplant stored skin as a bedside procedure Dissect pedicle up to axillary artery to rule out anomalies of the vascular system so that all components are nourished by one pedicle; there are anomalies, operative strategy has to be adjusted to perform additional micro-anastomoses Muscle flaps usually shrink and contouring is required in approximately 50% of cases; musculocutaneous flaps almost all tend to sag and need contouring; in the case of functional muscle transfers, re-adjusting muscle tension is sometimes required Coverage of large surface area defects; functional free muscle transfer for loss of forearm flexor and extensor systems; pedicle muscle transfer for restoration of biceps function

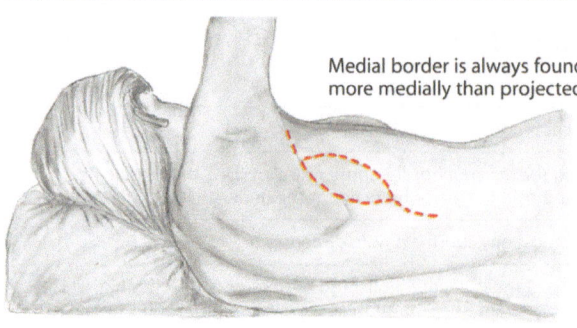

Medial border is always found
more medially than projected

Make skin island not too small
to allow reliable clinical monitoring

Identify pedicle first

Proceed with dissection along
the medial border. Divide
distally and move
towards the spine

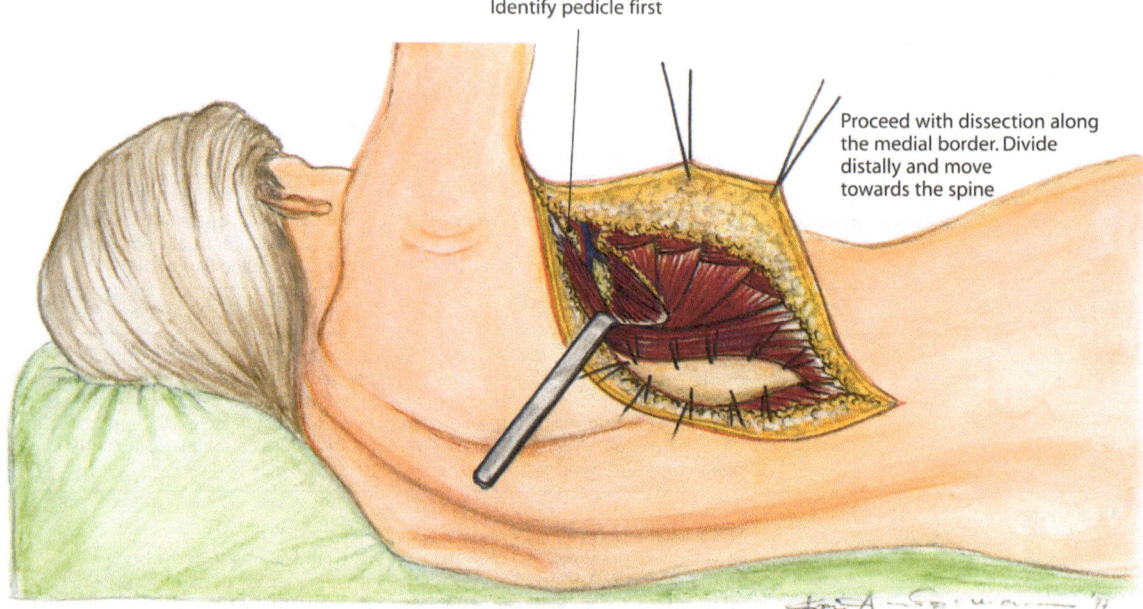

Leave tendon insertion intact until
the dissection is completed

Insert suction drain into the axilla and
lower donor site to prevent seromas

Coagulate all minor
perforators, clip or ligate
major perforators

Leave circumflex scapular artery
intact for possible future use

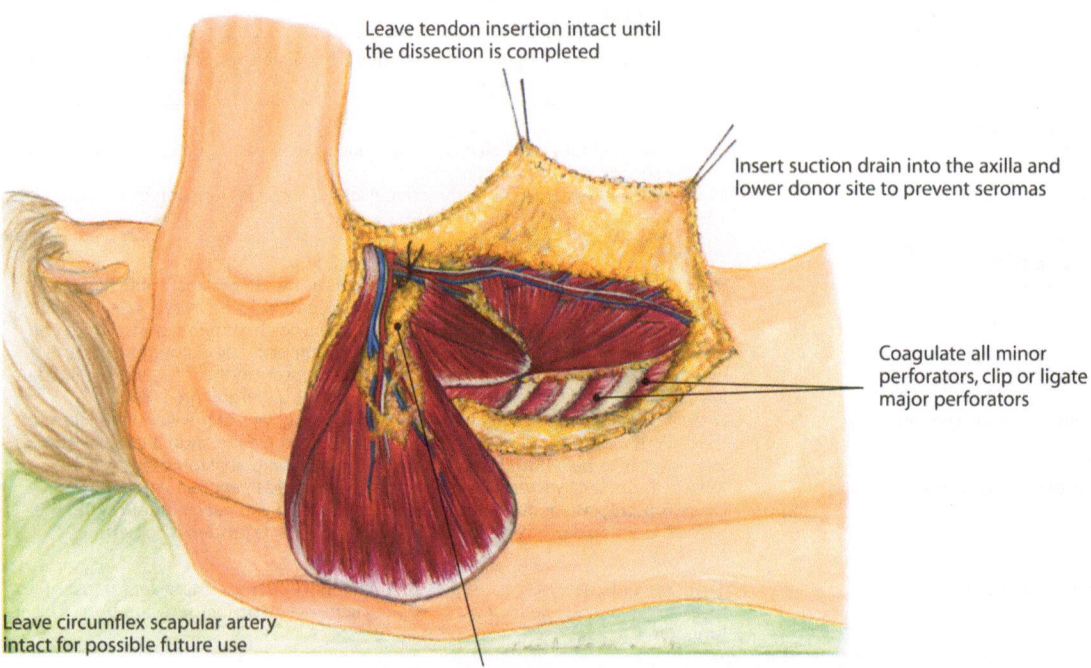

Mark nerve with 5–0 suture; this facilitates manipulation of the pedicle
during microsurgery
Clip branches of pedicle to avoid bleeding after vascular micro-
anastomosis

Flap	Seratus Muscle/Fascia Flap

Tissue	Muscle or fascia (lower three muscle slips)
Course of the vessels	On the muscle surface
Dimensions	10 × 15 cm (muscle flap) – 10 × 18 cm (fascia flap)
Extensions/combinations	Skin island – vacularized ribs

Anatomy
Neurovascular pedicle

Artery	Serrratus arcade es extension of thoraco-dorsal pedicle, direct serratus branches branch of the thoraco-dorsal artery in > 97 %
Veins	Vv. comitantes
Length	Up to 16 cm (when thoraco-dorsal pedicle is harvested)
Diameter	Artery: 3.5–4.5 mm, vein: 4–6 mm (when thoraco-dorsal pedicle is harvested), Artery: 1–1.5 mm, vein 1–1.5 mm (when only serratus arcade is taken)
Nerve	Long thoracic nerve (does not always have to be included into the flap)

Surgical technique

Preoperative examinations, markings	Mark anterior border of the latissimus dorsi muscle – tip of scapula; 5th–8th rib
Patient position	Patient in lateral position, arm elevated 90°

Dissection	**Muscle flap**
	Slightly curved incision along the border of the latissimus muscle; identification of muscle border and identification of serratus arcade; check if thoracodorsal pedicle is intact; determination of entrance points of motor fibers into the muscle; outline of flap size on the muscle surface; medial incision of muscle; ligation, coagulation or clipping of intercostal vessels to keep bleeding down; release the muscle from thoracic wall; preservation of three proximal slips to prevent wing scapula; dissection of thoracodorsal pedicle to the length required; check flap for perfusion; transfer flap
	Fascia flap
	Slightly curved incision along the border of the latissimus muscle; identification of muscle border and identification of serratus arcade; check if thoracodorsal pedicle is intact; determination of entrance points of motor fibers into the muscle; outline of flap size on the muscle surface; raise fascia from muscle surface; coagulate smaller vessels; preserve motor nerve; dissect thoracodorsal pedicle to the required length; check perfusion; transfer

Advantages

Vascular pedicle	Very long pedicle possible; extremely reliable
Flap size/shape	Thin and pliable as fascial flap; minimal donor morbidity
Combinations	Vascularized ribs can be harvested with the flap, a small skin island can be included as a monitor island; any combination with other flaps from the subscapular system possible

Disadvantages

Flap	Dissection can be tedious due to many small intercostal connections; injury to motor nerve may cause wing scapula; fascia is delicate and can easily be perforated
Bulkiness	Muscle flap can be bulky
Donor site morbidity	Acceptable – no funtional loss except when wing scapula occurs; donor scar is inconspicuous

Tricks/pitfalls

Dissection	Identify where motor fiber enters the muscle; avoid injury to the nerve; the nerve runs laterally from the vascular pedicle; preserve upper slips; flaps tend to bleed profusely as a fascial flap; delayed secondary skin grafting is recommended
Extensions/combinations	Bone defects can be simultaneously reconstructed with vascularized rig grafts
Contouring/corrections	Rarely required
Clinical applications	Perfect for mid-size defects requiring thin and pliable tissue; gliding tissue for tendon reconstruction; fascial flap mechanically stable: defects of the dorsum of the hand and forearm, exposed elbow joints

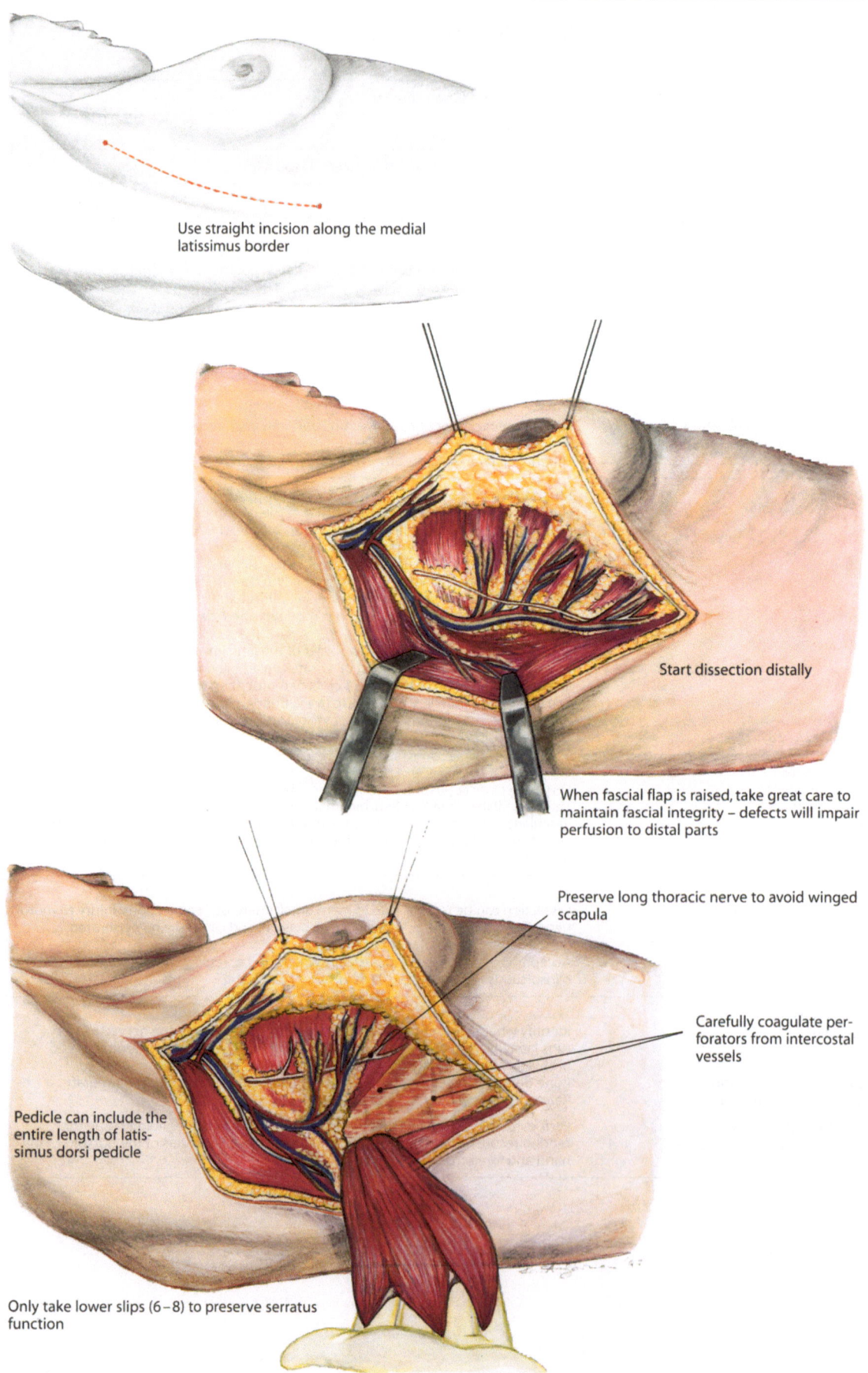

Use straight incision along the medial latissimus border

Start dissection distally

When fascial flap is raised, take great care to maintain fascial integrity – defects will impair perfusion to distal parts

Preserve long thoracic nerve to avoid winged scapula

Carefully coagulate perforators from intercostal vessels

Pedicle can include the entire length of latissimus dorsi pedicle

Only take lower slips (6 – 8) to preserve serratus function

Flap	**Temporal Fascia Flap**
Tissue	Fascia (thickness 1.5–3 mm)
Course of the vessels	Subcutaneously on the fascia from pre-auricular into the temporal fossa
Dimensions	8 × 15 cm
Extensions/combinations	Can be combined with the deep fascial layer or calvarian bone
Anatomy **Neurovascular pedicle** Artery Veins Length Diameter Nerve	 Common pedicle with deep fascia (proximal branch of STV/STA) – there are **no communicating vessels distal to common pedicle** Superficial temporal artery (STA-terminal branch of the carotid artery) Superficial temporal vein (STV) 2–4 cm without incising the parotid gland Artery: 1.5–2.7 mm; vein: 2.0–3.2 mm The auriculotemporal nerve is included in the fascial layer, but the flap is not innervated
Surgical technique **Preoperative examinations, markings**	 Doppler identification of the course of the vessels; marking of the incision line parallel to hair follicles; outline of flap dimensions
Patient position	Supine with head slightly tilted to the opposite side
Dissection	T-shape outline; start incision by raising a pretragal skin flap; identify and spare STV anterior and exterior to STA; identify STA; dissection proceeds cephalad deep to hair follicles; avoid damage to the very superficial vein!! use bipolar coagulation for terminal branches to subdermal plexus; do not damage frontal branch of facial nerve! after cephalad completion of dissection, incise flap; lift flap from deep fascial plane towards auricle; leave flap after completed dissection for observation of perfusion
Advantages Tissue Vascular pedicle Flap size/shape Donor site Combinations	 Flap is thin and pliable; cover without bulk Reliable pedicle with sufficient caliber and length Considerable flap size that can cover for example the entire dorsum of the hand without bulk Dissection of flap and donor site can be carried out simultaneously Donor site completely inconspicuous; no functional loss Can be combined with the deep temporal fascial layer. In this case the middle temporal vessel at the level of the zygoma has to be preserved. Possible combination with calvaria bone graft
Disadvantages Pedicle Flap Donor site	 Pedicle short; vein easy to damage due to it superficial location; sometimes vein is absent Capillary bleeding may jeopardize graft take Frontal nerve may be damaged during dissection Alopecia may result if superficial plane of dissection is too close to hair follicles
Tricks/pitfalls Dissection Extensions/combinations Contouring/corrections/flap Clinical applications	 Watch out for the superficial temporal vein When comined with deep layer; preserve middle temporal vessel Contour correction almost never indicated; delayed skin grafting recommended due to tendency for edema and capillary bleeding Dorsum of the hand; deep defects of the palm; degloving injuries of the digits; gliding tissue in scarred wound beds

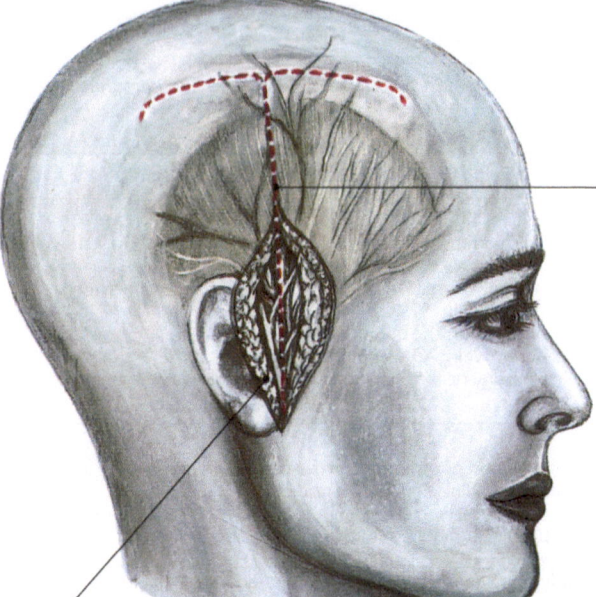

Define and mark the course of the pedicle by Doppler examination preoperatively

Inject the scalp donor site with xylocaine (¹/₂%) and epinephrine (1/2 000 000) prior to the dissection for better visualization and hemostasis

Alopecia may occur along incision line

Vascular anomalies can be found. Try to identify draining veins by placing a slight tourniquet around the head above the ear

Do not violate hair follicles to avoid alopecia

Identify fascular pedicle early in the dissection process

Stay in areolar layer above the fascia

Frontalis branch can be identified by nerve stimulator

Avoid excessively deep skin incisions to prevent damage of the superficial temporal vessels

Raise flap from cephalad to caudad

The deep temporal fascia can be harvested along with the tempo-parietal fascia to form a bilayer flap

Flap can be raised as a bilayer flap. Both flaps have a common pedicle, but no vascular connections after branching of the pedicle. A segment of calvarium can be raised with the flap, if the deep temporal layer is included

Pedicle can be dissected into the parotid gland

Flap	Groin Flap
	Can be used as pedicle or free flap – most common application as pedicle flap
Tissue	Skin or dermal fat flap
Course of the vessels	Superficial to Scarpa's fascia, branching in the overlying skin towards the iliac crest
Dimensions	10 × 25 cm
Extensions/combinations	Usually no combinations with this type of flap; very experienced surgeons may raise the superficial inferior epigastric artery (SIEA) flap as a second skin paddle
Anatomy **Neurovascular pedicle** Artery Veins Length Diameter Nerve	 Superficial circumflex iliac artery (SCIA) Two venous systems; one parallels the SCIA and drains into the saphenous bulb; the other vein runs deep directly into the femoral vein Artery: 1.5–2 cm; veins: 2.5–4 cm Artery: 0.8–1.8 mm; veins: 2–3 mm The flap is not innervated
Surgical technique **Preoperative examinations, markings**	 Outline of the flap so that one-third is above and two-thirds are below the inguinal ligament; dividing line is drawn from the anterior superior iliac spine to pubic tubercle
Patient position	Supine
Dissection	Lateral approach preferable for pedicle flap; flap is raised from lateral superficial to deep muscle fascia; care must be taken to avoid injury to the pedicle Medial approach for free flaps: identify SCIA approximately 5 cm below the inguinal line; medial incision; identification of superficial vein anterior to Scarpa's fascia; identification of femoral artery and definition of SIEA and SCIA; lateral skin incision; deep fascia is left intact; identify lateral border of sartorius muscle; ligate muscle branches of deep SCIA branch; lateral cutaneous nerve is divided; flap raising is completed and flap is checked for perfusion
Advantages Flap size/shape Donor site Combinations	 Large flap possible; non-hair-bearing Perfect inconspicuous donor site with primary wound closure when flap width does not exceed 10 cm Medial extensions for hair bearing flap
Disadvantages Flap Pedicle Bulkiness Donor site morbidity	 Poor color match in exposed areas Very short pedicle with variable arterial anatomy, arterial diameter is small, vein grafts frequently required Medial bulk Anesthesia in the lateral cutaneous nerve distribution area
Tricks/pitfalls Dissection Extensions/combinations Contouring/corrections Clinical applications	 Identification of pedicle should precede flap harvest when used as a free flap Correction and debulking are frequently indicated; color match Pedicle flap: dorsal hand and forearm defects in younger patients Free flap: dorsal hand and forearm defects in older patients where a short pedicle is possible; not recommended as a pedicle flap in older patients (risk of shoulder stiffness)

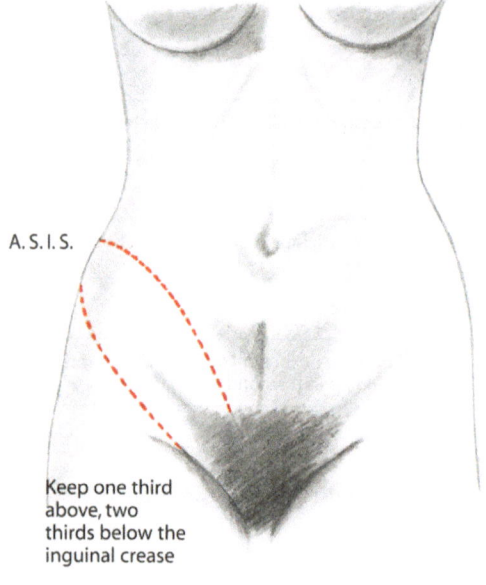

A. S. I. S.

Keep one third
above, two
thirds below the
inguinal crease

Vascular pedicle arises
deep to the deep fascia
below the inguinal ligament

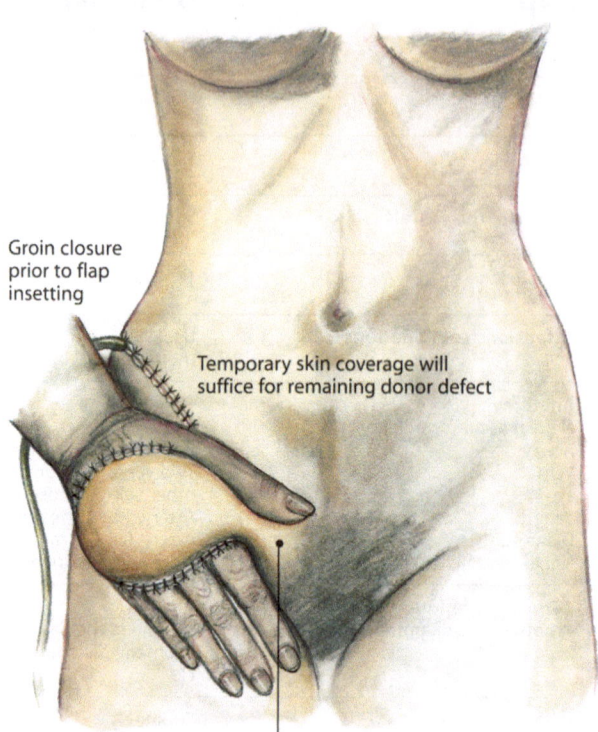

Groin closure
prior to flap
insetting

Temporary skin coverage will
suffice for remaining donor defect

Tube pedicle if possible

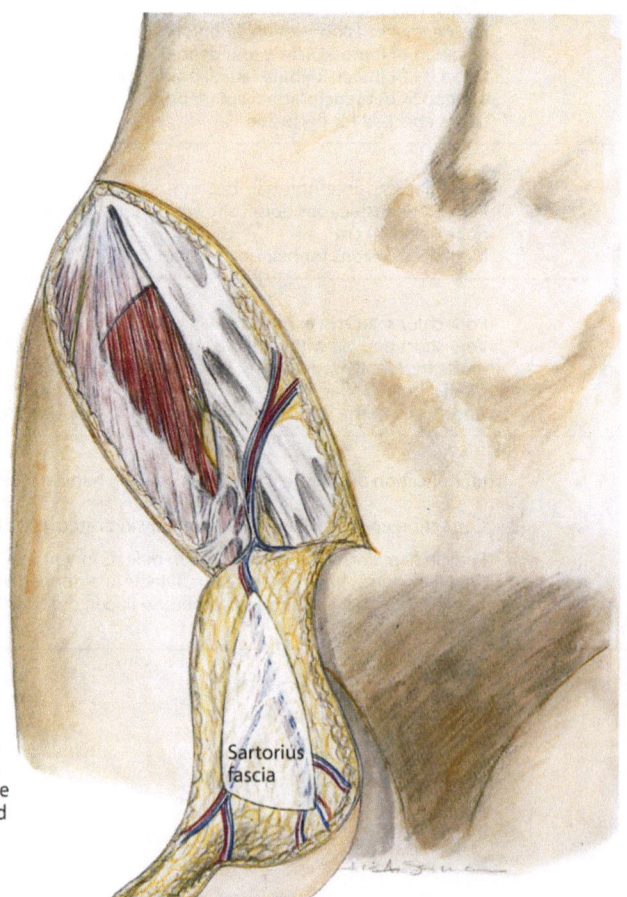

In free flaps, a medial
approach to identify
pedicle may be preferred.
In pedicle flaps, a lateral
approach is preferable

Identification and tracing
of the saphenous vein
will lead to the offspring
of the sup. circumflex
iliac vein

Do not inlude deep fascia
until the sartorius muscle
is encountered. From there
the deep fascia is included

Sartorius
fascia

Arterial anomalies are more
frequent than venous
irregularities

Ligate deep branch of SCIA
after certain identification of
the pedicle (superficial
branch)

Flap	Gracilis Muscle/Musculocutaneous Flap
Tissue	Muscle or muscle with skin paddle
Course of the vessels	Underneath the muscle distally after entering the muscle from laterally
Dimensions	4–6 × 20–25 cm (muscle); 6–8 × 10–12 cm (skin island)
Extensions/combinations	
Anatomy **Neurovascular pedicle** Artery Veins Length/arc of rotation Diameter Nerve	Terminal branch of medial femoral circumflex artery Concomitant veins of this artery 6–7 cm Artery: 1.2–1.8 mm; vein: 1.5–2.5 mm Anterior motor branch from the obturator nerve
Surgical technique **Preoperative examinations, markings**	Draw a line from the pubic tubercle to the medial condyle; prominence of the adductor magnus marks the superior border of the gracilis
Patient position	Supine, hip and knee flexed, leg abducted
Dissection	Incise 2 cm inferior and parallel to the line drawn preoperatively; do not violate the greater saphenous vein (anterior to the incision); incise fascia; identify gracilis muscle; divide muscle distally; ligate minor pedicle; proceed with dissection cephalad; retract adductor longus by moving proximally; expose pedicle 6–12 cm distal to pubic tubercle; protect medial cutaneous nerve on surface of adductor magnus; clip or ligate small branches; divide muscle superiorly; check perfusion; transfer flap Skin island: Center skin island over middle or proximal portion; incise down to fascia; include fascia lata in dissection; identify muscle; proceed as above
Advantages Vascular pedicle Flap size/shape Combinations Donor site	Short but reliable; vessel size sufficient, if pedicle is dissected to maximal length Long flat muscle with suitable cross-section area to serve as functional muscle transplant Skin island Minimal donor site morbidity with acceptable scar
Disadvantages Dissection Flap Donor site morbidity	Distal skin island is not reliable
Tricks/pitfalls Dissection Extensions/combinations Contouring/corrections Clinical applications	Do not confuse gracilis and sartorius muscles; dissect skin island not too anteriorly; the gracilis is always more dorsal than projected; good muscle excursion for functional replacement Rarely required, sometimes in bulky skin islands Long narrow defects for coverage alone; functional muscle transfer for loss of muscle groups

Plan incision line from pubic tubercle to medial femoral condyle in leg abduction

Center skin island over the gracilis muscle, not over the line separating the adductor muscle from the gracilis muscle

Distal skin paddle is not reliable

Incision always more dorsal than initially planned

Dissection proceeds proximally after distal division of the muscle

Ligate minor pedicles

Muscle inserts posteriorly to the sartorius muscle

Try to avoid violation of saphenous vein running anteriorly to the muscle

Pedicle has been dissected to maximum length

Motor nerve is included to facilitate re-neurotization in functional muscle transfer

Flap

Fibula Flap

Tissue	Bone – bone and skin paddle – bone, skin and muscle
Course of the vessels	Posterior to the fibula, through or beneath the flexor hallucis muscle
Dimensions	Bone length up to 26 cm; skin paddle 8 × 15 cm
Extensions/combinations	Parts of the soleus muscle can be included
Anatomy **Neurovascular pedicle** Artery Veins Length/arc of rotation Diameter	 Peroneal artery Peroneal veins 2–4 cm Artery: 1.5–2.5 mm; vein: 2–4 mm
Surgical technique **Preoperative examinations, markings**	Draw line from fibula head to lateral malleolus posterior to peroneal tendons; mark midpoint (approx. 15–17 cm from fibula head); identify skin perforators
Patient position	Supine with tourniquet on the thigh
Dissection	Lateral approach preferred for both flaps; anterior incision of designed skin paddle through crural fascia to the peroneus muscles; subfascial dissection towards posterior intermuscular septum; incision through posterior margin of skin paddle; subfascial dissection of the soleus muscle to the posterior intermuscular septum; septum is traced to the fibula; dissection proceeds anteriorly to detach the anterior septum from the fibula; posterior dissection towards flexor hallucis muscle; identify vessels (a cuff of flexor hallucis muscle may have to be incorporated); distal osteotomy (insert retractors close to the fibula to protect the vessels during osteotomy; distal end of the fibula is distracted cephalad with a clamp; divide interosseus membrane; expose peroneal vessels; proximal osteotomy; trace vessels back to origin; open tourniquet; check for perfusion
Advantages Vascular pedicle Flap size/shape Combinations Donor site	 Reliable vessels with large caliber; loss of donor vessels is usually tolerable Skin paddle is mobile, many defect variations can be reconstructed with a combined osteocutaneous flap; fibula provides ideal bone for replacement of radius, ulna and humerus Soleus muscle can be included to fill larger dead spaces Despite a slight torsion instability, minimal donor morbidity
Disadvantages Dissection Flap Donor site morbidity	 Dissection is tedious and technically difficult; pedicle is short Skin island may be too small in complex injuries with major soft tissue loss Donor scar is conspicuous; risk of nerve injury to peroneal nerve or to motor nerve of the flexor hallucis muscle, possible exposure of peroneal tendons
Tricks/pitfalls Dissection Extensions/combinations Contouring/corrections Clinical applications	 Do not confuse peroneal vessels with posterior tibial vessels; take muscle cuff (1–2 mm) to ensure bone perfusion; preserve proximal and distal 6 cm of the fibula to maintain stability; in children the distal 10 cm should be preserved When partial soleus muscle is included, be sure to include a muscle perforator; otherwise high risk of muscle necrosis Rarely required Complex segmental defects of wrist, forearm, humerus, shoulder (arthrodesis)

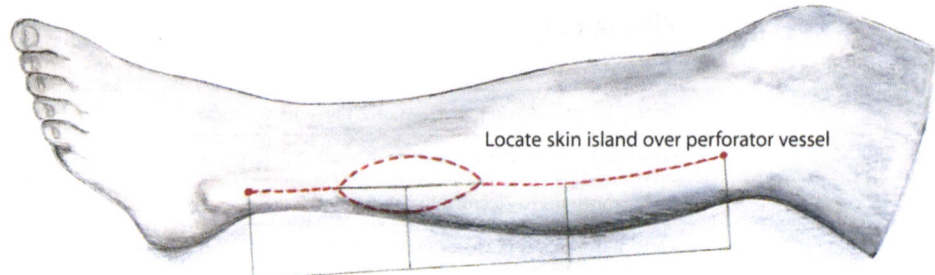

Locate skin island over perforator vessel

The proximal and distal 6 cm of the fibula have to be preserved to reduce donor site morbidity

Identify perforator vessels by preoperative Doppler examination

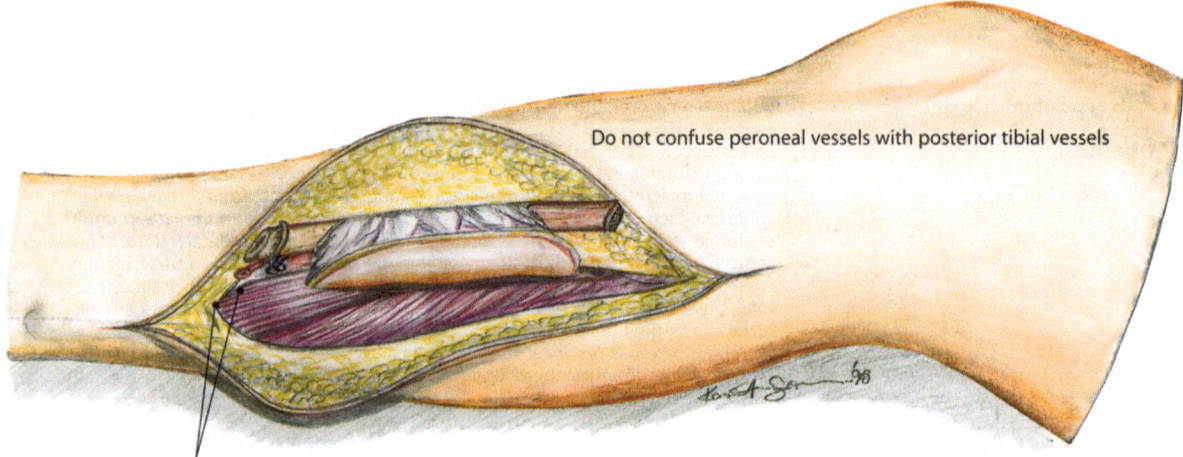

Do not confuse peroneal vessels with posterior tibial vessels

Distal pedicle is ligated

Dissection proceeds cephalad after distal osteotomy

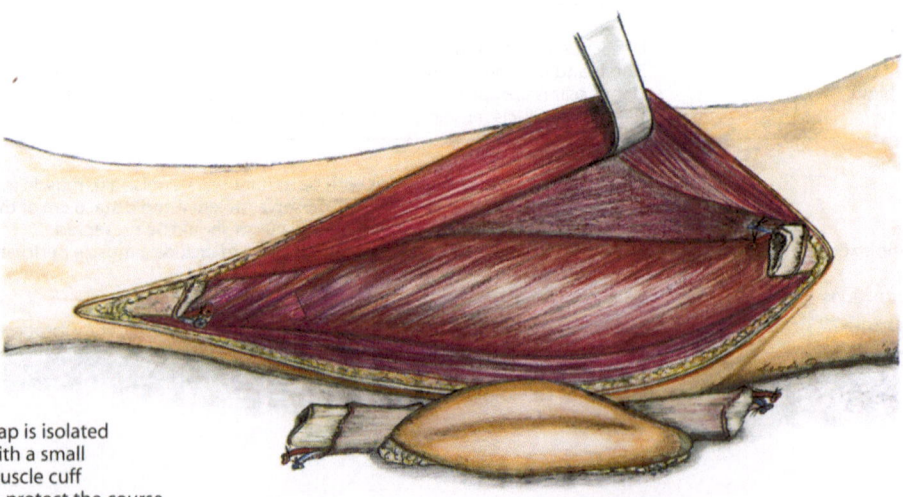

Flap is isolated with a small muscle cuff to protect the course of the vessels

Skin island is centered over perforator vessel

Rehabilitation Protocols

Repair of Thumb Flexor Tendon

Day 2 after surgery	Dorsal splint, wrist 30° flexion, MP joints extendable to 0°, IP joints extendable to 0°. Thumb should be positioned in slight opposition
Week 1	Active extension supported by hand therapist, passive flexion and extension by hand therapist. Patient's exercise: active extension 10 times/hour
Week 2	Same as week 1, every other day by hand therapist
Week 3, 4	Continuation of home exercises, 2–3/week controlled by hand therapist. When passive extension is free, no further support by hand therapist; in the case of extension lag, continuation of therapist support
Week 5	Active flexion followed by active extension within the limits of the splint. In the case of full flexion, remove rubber bands; splint remains. If full flexion is not achieved, rubber bands are left in place
Week 6	Modification of dorsal splint; wrist 0°; release of opposition position; home program comparable to week 5
Week 7	Removal of dorsal splint; start OT; no full stress
Week 8	Increasing stress, measure of grip strength, increasing weight loading – Discontinue treatment

Normal types: Ludwigshafen-Protocol
Italics: DUKE-Protocol

Repair of Long Finger Flexor Tendon

Washington Protocol (Chow et al. 1988)

Day 2 after surgery	Dorsal splint, wrist 20°–30° flexion, MP joints in 60° flexion, PIP and DIP joints extendable to 0°. Index finger involved – only index finger in rubber band system. In case of involvement of middle finger, ring finger, or little finger – all three digits in rubber band system no matter which finger is injured – during the night passive immobilization in extension of PIP and DIP *10° wrist flexion, 50–70° MP flexion, PIP and DIP full extension (0°)*
Week 1	Active extension supported by hand therapist, passive flexion and extension by hand therapist, Patient's exercise: active extension 10 times/hour *Under therapist supervision passive wrist tenodesis with digital flexion – passive tenodesis wrist flexion with digital extension*
Week 2	Same as week 1, every other day by hand therapist *Under therapist supervision passive wrist tenodesis with digital flexion – passive tenodesis wrist flexion with digital extension*
Week 3 and 4	Continuation of home exercises, 2–3 times/week controlled by hand therapist. When passive extension is free, no further support by hand therapist, in case of extension lag, continuation of therapist support; active flexion followed by active extension within the limits of the splint *Under therapist supervision passive wrist tenodesis with digital flexion; passive tenodesis wrist flexion with digital extension*
Week 5	In case of full flexion, removal of rubber bands If full flexion is not achieved, rubber bands are left in place *In case of PIP extension lag >30° – finger is strapped into full extension over night; MP in 45° continue rubber band traction*
Week 6	Modification of dorsal splint; wrist 0°, MP joints in 20° flexion; home program comparable to week 5 *MP in 45° continue rubber band traction*
Week 7	Removal of dorsal splint; Start OT; no full stress *Full tendon gliding program*
Week 8	Increasing stress; measure of grip strength, increasing weight loading Discontinue treatment

Extensor Tendon Repair – Central Slip (Zone 3 – 4)

Day 2 – Week 1	Manufacturing of Sandwich splint, 0° PIP and DIP; exercise splint allowing 15 or 30° flexion of PIP. Patient's exercise: active flexion and extension against exercise splint (10 times/hour). Immobilization in sandwich splint
Week 2	Same as week 1 (15° or 30°) *Conservative treatment: Immobilization of PIP at 0°*
Week 3	Alteration of volar exercise splint to PIP flexion of 40° *Conservative treatment: Immobilization of PIP at 0°*
Week 4	Alteration of volar exercise splint to PIP flexion of 50° *Conservative treatment: Immobilization of PIP at 0°* *Mobilization: MP 0°, PIP 30° flexion, active extension*
Week 5	Alteration of volar exercise splint to PIP flexion of 60° *Conservative treatment: Immobilization of PIP at 0°* *Mobilization: MP 0°, PIP 45 – 50°; active extension*
Week 6	Removal of splint; free active motion; Start with OT *Conservative treatment: Immobilization of PIP at 0°* *Mobilization: add 20° flexion for each week*
Week 6 – 10	Increasing stress loading

Extensor Tendon Repair – Zone 1 and 2

Osseus fixation	6 weeks of strict immobilization followed by gentle active exercise for two weeks until full stress loading after 8 weeks *Identical protocol*
Closed rupture – tendon suture – 8 weeks of splinting	
	6 – 8 weeks of continuous extension splinting

Extensor Tendon Repair – Zone 5–7

Reversed Flexor Tendon Protocol

Day 2 – Week 1 Dorsal splint, wrist 30° extension, MP joints, 10° hyperextension – PIP and DIP free.
Exercise: Active flexion to mark on the rubberband system (15° or 30°, depending on intraoperative situation)
Wrist 45° extension, MP and PIP 0°

Week 2 30° (45°) flexion
Wrist 45° extension, MP and PIP 0°

Week 3 45° or 60° flexion
Wrist 45° extension, MP and PIP 0°

Week 4 60° or 90° flexion; start of active extension of PIP and DIP with rubber band system in place
MP and PIP are moved to 30° flexion

Week 5 Flexion in all cases to 90°
Increasing MP and PIP flexion

Week 6 Removal of splint and rubber band system, start of OT

Week 7 – 10 Increased stress loading

Extensor Tendon Repair – Zone 5 – 7

Reversed Flexor Tendon Protocol

Day 2 – Week 4 Dorso-volar splint; wrist 30° extension, CMC joint 0° – MP 0°
Exercise: Active flexion of IP joint to mark on the rubber band system (60°). With Hand therapist support until end of 1st week, 10 times/hour by patient.

Week 5 Increase of range of active flexion 80 – 90°. Start of active extension

Week 6 Removal of splint and rubber band system, start of OT

Week 7 – 10 Increased stress loading

Injuries of Digital Joints (MP and PIP)

Joint	Type of Injury	Immobilization	Splint	Removal of splint	Stress loading
MP	I Volar plate	One week – splint in 30° MP flexion; wrist/PIP/DIP free	Resting periods: immobilization splint; exercise splint: 20°, 20°, 50°	6 weeks	7 weeks
	II Collateral ligaments with/ without volar plate involvement	One week – splint in 30° MP flexion; wrist/PIP/DIP free	Resting periods: immobilization splint; exercise splint: 20°, 20°, 50°; buddy taping to adjacent finger	6 weeks	7 weeks
	III Dorsal capsule; central slip	One week – splint in 30° MP flexion; wrist/PIP/DIP 0–10°	Resting periods: immobilization splint; exercise splint: limited flexion 30°; increase to 50° after 3 weeks	6 weeks	7 weeks
PIP	I Volar plate	One week – sandwich splint in 25° flexion	Exercise splint: limited extension 20°; free flexion	6 weeks	7 weeks
	II Volar plate + collateral ligaments and/or central slip	One week – sandwich splint in 25° flexion	Exercise splint: 20°, 20°, 50°; after 3 weeks 20°, 20°, 70°	6 weeks	7 weeks
	III Collateral ligaments	One week – sandwich splint in 25° flexion	Ligament splint	5 weeks	7 weeks
	IV Dorsal capsule; central slip	3 days – sandwich splint in 25° flexion	Sandwich splint; exercise splint: 30°, 40°, 50°, 60° (central slip)	6 weeks	7 weeks

References

General Considerations – Trauma – Tumor

Adani R, Castagnetti C, Landi A (1995) Degloving injuries of the hand and fingers. Clin Orthop 19–25

Baack BR, Osler T, Nachbar JM, Harris V (1993) Steam press burns of the hand. Ann Plast Surg 30 : 345–349

Biemer E (1979) Experience in replantation surgery in the upper extremity. Ann Acad Med Singapore 8 (4): 393–397

Brown H (1970) Closed crush injuries of the hand and forearm. Orthop Clin North Am 1 : 253–259

Büchler U (1990) Traumatic soft-tissue defects of the extremities. Implications and treatment guidelines. Arch Orthop Trauma Surg 109 : 321–329

Burke FD, Mc Grouther AD, Smith PJ (1990) Principles of hand surgery. Churchill Livingstone, Edinburgh

Chen SH, Wei FC, Noordhoff SM (1992) Free vascularized joint transfers in acute complex hand injuries: case reports. J Trauma 33 : 924–930

Chow SP, So YC, Pun WK, Luk KD, Leong JC (1988) Thenar crush injuries. J Bone Joint Surg Br 70 : 135–139

Campbell DA, Kay PJ (1996) The hand injury severity scoring system. J Hand Surg 21 (B) : 295–298

Cooney WP, Linscheid RL, Dobyns JH (eds) (1998) The wrist – diagnosis and operative treatment. Mosby, St. Louis

Garcia Elias M, Abanco J, Salvador E, Sanchez R (1985) Crush injury of the carpus. J Bone Joint Surg Br 67 : 286–289

Green DP (1998) Operative hand surgery (4th edn). Churchill Livingstone, New York

Lister G (1993) The hand. Churchill Livingstone, Edinburgh

Mahoney J, Bell RH, Hudson AR, O'Sullivan B, Davis A (1994) Aggressive fibrous tissue lesions in the upper extremity: treatment and results. J Hand Surg Am 19 : 686–693

Nettelblad H, Karlander LE, Nylander G (1989) Pain relief after free flap reconstruction in adriamycin necrosis on the dorsum of the hand. A case report. J Hand Surg Br 14 : 45–46

Simpson SG (1984) Farm machinery injuries. J Trauma 24 : 150–152

Weiland AJ, Villarreal-Rios A, Kleinert HE, Kutz J, Atasoy E, Lister G (1977) Replantation of digits and hands: analysis of surgical techniques and functional results in 71 patients with 786 replantations. J Hand Surg 2 (1) : 1–12

Wintman BI, Gelberman RH, Katz JN (1995) Dynamic scapholunate instability: results of operative treatment with dorsal capsulodesis. J Hand Surg 20 (6): 971–979

Burns

Barisoni D, Bortolani A, Sanna A, Lorenzini M, Governa M (1996) Free flap cover of acute burns and post-burn deformity. Eur J Plast Surg 19 : 257–261

Muuronen E, Asco-Seljavaara S, Tukiainen E, Härmä H (1997) Free flap reconstruction in massive upper extremity burns. Eur J Plast Surg 20 : 7–10

Fracture Treatment

Chen SH, Wei FC, Chen HC, Chuang CC, Noordhoff S (1994) Miniature plates and screws in acute complex hand injury. J Trauma 37 (2) : 237–242

Cooney, WP (ed) (1998) The wrist. Mosby, St. Louis

Fernandez DL, Jupiter JB (1996) Fractures of the distal radius. Springer, Berlin Heidelberg New York

Heim U (1973) Indications and technique of AO osteosynthesis in the treatment of the fractures of the hand. Acta Orthop Belg 39 (6) : 957–972

Herbert TJ, Fischer WE, Leicester AW (1992) The Herbert bone screw: a ten year perspective. Hand Surg 17 (4) : 415–419

Herbert TJ (1990) The fractured scaphoid. Quality Medical Publishers, St. Louis

Saffer P (1990) Carpal injuries: anatomy, radiology, current treatment, Springer, Berlin Heidelberg New York

Tendon Repair

Beng HL, Tsai TS (1996) The six strand technique for flexor tendon repair. In: Taras, JS, Schneider LM (eds) 65–76. WB Sanders, Boston

Bruner JM (1967) The zig-zag volar digital incision for flexor tendon surgery. Plast Reconstr Surg 40 : 571–574

Bunnell S (1918) Repair of tendons in fingers and description of two new instruments. Surg Gynecol Obstet 26 : 103–110

Chow JA, Thomes LJ, Dovelle S, Milnor WH, Syfer AE, Smith AC (1988) A combined regimen of controlled motion following flexor tendon repair in "no man's land". Plast Reconstr Surg 79:447–453

Gelberman RH, Steinberg D, Amiel D, Akeson W (1991) Fibroblast chemotaxis after tendon repair. J Hand Surg 16(4):686–693

Gelberman RH, Chu CR, Williams CS, Seiler JG, Amiel D (1992) Angiogenesis in healing autogenous flexor-tendon grafts. J Bone Joint Surg 74(8):1207–1216

Ibaraki K, Kanaya F (1995) Free vascularized medial plantar flap with functioning abductor hallucis transfer for reconstruction of thenar defects. Plast Reconstr Surg 95:108–113

Kessler I (1973) The "grasping" technique for tendon repair. Hand 5:253–255

Kirchmayr L (1917) Zur Technik der Sehnennaht. (The technique of tendon repair.) Zbl Chir 44:906–907

Krimmer H, Hahn P, Lanz U (1995) Free gracilis muscle transplantation for hand reconstruction. Clin Orthop 13–18

Manske PR, Gelberman RH, Lesker PA (1985) Flexor tendon healing. Hand Clin 1(1):25–34

Noguchy M, Seiler JG, Gelberman RH, Sofranko RA, Woo SL (1993) In vitro biomechanical analysis of suture methods for flexor tendon repair. J Orthop Res 11(4):603–611

Lister GD, Kleinert HE (1977) Primary flexor tendon repair followed by immediate controlled mobilisation. J Hand Surg 2:441–451

Pulvertaft RG (1977) Reconstruction of the mutilated hand. Eric Moberg Lecture. Scand J Plast Reconstr Surg 11(3):219–224

Taylor GI, Townsend P (1979) Composite free flap and tendon transfer: an anatomical study and a clinical technique. Br J Plast Surg 32(3):170–183

Strickland JW (1985) Results of flexor tendon surgery in zone II. Hand Clin 1(1):167–179

Verdan C (1979) Tendon surgery of the hand. Churchill Livingstone, Edinburgh

Yajima H, Inada Y, Shono M, Tamai S (1996) Radial forearm flap with vascularized tendons for hand reconstruction. Plast Reconstr Surg 98:328–333

Vascular Repair

Buncke HJ (1981) The role of microsurgery in hand surgery. J Hand Surg 6(6):533–536

Buncke HJ, Alpert B, Shah KG (1978) Microvascular grafting. Clin Plast Surg 5(2):185–194

Goldner RD, Urbaniak JR (1989) Indications for replantation in the adult upper extremity. Occup Med 4(3):525–538

Harashina, T (1977) Use of untied suture in microvascular anastomoses. Plast Recon Surg 59:134–135

Kaplan EN, Buncke HJ, Murrey DE (1973) Distant transfer of cutaneous island flaps in humans by microvascular anastomosis. Plast Reconstr Surg 52(3):301–305

O'Brien BM (1976) Replantation and reconstructive microvascular surgery. Part II. Ann R Coll Surg Engl 58(3):171–182

Richards RR, Urbaniak JR (1986) The surgical and rehabilitation management of vascular injury to the hand. Hand Clin 2(1):171–178

Schenkk RR, Derman DH (1977) An intraluminal silastic stent for small vessel repair. Orthop Clin North Am 8(2):265–271

Taras JS, Nunley JA, Urbaniak JR, Goldner RD, Fitch RD (1991) Replantation in children Microsurgery 12(3):216–220

Nerve Repair

Berger A, Mailander P (1991) Advances in peripheral nerve repair in emergency surgery of the hand. World J Surg 15(4):493–500

Millesi H (1977) Healing of nerves. Clin Plast Surg 4(3):459–473

Millesi H (1979) Nerve suture and grafting to restore the extratemporal facial nerve. Clin Plast Surg 6(3):333–341

Millesi H (1988) Brachial plexus injuries. Nerve grafting. Clin Orthop 237:36–42

Millesi H (1993) Forty-two years of peripheral nerve surgery. Microsurgery 14(4):228–233

Weinstein SM, Herring SA (1992) Nerve problems and compartment syndroms in the hand, wrist and forearm. Clin Sports Med 11(1):161–188

Skin and Soft Tissue

Bertelli JA, Pagliei A (1994) Direct and reversed flow proximal phalangeal island flaps. J Hand Surg Am 19A:671–680

Buncke HJ (1991) Microsurgery: transplantation – replantation. Lea and Febiger, Philadelphia

Chen C-L, Chiu H-Y, Lee J-W, Yang J-T (1994) Arterialized tendocutaneous venous flaps for dorsal finger reconstruction. Microsurgery 15:886–890

Flemming AF, Stilwell JH (1991) Cross-arm dermis flaps for repair of dorsal finger defects. J Hand Surg Br 16:339–341

Fukui A, Inada Y, Maeda M (1989) Pedicled and "flow through" venous flaps: clinical applications. J Reconstr Microsurg 5:235–243

Germann G, Levin S (1997) Intrinsic flaps in the hand; new concepts in skin coverage. Techniques in hand and upper extremity surgery 1:48–61

Gilbert A, Masquelet AC, Hentz VR (1992) Pedicle flaps of the upper limb. Dunitz, London

Goffin D, Brunelli F, Galbiatti A, Sammut D, Gilbert A (1992) A new flap based on the distal branches of the radial artery. Ann Chir Main Memb Super 11:217–225

Hsu WM, Wei FC, Lin CH, Chen HC, Chuang CC, Chen HT (1996) The salvage of a degloved hand skin flap by arteriovenous shunting. Plast Reconstr Surg 98:146–150

Inoue T, Ueda K, Kurihara T, Harada T, Harashina T (1993) A new cutaneous flap: snuff-box flap. Br J Plast Surg 46:252–254

Katsaros J (1992) Indications for free soft-tissue flap transfer to the upper limb and the role of alternative procedures. Hand Clin 8:479–507

Lee WP, May JW Jr (1992) Neurosensory free flaps to the hand. Indications and donor selection. Hand Clin 8:465–477

Levin LS, Germann G (eds) (1998) Atlas of the Hand Clinics – Local flap coverage about the hand. WB Saunders, Philadelphia

Milford L (1966) Resurfacing hand defects by using deboned useless fingers. Am Surg 32:196–200

Moiemen N, Elliot D (1994) Palmar V-Y reconstruction of proximal defects of the volar aspect of the digits. Br J Plast Surg 47:35–41

Morrison WA, Cavallo AV (1993) Revascularization of an ischemic replanted thumb using a lateral arm free fascial flap. Ann Plast Surg 31:467–470

O'Brien B (1968) Neurovascular island pedicle flaps for terminal amputations and digital scars. Br J Plast Surg 21(3):258–261

Omokawa S, Mizumoto S, Iwai M, Tamai S, Fukui A (1996) Innervated radial thenar flap for sensory reconstruction of fingers. J Hand Surg Am 21:373–380

Onishi K, Maruyama Y, Yoshitake M (1996) Transversely designed dorsal metacarpal V-Y advancement flaps for dorsal hand reconstruction. Br J Plast Surg 49:165–169

Rockwell WB, Lister GD (1993) Soft tissue reconstruction. Coverage of hand injuries. Orthop Clin North Am 24:411–423

Rose EH (1989) Small flap coverage of hand and digit defects. Clin Plast Surg 16:427–442

Serafin D (1996) Atlas of microsurgical composite tissue transplantation. Saunders, Philadelphia

Shibu MM, Tarabe MA, Graham K, Dickson MG, Mahaffey PJ (1997) Fingertip reconstruction with a dorsal island homodigital flap. Br J Plast Surg 50:121–124

Smith CB, O'Brien BM (1991) Free flap from a non-replantable digit for microvascular digital reconstruction in a multi-digital hand injury. Aust NZ J Surg 61:699–702

Stice RC, Wood MB (1987) Neurovascular island skin flaps in the hand: functional and sensibility evaluations. Microsurgery 8:162–167

Strauch B, Vasconez LO, Hall-Findlay EJ (eds) (1990) Grabb's enzyclopedia of flaps. Little, Brown, Boston

Tsai TM, Matiko JD, Breidenbach W, Kutz JE (1987) Venous flaps in digital revascularization and replantation. J Reconstr Microsurg 3:113–119

Woo SH, Jeong JH, Seul JH (1996) Resurfacing relatively large skin defects of the hand using arterialized venous flaps. J Hand Surg Br 21:222–229

Thumb Reconstruction

Biemer E, Stock W (1983) Total thumb reconstruction: a one-stage reconstruction using an osteocutaneous forearm flap. Br J Plast Surg 36(1):52–55

Iglesias M, Butrun P, Serrano A (1995) Thumb reconstruction with extended twisted toe flap. J Hand Surg Am 20:731–736

Kumta SM, Yip KMH, Pannozzo SL, Fong SL, Leung PC (1997) Resurfacing of thumb pulp loss with a heterodigital neurovascular island flap using a nerve disconnnection-reconnection technique. J Reconstr Microsurg 13:117–123

Morrison WA, O'Brien BMcC, Mac Leod AM (1980) Thumb reconstruction with a free neurovascular wrap-around flap from the bit toe. J Hand Surg 5:575–577

Morrison WA (1992) Thumb and fingertip reconstruction by composite microvascular tissue from the toes. Hand Clin 8:537–550

Tubiana R, Duparc J (1961) Restoration of sensibility in the hand by neurovascular skin island transfer. J Bone Joint Surg Br 43b:474–480

Wei FC, Chen HC, Chuang CC, Chen SH (1994) Microsurgical thumb reconstruction with toe transfer: selection of various techniques. Plast Reconstr Surg 93:345–351

Cross-Finger Flap

Atasoy E (1982) Reversed cross-finger subcutaneous flap. J Hand Surg 7:481–483

Cronin TD (1951) The cross-finger flap – a new method of repair. Am Surg 17:419–425

Mutaf M, Sensoz O, Ustuner ET (1993) A new design of the cross-finger flap: The C-ring flap. Br J Plast Surg 46:97–104

Pakiam IA (1978) The reversed dermis flap. Br J Plast Surg 31:131–135

V-Y Flap (Volar V-Y, Lateral V-Y)

Atasoy E, Ioakimidis E, Kasdan ML, Kutz JE, Kleinert HE (1970) Reconstruction of the amputated finger tip with a triangular volar flap. A new surgical procedure. J Bone Joint Surg 52A:921–926

Geissendörffer H (1943) Beitrag zur Fingerkuppenplastik. [Thoughts on fingertip plasty – first description of a lateral V-Y flap] Zbl Chir 70:1107–1108

Kutler W (1947) A new method for fingertip amputation. JAMA 133:29–30

Tranquilli-Leali, LE (1935) Ricostruzione dell'apice delle falangi ungeali mediante autoplastica volare peduncolata per scorrimento. (Reconstruction of the fingertip by a medial volar flap), Infort Traum Lavoro 1:186–193

Axial Digital Island Flap

Büchler U, Frey HP (1988) The dorsal middle phalangeal finger flap. Handchir Mikrochir Plast Chir 20:239–243

Niranjan NS, Armstrong JR (1994) A homodigital reverse pedicle island flap in soft tissue reconstruction of the finger and the thumb. J Hand Surg Br 19:135–141

Schuind F, Van Genechten F, Denuit P, Merle M, Foucher G (1985) Homodigital neurovascular island flaps in hand surgery. A study of sixty cases. Ann Chir Main 4:306–315

Reverse Axial Digital Island Flap

Bene MD, Petrolati M, Raimondi P, Tremolada C, Muset A (1994) Reverse dorsal digital island flap. Plast Reconstr Surg 93:552–557

Germann G, Rütschle S, Kania N, Raff T (1997) The reverse pedicle heterodigital cross-finger island flap. Br J Hand Surg 22:25–29

Kojima T, Tsuchida Y, Hirase Y, Endo T (1990) Reverse vascular pedicle digital island flap. Br J Plast Surg 43:290–295

Lai CS, Lin SD, Tsai CC, Tsai CW (1995) Reverse digital artery neurovascular cross-finger flap. J Hand Surg Am 20:397–402

Dorsal Metacarpal Artery Flaps

Chang L-Y, Yang J-Y, Wei F-C (1994) Reverse dorsometacarpal flap in digits and web-space reconstruction. Ann Plast Surg 33:281–289

Early MJ, Milner RH (1987) Dorsal metacarpal flaps. Br J Plast Surg 40:333–341

Earley MJ (1989) The second dorsal metacarpal artery neurovascular island flap. J Hand Surg Br 14:434–440

Maruyama Y (1990) The reverse dorsal metacarpal flap. Br J Plast Surg 43:24–27

Quaba AA, Davison PM (1990) The distally-based dorsal hand flap. Br J Plast Surg 43:28–29

Sapp JW, Allen RJ, Dupin C (1993) A reversed digital artery island flap for the treatment of fingertip injuries. J Hand Surg AM 18:528–534

Schoofs M, Chambon E, Leps P, Millot F, Bahm J, Lambert F (1993) The reverse dorsal metacarpal flap from the first web. Eur J Plast Surg 16:26–29

Sherif MM (1994) First dorsal metacarpal artery flap in hand reconstruction. II. Clinical application. J Hand Surg Am 19:26–31

Yousif NJ, Ye Z, Sanger JR, Arria P, Gilbert A, Matloub HS (1992) The versatile metacarpal and reverse metacarpal artery flaps in hand surgery. Ann Plast Surg 29:523–531

First Dorsal Metacarpal Artery Flap ("Kite Flap")

Foucher G, Braun JB (1979) A new island flap transfer from the dorsum of the index to the thumb. Plast Reconstr Surg 63:344–349

Williams RL, Nanchahal J, Sykes PJ, O'Shaughnessy M (1995) The provision of innervated skin cover for the injured thumb using dorsal metacarpal artery island flaps. J Hand Surg Br 20:231–236

Yang JY (1991) The first dorsal metacarpal flap in first web space and thumb reconstruction. Ann Plast Surg 27:258–264

Moberg Flap (Volar Advancement) – O'Brien Modification

Moberg E (1964) Aspects of sensation in reconstructive surgery of the upper limb. J Bone Joint Surg 1964, 46A:17–825

O'Brien BM (1968) Neurovascular island pedicle flap for terminal amputations and digital scars. Br J Plast Surg 21:258–261

Lateral Advancement Flap

Venkataswami R, Subramanian N (1980) Oblique triangular flap: a new method of repair for oblique amputation of the finger tip and thumb. Plast Reconstr Surg 66:296–300

Distal Ulnar Perforator Flap

Becker C, Gilbert A (1988) Le lambeau cubital. Ann Chir Main 7:136–142

Radial Forearm Flap

Braun RM, Rechnic M, Neill Cage DJ, Schorr RT (1995) The retrograde radial fascial forearm flap: surgical rationale, technique, and clinical application. J Hand Surg Am 20:915–922

Gang RK (1990) The Chinese forearm flap in reconstruction of the hand. J Hand Surg Br 15:84–88

Govila A, Sharma D (1990) The radial forearm flap for reconstruction of the upper extremity. Plast Reconstr Surg 86:920–927

Holevich Madjarova B (1990) The Chinese flap in hand surgery. Acta Chir Plast 32:1–10

Hulsbergen Kruger S, Muller K, Partecke BD (1996) Donor site defect after removal of free and pedicled forearm flaps: functional and cosmetic results. Handchir Mikrochir Plast Chir 28:70–75

Swanson E, Boyd JB, Manktelow RT (1990) The radial forearm flap: reconstructive applications and donor site defects in 35 consecutive patients. Plast Reconstr Surg 85:258–266

Timmons MJ (1986) The vascular basis of the radial fore-arm flap. Plast Reconstr Surg 77:80–92

Posterior Interosseous Flap

Costa H, Comba S, Martins A, Rodrigues J, Reis J, Amarante J (1991) Further experience with the posterior in-terosseous flap. Br J Plast Surg 44:449–455

Mazzer N, Barbieri CH, Cortez M (1996) The posterior interosseous forearm island flap for skin defects in the hand and elbow. A prospective study of 51 cases. J Hand Surg Br 21:237–243

Wang Y, Li X, Yuan Z, Seiler H (1994) Anatomy and clinical use of posterior interosseous island forearm flap. Unfallchirurg 97:541–544

Zancolli EA, Angrigiani C (1988) Posterior interosseous island forearm flap. J Hand Surg Br 13:130–135

Lateral Arm Flap

Katsaros J, Schusterman M, Beppu M, Banis JC, Acland RC (1984) The lateral upper arm flap: anatomy and clinical applications. Ann Plast Surg 12:489–500

Scheker LR, Kleinert HE, Hanel DP (1987) Lateral arm composite tissue transfer to ipsilateral hand defects. J Hand Surg 12:665

Shibata M, Hatano Y, Iwabuchi Y, Matsuzaki H (1995) Combined dorsal forearm and lateral arm flap. Plast Reconstr Surg 96:1423–1429

Parascapular/Scapular Flap

Dos Santos LF (1984) The vascular anatomy and dis-section of the free scapula flap. Plast Reconst Surg 73:599

Nassif T, Vidal L, Bovet JL, Baudet J (1982) The parascapu-lar flap: a new cutaneous microsurgical free flap. Plast Reconst Surg 65:1982

Urbaniak JR, Koman LA, Goldner RD, Armstrong NB, Nunley JA (1982) The vascularized cutaneous scapu-lar flap. Plast Reconstr Surg 69:772–778

Tempoparietal Fascia Flap

Abdul Hassan HS, v Drasek-Ascher G, Acland RC (1986) Surgical anatomy and blood supply of the fascial layers of the temporal region. Plast Reconstr Surg 77:17–24

Rose EH, Norris MS (1990) The versatile temporoparietal fascial flap: adaptability to a variety of composite defects. Plast Reconstr Surg 85:224–232

Upton J, Rogers C, Durham-Smith G, Swartz WM (1986) Clinical application of tempo-parietal flaps in hand reconstruction. J Hand Surg 11A:475

Serratus Muscle/Fascia Flap

Rousell AR, Davies DM, Eisenberg N, Taylor GI (1984) The anatomy of the subscapular – thoraco-dorsal arterial system: study of 100 cadaver dissections. Br J Plast Surg 37:574

Takayanagi S, Maeda T, Tsuki T (1988) Use of the latis-simus dorsi and the serratus anterior muscles as a combined flap. Ann Plast Surg 20:333

Latissimus Dorsi Muscle/Musculocutaneous Flap

Baudet J, Guimberteau JS, Nascimento E (1976) Success-ful clinical transfer of two free thoracodorsal axillary flaps. Plast Reconst Surg 58:680

Franceschi N, Yim KK, Lineaveaver WC, Siko PP, Alpert BS, Buncke GM, Buncke HJ (1991) Eleven consecutive combined latissimus dorsi and serratus anterior free muscle transplantations. Ann Plast Surg 27(2): 121–125

Fibula Flap

Gilbert A (1981) Free vascularized bone grafts. Int Surg 66:27

Taylor GI (1983) The current status of free vascularized bone grafts. Clin Plast Surg 10:185

Gracilis Flap

Manktelow RT, Mc Knee NH (1978) Free muscle trans-plantation to provide active finger flexion. J Hand Surg 3:416

O'Brien BM, Morrison WA, Mac Leod AM, Weiglein OV (1982) Free microneurovascular muscle transfer in limbs to provide motor power. Ann Plast Surg 9:381

Groin Flap

Boo Chai K (1977) John Wood and his contributions to plastic surgery: the first groin flap. Br J Plast Surg 30:9–13

Daniel RK, Taylor GI (1973) Distant transfer of an island flap by microvascular anastomoses. A clinical tech-nique. Plast Reconstr Surg 52:111–117

McGregor IA, Jackson IT (1972) The groin flap. Br J Plast Surg 25:3

Subject Index